Israel's Destiny

Israel's Destiny

Fertility and Mortality in a Divided Society

Edited by
Jona Schellekens
& Jon Anson

Schnitzer Studies in Israeli Society • Volume 12

Publication Series of the Israel Sociological Society
Series Editor Eva Etzioni-Halevy

Routledge
Taylor & Francis Group
LONDON AND NEW YORK

First published 2007 by Transaction Publishers

Published 2017 by Routledge
2 Park Square, Milton Park, Abingdon, Oxon OX14 4RN
711 Third Avenue, New York, NY 10017, USA

Routledge is an imprint of the Taylor & Francis Group, an informa business

Sponsored by the Schnitzer Foundation for Research on the Israeli Economy and Society-Bar-Ilan University.

Library of Congress Catalog Number: 2006044575

Library of Congress Cataloging-in-Publication Data

Israel's destiny : fertility and mortality in a divided society / Jon Anson, Jona Schellekens, editors.
p. cm.—(Schnitzer studies in Israeli society ; v. 12)
Includes bibliographical references and index.
ISBN 978-0-7658-0369-6 (cloth : alk. paper)—ISBN 978-1-4128-0626-8 (pbk.: alk. paper)
1. Fertility, Human—Israel. 2. Marriage—Israel. 3. Mortality— Israel. 4. Israel—Population policy. 5. Israel—Social conditions. I. Anson, Jon. II. Schellekens, Jona. III. Series.

HB1044.A3177 2006
304.6095694—dc22

ISBN 13: 978-1-4128-0626-8 (pbk)

Contents

Sources vii

1. Introduction 1
   Jona Schellekens and Jon Anson

Part 1: Fertility

2. The Modern Shift to Below-Replacement Fertility: Has Israel's Population Joined the Process? 15
   Dov Friedlander and Carole Feldmann
3. Religiosity, Nationalism and Fertility in Israel 29
   Jon Anson and Avinoam Meir
4. Innovation and Adaptation in Fertility Transition: Jewish Immigrants to Israel from Muslim North Africa and the Middle East 53
   Barbara S. Okun
5. Fertility Behavior of Recent Immigrants to Israel: A Comparative Analysis of Immigrants from Ethiopia and the Former Soviet Union 83
   Petra Nahmias
6. The Predecline Rise in Israeli Muslim Fertility 113
   Jona Schellekens and Zvi Eisenbach

Part 2: Nuptiality and Contraception

7. Age at Marriage, Sex-Ratios, and Ethnic Heterogamy 131
   Haya Stier and Yossi Shavit
8. Insight into Ethnic Flux: Marriage Patterns among Jews of Mixed Ancestry in Israel 145
   Barbara S. Okun
9. Religiosity and Contraceptive Method Choice: The Jewish Population of Israel 165
   Barbara S. Okun
10. Socioeconomic and Cultural Determinants of Abortion Among Jewish Women in Israel 189
    Esther I. Wilder

Part 3: Mortality

11. Old-Age Mortality in Israel: Analysis of Variation and Change — 217
    Dov Friedlander, Jona Schellekens and Refaela Sharashov Cohen
12. Does Religious Observance Promote Health? Mortality in Secular vs. Religious Kibbutzim in Israel — 243
    Jeremy D. Kark, Galia Shemi, Yechiel Friedlander, Oz Martin, Orly Manor and S. H. Blondheim
13. Death Rests a While: Holy Day and Sabbath Effects on Jewish Mortality in Israel — 257
    Jon Anson and Ofra Anson
14. Mortality Differentials among Women: The Israel Longitudinal Mortality Study — 281
    Orly Manor, Zvi Eisenbach, Avi Israeli and Yechiel Friedlander
15. Mortality after Spousal Loss: Are There Socio-Demographic Differences? — 303
    Orly Manor and Zvi Eisenbach
16. Mortality in Two Jewish Populations—Montreal and Israel: Environmental Determinants of Differences — 319
    Bryna Shatenstein and Jeremy D. Kark

Part 4: Related Issues

17. The Extra Burden of Muslim Wives: Clues from Israeli Women's Labor Supply — 339
    Shoshana Grossbard-Shechtman and Shoshana Neuman
18. From Pronatalism to Social Welfare? Extending Family Allowances to Minority Populations in France and Israel — 365
    Leslie King
19. Jerusalem's Population, 1995-2020: Demography, Multiculturalism and Urban Policies — 383
    Sergio DellaPergola

Sources

We wish to gratefully acknowledge the permission to use copyrighted material granted by journals and publishers.

Chapter 2 is reprinted from D. Friedlander and C. Feldmann (1993), "The Modern Shift to Below-replacement Fertility: Has Israel's Population Joined the Process?" *Population Studies*, 47, 295-306, with permission from Taylor & Francis Ltd., http://www.tandf.co.uk/journals.

Chapter 3 is reprinted from J. Anson and A. Meir (1996), "Religiosity, Nationalism and Fertility in Israel," *European Journal of Population*, 12, 1-25, with kind permission from Springer Science and Business Media. Copyright © 1996 Kluwer Academic Publishers.

Chapter 4 is reprinted from B. Okun (1997), "Innovation and Adaptation in Fertility Transition: Jewish Immigrants to Israel from Muslim North Africa and the Middle East," *Population Studies,* 51, 317-335, with permission from Taylor & Francis Ltd., http://www.tandf.co.uk/journals.

Chapter 5 is reprinted from P. Nahmias (2004), "Fertility Behavior of Recent Immigrants to Israel: A Comparative Analysis of Immigrants from Ethiopia and the Former Soviet Union," *Demographic Research*, 10-4, http://www.demographic-research.org/volumes/vol10/4/, with permission from the Max Planck Institute for Demographic Research.

Chapter 6 is reprinted from J. J. Schellekens and Z. Eisenbach (2002), "The Predecline rise in Israeli Muslim fertility," *Economic Development and Cultural Change*, 50, 541-555. Copyright © 2002 The University of Chicago. Reprinted with permission.

Chapter 7 is reprinted from H. Stier and Y. Shavit (1994), "Age at Marriage, Sex-Ratios, and Ethnic Heterogamy," *European Sociological Review*, 10, 79-87, with permission of the Oxford University Press.

Chapter 8 is reprinted from B. S. Okun (2004), "Insight into Ethnic Flux: Marriage Patterns among Jews of Mixed Ancestry in Israel," *Demography*, 41, 173-187, with permission of the Population Association of America.

Chapter 9 is reprinted from B.S. Okun (2000), "Religiosity and Contraceptive Method Choice: the Jewish Population of Israel," *European Journal of Population*, 16, 109-132. Copyright © 2000 Kluwer Academic Publishers. With kind permission from Springer Science and Business Media.

Chapter 10 is reprinted from E. I. Wilder (2000), "Socioeconomic and Cultural Determinants of Abortion among Jewish Women in Israel," *European Journal of Population*, 16, 133-162. Copyright © 2000 Kluwer Academic Publishers. With kind permission from Springer Science and Business Media.

Chapter 11 is reprinted from D. Friedlander, J. J. Schellekens and R. S. Cohen (1995), "Old-age Mortality in Israel: Analysis of Variation and Change," *Health Transition Review*, 5, 59-83. Reprinted with permission.

Chapter 12 is reprinted from J. D. Kark, G. Shemi, Y. Friedlander, O. Martin, O. Manor and S. H. Blondheim (1996), "Does Religious Observance Promote Health? Mortality in Secular vs. Religious Kibbutzim in Israel," *American Journal of Public Health*, 86, 341-6. Reprinted with permission from the American Public Health Association.

Chapter 13 is reprinted from J. Anson and O. Anson (2001), "Death Rests a While: Holy Day and Sabbath effects on Jewish Mortality in Israel," *Social Science and Medicine*, 52, 83-97. Copyright © 2001 with permission from Elsevier.

Chapter 14 is reprinted from O. Manor, Z. Eisenbach, A. Israeli and Y. Friedlander (2000) "Mortality Differentials among Women: The Israel Longitudinal Mortality Study," *Social Science and Medicine*, 51, 1175-1188. Copyright © 2000 with permission from Elsevier.

Chapter 15 is reprinted from O. Manor and Z. Eisenbach (2003), "Mortality after Spousal Loss: Are there Socio-demographic Differences?" *Social Science and Medicine*, 56, 405-413. Copyright © 2003 with permission from Elsevier.

Chapter 16 is reprinted from B. Shatenstein and J. D. Kark (1995), "Mortality in Two Jewish Populations—Montreal and Israel: Environmental Determinants of Differences," *International Journal of Epidemiology*, 24, 730-9, with permission of the Oxford University Press.

Chapter 17 is reprinted from S. Grossbard-Shechtman and S. Neuman (1998), "The Extra Burden of Muslim Wives: Clues from Israeli Women's Labor Supply," *Economic Development and Cultural Change*, *46*, 491-517. Copyright © 1998 The University of Chicago. Reprinted with permission.

Chapter 18 is reprinted from by L. King (2001), "From Pronatalism to Social Welfare? Extending Family Allowances to Minority Populations in France and Israel," *European Journal of Population*, 17, 305-322. Copyright © 2001 Kluwer Academic Publishers. With kind permission from Springer Science and Business Media.

Chapter 19 is reprinted from Sergio DellaPergola (2001), "Jerusalem's Population, 1995-2020: Demography, Multiculturism and Policy," *European Journal of Population*, 17, 165-199. Copyright © 2001 Kluwer Academic Publishers. With kind permission from Springer Science and Business Media.

1

Israel's Destiny: Fertility and Mortality in a Divided Society

Jona Schellekens and Jon Anson

Introduction

In Israeli public discourse, demography is associated more than anything else with the relative size of different ethnic groups, and population forecasts. This is a frustrating view of the subject for many academic demographers, who devote so much of their time in an effort to understand a specific domain of human behavior. Counting the population of Israel and making population forecasts are mostly the task of the Central Bureau of Statistics, but this is only a small and very applied part of demography. Most demographers doing scientific research are far more interested in studying the determinants and implications of demographic behavior than in undertaking technical surveys and forecasts.

This stereotype of the demographer as a kind of population accountant is not limited to public discourse. In Israeli academia too, demography is treated as a minor, largely technical side-issue in the social sciences, with little theoretical consideration given to population processes as social processes. This is a reflection of the more general sociological view of society as based on current relations between socially identified roles, with little attention given to the people who fulfill these roles, and even less to their reproduction. The purpose of this book is to correct this lacuna. It is self evident that all societies are made up of people who have been conceived and born, and all of who must die, yet it would appear less self-evident that conception, birth and death are all socially patterned. In this book we focus on work that has been published in the past decade, in particular articles reporting research on the influence of social class, religion, religiosity, nationalism, and ethnicity on fertility and mortality in Israel.

More than any other social institution, the family is at the heart of sociology. Demographers are well positioned to contribute to empirical research on the family because the census, vital statistics, and fertility surveys are the primary sources for studies of the family. In the past, different names were used by sociologist demographers to describe their area of specialization, including *social* as well as *sociological demography* (Goldscheider 1971; and Matras 1977). Today, however, social demography is accepted by most sociologist demographers to describe their area of specialization (Hirschman and Tolnay 2005). Social demography covers a wide range of topics, including fertility and nuptiality, household and family structure, morbidity and mortality, senescence, population aging, education, income inequality, and migration.

The substantive areas selected over time for the main focus in the study of fertility have changed with the historical circumstances and with the theoretical perspectives that guide research. After World War II, Demographic Transition Theory was the dominant paradigm in fertility studies. It attributed the decline in fertility that had occurred in the developed countries before the war to social and economic changes including the spread of education and rational thought, changes in the economic benefits and costs of children and the emergence of new economic roles for women that were incompatible with childbearing. Considerable stimulus to the development of transition theory came with the Cold War. In most developing countries mortality was declining, while fertility remained high, and the political implications of this disequilibrium was reflected in an academic concern that the high rates of natural increase resulting from such levels of mortality and fertility would interfere with economic development (Coale and Hoover, 1958).

Explanations of the fertility decline fall into two major categories: adjustment and innovation. The view of fertility decline as an adjustment states that fertility control reflects an adjustment to economic and social change. The view of the decline as a process of innovation, on the other hand, states that the adoption of fertility control represents new behavior due to changes in the acceptability of fertility control on moral grounds. Empirical tests have failed to settle the dispute so far and a consensus view is not yet in sight (Hirschman 1994). This book contains a relatively recent contribution to this debate by Barbara Okun in chapter 4.

In the last thirty years, fertility in most developed countries has declined below replacement level, or below the number of children that is needed to keep a closed population from declining in the long run, which is approximately 2.1 births per woman in low-mortality countries. Three major categories of explanations have been suggested for the recent decline in fertility: economic factors, especially those concerned with women's employment opportunities and relative incomes (e.g., Engelhardt et al. 2004); cultural or attitudinal change, particularly associated with assertive individualism and secularization (Lesthaeghe and Surkyn 1988); and contraceptive and related technological factors such as improved contraceptive methods, induced abortion, and sterilization pills (Murphy 1993).

Early mortality decline, particularly in today's more developed countries, was closely associated with improvement in living standards and public health (Harris 2004; Cutler and Miller, 2005). Following a decade of stagnation in the 1960s, adult mortality in many developed countries started to decline faster in the 1970s, mainly as a result of delayed cardiovascular disease (Olshansky and Ault, 1986). However, more recent analyses indicate that there may also be counter-tendencies at work, limiting mortality decline (Olshansky et al. 2000). These findings raise an old debate about the contribution of living standards to mortality decline. Investigating the period 1850-1970, McKeown (1979) had shown that medical technology only played a very minor role in the decline in mortality in today's developed countries. Instead, McKeown suggested that improved living standards explain most of the decline in mortality. Obviously, this hypothesis needs reassessment in the light of recent developments. Today, the correlation between per capita income and life expectancy at birth among developed countries is very weak. Life expectancy in Israel, for example, is higher than in the United States and, indeed, life expectancy at birth for Israeli men is among the highest in the world. That of Israeli women, however, ranks near the middle of developed countries.

One of the explanations for the poor performance of the United States is the degree of income inequality. Kawachi et al. (1997) show that income inequality is strongly correlated with both per capita group membership and lack of social trust, both of which are associated with high mortality. However, while early analyses suggested a clear positive relation between income inequality and mortality rates (Rodgers 1979), recent analyses suggest that this may not longer be the case in very high income countries. The changing age distribution of relative poverty may have affected the way income inequality in these countries impacts on mortality measured across all ages (Lobmayer and Wilkinson 2000).

A Concise Population History of the State of Israel

This is not the place to expand on Israel's immigration history. The story of the different waves of Jewish immigrants has already been told elsewhere many times. Neither is this the place to discuss the (forced) emigration of Arabs.

The renewal of family-building activity by European Jews after the Holocaust is evident in the population pyramid of the Jewish population in Israel, which shows a growing base starting in the late 1940s. Many children were born to European parents in those days, raising the percent of children relative to other age groups. However, the rise in fertility among European Jews is not the only explanation for the growing base of the population pyramid of the Jewish population in Israel. Immigrants from the Near East and North Africa who were starting to arrive at about the same time also contributed to the peculiar shape of the Israeli Jewish population pyramid by an increase in the survival rate of infants and young children (Friedlander 1975). Before immigration, they had suffered from relatively high levels of infant and early childhood mortality. Immediately upon their arrival, improved medical care and sanitary conditions caused their mortality levels to plummet, raising the percentage of infants and young children in the population. Immigrants from the Near East and North Africa also arrived with relatively high levels of fertility. Although fertility decline among these immigrants started within a few years after immigration, its pace was much slower than that of their mortality decline.

Demographic Transition Theory lists infant mortality decline as one of the causes of fertility decline (Caldwell and Caldwell 1997). However, fertility decline among Israeli Arab Muslims only started in the early 1970s, long after infant mortality had started to decline. The reason for this late fertility decline remains an issue of debate (Schellekens and Eisenbach 2006). In many populations, there was a pre-decline rise in fertility (Dyson and Murphy 1985). This can also be observed among Israeli Arab Muslims. Jona Schellekens and Zvi Eisenbach in chapter 6 discuss this episode in Israeli population history.

Today, Israel has the highest fertility level among developed countries and is one of the few to have a fertility level that is still above replacement level. This is true for both major ethnic groups, Arabs and Jews. Part of the decline in fertility is due to a decline in nuptiality. Age at first marriage among Israeli Jews has increased among both sexes in the last thirty years. Celibacy rates, however, are still low compared with most other developed countries.

Fertility and Mortality in a Divided Society

Ethnic and religious identities play an important role in Israeli society, indeed, as Al-Haj (2004) has recently argued, Israel remains a deeply divided society and the recent wave of immigration from the former USSR has probably added to this division. Ethnic identities are relatively easy to ascertain from the census and vital registration and ethnicity has always figured as an important categorical variable in demographic studies of Israeli society. Information on religiosity, on the other hand, needs to be collected from surveys, although a few macro-level studies have measured religiosity indirectly by using voting patterns. Hence, there are fewer studies of the effect of religiosity on fertility and mortality. Papers on the effect of religiosity on fertility are not new (e.g., Matras 1964), but the study of the effect of religiosity on mortality is relatively new. This book includes much of the recent output in research on the effects of religiosity on demographic behavior in Israel.

Fertility

Studies of Israeli fertility in the 1970s and 1980s dealt with issues related to the fertility decline among Asian and African immigrants and the Arab population, such as the convergence of fertility patterns among immigrants (Friedlander and Goldscheider 1978), and the relationship between socio-economic development and fertility decline (Friedlander, Eisenbach and Goldscheider 1979 and Friedlander, Eisenbach and Goldscheider 1980).

Although Israel is a society with characteristics that place it among the developed countries of the world, its fertility history is unlike that of any other developed country. Take, for example, the modern shift to below-replacement fertility, which has been the most significant demographic development in developed countries in the last forty years. Although fertility levels among Israeli Jews have declined, they still remain well above replacement level. The recent immigration wave from the former Soviet Union, where fertility levels are extremely low, has not changed this. Actually, former Soviet Union immigrants are raising their fertility, although the increase is small, as shown in chapter 5 by Petra Nahmias.

One of the explanations for Israeli Jewish fertility being so different may be their religiosity. Dov Friedlander and Carole Feldmann in chapter 2 test this hypothesis. They use regression estimates to show that fertility among secular European Jews is below-replacement level. They control for socio-economic characteristics. Hence, in theory the effect of religiosity could be due to specific doctrines. However, it is unlikely that religiosity in Judaism implies the simple connection between doctrine and fertility, since there is neither a known, clear doctrine in Judaism on family size nor a clear-cut prohibition on the use of all forms of contraception (Goldscheider 2002: 227).

Another hypothesis proposed by Goldscheider (1967) focuses on minority-group status. If a group feels threatened, minority-group status may encourage higher fertility to ensure group preservation and strength in numbers. Resistance may encourage group integration and identification. It may also encourage a greater commitment to religious ideology and to norms particular to the minority group. Jon Anson and Avinoam Meir in chapter 3 follow up on this lead and test the hypothesis that nationalist sentiments mediate the influence of religiosity. They argue that Israel's high fertility stems from the salience of nationalist sentiments due to its special position in the Middle East. Using voting returns from the 1984 elections, they classified census statistical areas by religiosity and their support for radical nationalist parties. They show that once nationalist support is controlled the effect of religiosity is insignificant, and suggest that both high fertility *and* religiosity derive from the particular form of national conflict in which Israel is engaged.

Israeli Arab Muslim fertility is even higher than that of Israeli Jews. In the 1960s it had reached levels that are among the highest on record. Jona Schellekens and Zvi Eisenbach in chapter 6 show that the most likely explanation for this unique episode in the demographic history of Israel is a decline in breastfeeding. Arab Israeli fertility started to decline in the early 1970s, but its pace slackened from the mid 1980s. Fargues (2000) suggests that a version of Goldscheider's minority-group status hypothesis may help us understand what happened to Israeli Arab fertility. He argues that the Israeli-Palestinian conflict shaped ideational change related to fertility sharpening identities and the vision of the nation as a quasi-biological body whose vitality is closely linked to reproduction (see also Kanaaneh 2002). Child allowances may also have contributed to a slackening of the pace of decline among Israeli Muslims (Friedlander, Eisenbach and Goldscheider 1979).

Nuptiality and contraception

Nuptiality and contraception are major proximate determinants (Bongaarts, 1978) of fertility. As in other developed countries, nuptiality is declining while cohabitation is spreading. A comparison between total fertility rates and total marital fertility rates using published data in the Statistical Abstracts of Israel suggests the decline in marriage has contributed to the decline in fertility in the past thirty years.

Besides a paper that focuses on the effects of a marriage squeeze in the early 1970s (Ben-Moshe 1989), the question why marriage is declining has received little attention. There are more publications on ethnic intermarriage. As in other immigrant countries, research on ethnic intermarriage in Israel is motivated by the question of whether the various ethnic groups will integrate with one another (Kalmijn 1998). The general expectation is that intermarriage will reduce the salience of ethnicity. Goldscheider (2002: 204) warns, however, that selective out-marriage of those who are marginal to the ethnic group may result in a core of more committed ethnic group members. Assimilation theories predict that education will weaken ethnic attachments and will lead to a loss of ethnic identity among the upwardly mobile members of disadvantaged ethnic groups. In the Israeli context, the assimilation hypothesis suggests that the greater contact of educated Mizrahim with Ashkenazim will lead to the erosion of their Mizrahi ethnic consciousness, more frequent intermarriage, and the consequent concentration of Mizrahi ethnicity in the lower classes. Barbara Okun in chapter 8 tests this hypothesis and finds that it fits the data. She also shows that more-educated people of mixed ethnicity tend to marry Ashkenazim, while less-educated people of mixed ethnicity tend to marry Mizrahim. Thus, there is no evidence for the emergence of a new national Israeli ethnicity.

Although ethnicity continues to play a central role in mate selection, all agree that ethnic homogamy is decreasing. However, this is not due to educational homogamy which shows little evidence of overall increases (Okun 1997). Thus the reasons for the decline in ethnic homogamy must be sought elsewhere. Haya Stier and Yossi Shavit in chapter 7 discuss the influence of the marriage squeeze and the rise in the age at first marriage on ethnic homogamy. They conclude that intermarriage between ethnic groups was partly a result of uneven sex-ratios (see also Ben-Moshe 1989).

While little has been written about the effect of religiosity on age at marriage, there are a few articles on the effect of religiosity on two other major proximate determinants of fertility (for contraceptive behavior see Barbara Okun in chapter 9 and for abortions see Esther Wilder in chapter 10). One of the main issues in the study of the effect of religion is *how* it affects reproductive behavior. Thus, Barbara Okun in this volume tries to go beyond simply measuring the effect of religiosity on contraceptive behavior using an analytic framework, which builds on previous work of Goldscheider (1971).

Mortality

Differentials in mortality by socio-economic status and the nature of social ties have been well established (Black et al., 1980; for a review see Goldman 2000). Although the study of socio-economic differentials in morbidity and mortality is not a new area of research (e.g., Antonovosky 1967), the debate over the causes of socio-economic differentials in Israel has received much attention in the last ten years. Health policy has commonly focused on the organization and funding of health services. Concern with prevention of the major chronic diseases has tended to focus on lifestyles, such as smoking. The Whitehall Studies of British civil servants (Marmot et al. 1991) have been in the lead in showing that the circumstances in which people live and work are major influences on their health. The studies showed that big differences in health between people in different social groups remain even after correcting for factors such as differences in smoking. The studies showed that the social gradient is not only related to poverty, it is related to where you are in the hierarchy. Those at one step from the top, professionals and executives in the British Civil Service, doctors and lawyers, have rates twice as high as those at the very top.

The first thing Michael Marmot and his group did was try to explain this gradient by reference to the important risk factors that we know about. They adjusted for diet, smoking, blood pressure, physical activity, obesity, social support, and hundreds of other variables. But the gradient remained even after adjusting for these factors. The risk factors explain something like a quarter to a third of the gradient, but the rest remained a mystery. Wilkinson has argued that perceptions of place in the social hierarchy produce negative emotions such as shame and distrust that are translated inside the body into poor health via psycho-neuro-endocrine mechanisms and stress-induced behaviors such as smoking (Lynch et al. 2000; Marmot and Wilkinson 2001).

Anson (1988) was among the first to report socio-economic differentials in mortality in Israel, while Dov Friedlander et al. in chapter 11 showed that these differentials were on the increase. They also found ethnic differentials in mortality that could not be explained by the socio-economic differentials, in particular among North-African immigrants. Two later micro-level studies by Orly Manor et al. (1999) and by Orly Manor et al. in chapter 14 were able to eliminate the excess mortality among North African men and women after allowing for several socio-economic indicators. Unfortunately, data-quality problems have so far prevented mortality studies from including Israeli Arabs.

A related area of research has examined the association between social ties and morbidity and mortality. People who are less socially integrated have higher rates of morbidity and mortality (Berkman and Syme 1979). The earliest research on the effects of social connection on morbidity and mortality focused on marital status. It demonstrated that married people have lower rates of morbidity and mortality than unmarried people. Although some of this effect may be due to selection, most of it is now thought to be due to health-related behavior and social ties (Hu and Goldman 1990). Part of the differentials in mortality between the widowed and the married is due to the so-called bereavement effect. Evidence for this effect has also been documented in Israel. Orly Manor and Zvi Eisenbach in chapter 15 found that the effect of bereavement on mortality varied by duration of bereavement, age, and education.

Research has demonstrated that religious attendance is associated with lower morbidity and mortality. Again, some of this effect is due to selectively, but most must be due to health-related behavior and social ties (Hummer et al. 1999; McCullough et al. 2000). Chapter 13 by Jon Anson and Ofra Anson supports a psychosocial explanation for the effect of religiosity on mortality. They found a clear and significant dip-peak pattern in the number of deaths around the Sabbath for all men, and for younger women. This pattern was stronger for men than for women. Dov Friedlander et al. in chapter 11 and Jaffe et al. (2005) also found that the religiosity effect among Jewish men is stronger. However, Jeremy Kark et al. in chapter 12 found an apparently stronger protective effect of religiosity in women than in men in a comparison between secular and religious kibbutzim. It should be noted, however, that the kibbutz study does not include any ultra-orthodox, while the studies of Dov Friedlander et al. in this volume and of Jaffe et al. (2005) do. Hence, it is possible that the different results are somehow related to differences in the status of women between the modern-orthodox and ultra-orthodox.

A great deal of research has been conducted on the subject of sex-specific mortality differences. The hypotheses advanced to explain male excess mortality fall into two basic categories; the biological approach and the behavioral approach. According to the biological approach, women are less prone to disease for anatomic and physiological reasons. Advocates of the behavioral approach argue that society and culture influence men to lead more dangerous lifestyles, that men are subjected to greater health risks at work, and that men are generally more exposed to, and susceptible to, social and psychological stress (Luy 2003). Men also appear to be more sensitive to deprivations, both of a material and emotional nature (Anson 2003). Sex differentials in mortality among the Jewish population of Israel are the smallest among developed countries. The reason for this remains unclear, but this phenomenon does not appear to be limited to

Jews living in Israel (Shkolnikov et al. 2005). Bryna Shatenstein and Jeremy Kark in chapter 16 compared mortality in the Jewish populations of Montreal and Israel and the overall Canadian population, to investigate whether the Israeli pattern of low male mortality and relatively high female mortality is replicated among Jews living elsewhere. Their findings suggest that the mortality pattern characteristic of Israeli Jews is not a universal Jewish phenomenon.

Related Issues

The study of fertility and mortality and their determinants are at the core of the research effort of demographers. We conclude with three articles dealing with related issues.

The participation of women in the labor force is a key variable in many economic models of fertility. The effect of this variable on fertility is difficult to measure, however, because there is also a reverse effect of fertility on the labor-force participation of married women. Labor-force participation rates in Israel differ across religious groups. Participation rates of Muslim women are lower than those of Christian or Jewish—including ultra-orthodox—women. Shoshana Grossbard-Shechtman and Shoshana Neuman in chapter 17 show that the effect of the number of children is weaker on Muslim women's labor supply than that of Jewish women, in spite of the higher fertility of Muslims.

In 1975 Israel instituted a generous non-income tested family allowance program, replacing a complex system of benefits for children. This population policy grew out of a concern for the socioeconomic conditions of disadvantaged social groups in general, and of the large Oriental Jewish families in particular, on the one hand, and for the low fertility rates of Jews compared with Israeli Arab Muslims, on the other. Symptomatic of the latter concern is the initiative of Israel's first Prime-minister David Ben-Gurion to pay a cash prize to every woman who gave birth to a tenth child. The Ben-Gurion prize was finally abolished in 1959, one of the reasons apparently being that many Arab women received it (Friedlander 1974).

Micro-economic theory predicts that cash benefits will increase fertility. However, studies involving econometric modelling of aggregate and individual data generally find a weak, although positive, relationship between cash benefits and fertility (Gauthier and Hatzius 1997; Schellekens 2006). When governments contemplate population policies, they do not seem to consult experts on the efficiency of child allowances in raising the birth rate. As Leslie King in chapter 18 shows, government policies in Israel and in other countries are more likely to be influenced by demographic trends and nationalist ideologies.

How to make population forecasts is not a substantive question, but a methodological one. Nonetheless, it is a central question for demography. Without them, future demographic trends cannot be assessed. Unfortunately, it receives very little serious attention from demographers these days who tend to regard it as a mechanical exercise with little or no intellectual content (Lee 2001). But some demographers still make forecasts, such as Sergio DellaPergola in chapter 19. He presents population forecasts for Jerusalem in the year 2020 by major ethnic group—Arab and Jewish—and by religiosity (Jews only). Jerusalem has a very large minority of ultra-orthodox Jews, who have very high fertility levels. The average number of births an ultra-orthodox woman has may be as high as 7.5 (Friedlander and Feldmann in this volume). Manski and Mayshar (2003) argue that the generous child allowances are one explanation for the relatively high fertility of ultra-orthodox couples. The high fertility of the ultra-orthodox dominates the population forecast scenarios for Jerusalem by DellaPergola.

References

Al-Haj, Majid. 2004. *Immigration and Ethnic Formation in a Deeply Divided Society: The Case of the 1990s Immigrants from the Former Soviet Union in Israel.* Leiden: Brill.

Anson, J. 1988. "Mortality and living conditions: Relative mortality levels and their relation to the physical quality of life in urban populations." *Social Science and Medicine* 27: 901-910.

Anson, J. 2003. "Sex differences in mortality at the local level: An analysis of Belgian municipalities." *European Journal of Population* 19: 1-28.

Antonovsky, A. 1967. "Social class, life expectancy and overall mortality." *Millbank Memorial Fund Quarterly* 45: 151-193.

Ben-Moshe, Eliahu. 1989. "Marriage squeeze and marriage patterns in Israel." In U. O. Schmelz and S. DellaPergola (eds.), *Papers in Jewish Demography 1985*, 87-95. Jerusalem: The Institute of Contemporary Jewry.

Berkman, Lisa F., and S. Leonard Syme. 1979. "Social networks, host resistance, and mortality: A nine-year follow-up study of Alameda county residents." *American Journal of Epidemiology* 109: 186-204.

Bongaarts, John. 1978. "A framework for analyzing the proximate determinants of fertility." *Population and Development Review* 4: 105-132

Caldwell, John. C., and Pat Caldwell. 1997. "What do we need to know about fertility transition." In G. W. Jones, R. M. Douglas, J. C. Caldwell and R. M. D'Souza (eds.), *The Continuing Demographic Transition*, 15-25. Oxford: Clarendon Press.

Coale, Ansley J. and Edgar M. Hoover. 1958. *Population Growth and Economic Development in Low-Income Countries: A Case Study of India's Prospects.* Princeton, NJ: Princeton University Press

Cutler, David and Grant Miller. 2005. "The role of public health improvements in health advances: The twentieth-century United States." *Demography* 42: 1-22.

Dyson, Tim, and Mike Murphy. 1985. "The onset of fertility transition." *Population and Development Review* 11: 399-440.

Engelhardt, Henriette, Tomas Kögel and Alexia Prskawetz. 2004. "Fertility and women's employment reconsidered: A macro-level time-series analysis for developed countries, 1960-2000." *Population Studies* 58: 109-120

Fargues, Philippe. 2000. "Protracted national conflict and fertility change among Palestinians and Israelis." *Population and Development Review* 26: 441-82.

Friedlander, Dov. 1974. "Population Policy in Israel." In Bernard Berelson (eds.), *Population Policy in Developed Countries*, 42-97. New York: McGraw-Hill.

Friedlander, Dov. 1975. "Mass immigration and population dynamics in Israel." *Demography* 12: 581-599.

Friedlander, Dov, Zvi Eisenbach, and Calvin Goldscheider. 1979. "Modernization patterns and fertility change: The Arab populations of Israel and the Israel-administered territories." *Population Studies* 33: 239-254.

Friedlander, Dov, Zvi Eisenbach, and Calvin Goldscheider. 1980. "Family-size limitation and birth spacing: The fertility transition of African and Asian immigrants in Israel." *Population and Development Review* 6: 581-593.

Friedlander, Dov, and Calvin Goldscheider. 1978. "Immigration, social change and cohort fertility in Israel." *Population Studies* 32: 299-317.

Gauthier, Anne Hélène, and Jan Hatzius. 1997. "Family benefits and fertility: An econometric analysis." *Population Studies* 51: 295-306.

Goldman, Noreen. 2001. "Mortality differentials: Selection and causation." In Neil J. Smelser and Paul B. Baltes (eds.), *International Encyclopedia of the Social and Behavioral Sciences*, 10068-10070. Amsterdam: Elsevier.

Goldscheider, Calvin. 1967. "Fertility of the Jews." *Demography* 4: 196-209.

Goldscheider, Calvin. 1971. *Population, Modernization, and Social Structure*. Boston, MA: Little Brown and Company.

Goldscheider, Calvin. 2002. *Israel's Changing Society: Population, Ethnicity, and Development*, second edition. Boulder, CO: Westview Press.

Harris, Bernard. 2004. "Public health, nutrition, and the decline of mortality: The McKeown thesis revisited." *Social History of Medicine* 17: 379-407.

Hirschman, Charles. 1994. "Why fertility changes." *Annual Review of Sociology* 20: 203-233.

Hirschman, Charles, and Stewart E. Tolnay. 2005. "Social demography." In Dudley L. Poston, Jr., and Michael Micklin (eds.), *Handbook of Population*, 419-449. New York: Springer Publishers.

Hu, Yuanreng, and Noreen Goldman. 1990. "Mortality differentials by marital status: An international comparison." *Demography* 27: 233-50.

Hummer, R., R. Rogers, C. Nam and C. G. Ellison. 1999. "Religious attendance and mortality in the US adult population." *Demography* 36: 273-85.

Jaffe, Dena H., Zvi Eisenbach, Yehuda D. Neumark, and Orly Manor. 2005. "Does living in a religiously affiliated neighborhood lower mortality?" *Annals of Epidemiology* 15: 804-810.

Kalmijn, Matthijs. 1998. "Intermarriage and homogamy: Causes, patterns, trends." *Annual Review of Sociology* 24: 395-421.

Kanaaneh, Rhoda Ann. 2002. *Birthing the Nation: Strategies of Palestinian Women in Israel*. University of California Press.

Kawachi, Ichiro, Bruce P. Kennedy, Kimberly Lochner and Deborah Prothrow-Stith, 1997. "Social capital, income inequality, and mortality." *American Journal of Public Health* 87: 1491-98.

Lee, Ron. 2001. "The decline of formal and aggregate analysis: Demography abandons its core." http://www.ceda.berkeley.edu/papers/rlee/FormalDemog.pdf (accessed 31/8/06).

Lesthaeghe, R. and J. Surkyn. 1988. "Cultural dynamics and economic theories of fertility change." *Population and Development Review* 14: 1-45.

Luy, Marc. 2003. "Causes of male excess mortality: Insights from cloistered populations." *Population and Development Review* 29: 647-676

Lobmayer, Peter and Richard Wilkinson. 2000. "Income, inequality and mortality in 14 developed countries." *Sociology of Health and Illness* 22: 401-414.

Lynch, John W., George Davey Smith, George A. Kaplan, and James S. House. 2000. "Income inequality and mortality; Importance to health of individual income, psychosocial environment, or material conditions." *British Medical Journal* 320: 1200-1204.

Manor, Orly, Zvi Eisenbach, Eric Peritz and Yechiel Friedlander. 1999. "Mortality differentials among Israeli men." *American Journal of Public Health* 89: 1807-1813.

Manski. Charles F., and Joram Mayshar. 2003. "Private incentives and social interactions: Fertility puzzles in Israel." *Journal of the European Economic Association* 1: 181-211.

Marmot, Michael G., G.D. Smith, S. Stansfeld, C. Patel, F. North, J. Head, I. White, E. Brunner, A. Feeney. 1991. "Health inequalities among British civil servants: The Whitehall II Study." *Lancet* 337: 1387-93.

Marmot, Michael, and Richard G. Wilkinson. 2001. "Psychosocial and material pathways in the relation between income and health: A response to Lynch et al." *British Medical Journal* 322: 1233-1236.

Matras, Judah. 1964. "Religious observance and family formation in Israel: Some intergenerational changes." *The American Journal of Sociology* 69: 464-475.

Matras, Judah. 1977. *Introduction to Population: A Sociological Approach*. Englewood Cliffs, NJ: Prentice Hall.

McCullough, Michael E., William T. Hoyt, David B. Larson, Harold G. Koenig, Carl Thoresen. 2000. "Religious involvement and mortality: A meta-analytic review." *Health Psychology* 19: 211-222.

McKeown, Thomas. 1979. *The Role of Medicine: Dream, Mirage or Nemesis*. Princeton, NJ: Princeton University Press.

Murphy, Michael. 1993. "The contraceptive pill and female employment as factors in fertility change in Britain 1963-80: A challenge to the conventional view". *Population Studies* 47: 221-43.

Okun, Barbara. 2001. "The effects of ethnicity and educational attainment on Jewish marriage patterns: Changes in Israel, 1957-1995." *Population Studies* 55: 49-64.

Olshansky, S.Jay. and A. Brian Ault. 1986. "The fourth stage of the epidemiologic transition: The age of delayed degenerative diseases." *The Milbank Quarterly* 64: 355-391.

Olshansky, S. Jay, B. A. Carnes, R. G. Rogers and L. Smith. 2000. "Emerging infectious diseases: The fifth stage of the epidemiologic transition." *World Health Statistical Quarterly* 51: 207-217.

Rodgers, G B. 1979. "Income and inequality as determinants of mortality: An international cross-section analysis." *Population Studies* 33: 343-351

Shkolnikov, Vladimir M., Evgueni M. Andreev, Jon Anson and France Meslé. 2004. "The peculiar pattern of mortality of Jews in Moscow, 1993 – 1995." *Population Studies* 58: 311-329.

Part 1

Fertility

2

The Modern Shift to Below-Replacement Fertility: Has Israel's Population Joined the Process?

Dov Friedlander and Carole Feldmann

Introduction

The modern shift to "below replacement" fertility levels has been the most significant demographic development in industrial societies since the fertility transitions of the nineteenth and early twentieth centuries. These transformations reduced total fertility of 2.5-3.0 during the 1950s to low levels of 1.4-1.9 during the late 1970s and 1980s.[1] An examination of cohort marital fertility shows similar patterns. Hence, although a delay in marriage, or a shift of reproduction to later marriage durations, could have affected current total fertility in these societies, they cannot possibly provide the whole explanation. This transition to very low fertility levels has been explained by the general rise in the status of women, the large variety of substitutes for children and family in modern society, and the increasing costs of raising "quality" children (Davies 1986).

Israel's Jewish population is a modern, urban, industrial society. In terms of education levels, occupational distribution, women's participation in the labor force, consumption patterns, and aspirations it resembles European societies, though not the richest among them. Therefore, it would be expected that its characteristics should also result in low fertility levels in Israel. Nevertheless, total fertility in 1989 was 2.77 births per woman (Central Bureau of Statistics)!

The major questions raised in this chapter are: Is Israel's population an exception? If so, an explanation is needed. Alternatively, does the great heterogeneity of Israel's population disguise fertility declines that might have occurred in some population subgroups while others are characterized by high fertility?

Ethnic and Religiosity Differences in Israel's Jewish Population

The Jewish population in Israel can be divided into immigrants and Israeli-born, and also by origin, namely Asia-Africa and Europe. We define individuals as being of Asian-African and European ethnicity, respectively, if they had immigrated from these continents or are first-generation Israeli-born descendants of such immigrants. A previous study has demonstrated the strong association between marital fertility and ethnicity. It has been shown that fertility of the European group has been moderately low for several decades (Friedlander and Goldscheider 1978). We now ask whether this group has joined the new European "below-replacement fertility pattern." The total fertility of this ethnic group was 2.60 in 1989, compared with 2.83 between 1970 and 1974. Although this is a significant decline, the level of 1989 does not, on the face of it, seem to support the hypothesis that members of the European ethnic group have joined, or are about to join, the new low European fertility pattern. The same conclusion is reached when the decline in cohort marital fertility rates is considered.

Fertility in the Asian-African ethnic group was high during the early 1950s, shortly after the mass immigration wave when their total fertility was 5.5 births per woman. However, with increased length of stay in Israel, fertility declined fairly rapidly, so that their total fertility in 1989 was 2.84 births per woman (Central Bureau of Statistics).

Differentiation between the two major ethnic groups of Israel's heterogeneous population cannot identify a major sub-population with below-replacement fertility. However, another source of fertility variation in Israel's population, apparently much more significant than ethnicity, is religiosity. Heilman and Friedman (1991), have described the characteristics of Israel's religious population. According to them, the origin of Israel's current religiosity division dates back to the period of emancipation and enlightenment. There were three responses to this movement. The first was assimilation—the complete adoption of the culture of the larger society. The second was acculturation—the promotion of cultural contact with the outer world, whilst retaining Jewish culture and beliefs. The third was contra-acculturation—turning away from the contemporary way of life in order to preserve traditional ways. Israel's *national religious* population forms a continuous link with the acculturation stream, while Israel's *ultra-orthodox* groups originate from the contra-acculturation group. Indeed, the ultra-orthodox in Israel, as in the diaspora, "strived to separate themselves not only from every aspect of the outside culture, but also from people or things that, having passed near or through that world, carried contaminating elements of it" (Heilman and Friedman 1991: 9). Rough estimates suggest that total fertility in the ultra-religious population is of around 7, whereas in the national religious population it is about 4.5 births per woman.

In the 1984 elections some 15 percent of the total electorate voted for the religious parties, which should be considered a minimum estimate of the religious population, because an unknown, though significant proportion of the ultra-orthodox community, ban the elections on ideological grounds. Additionally, a proportion among the remaining orthodox population vote for right-wing national non-religious parties, while the opposite voting behavior is rare. Hence, 20 percent would be a more realistic estimate of the religious part of Israel's population. The very high fertility of the religious groups and their weight in the population lead us to the hypothesis that fertility of the non-religious part of the European ethnic group must have been much lower than the average for this ethnic group, possibly "below replacement level." A similar argument, though not as forceful, may also be valid for the Asian-African ethnic group.

The following sections deal mainly with the fertility patterns of the European population, attempting to control religiosity at low levels. The purpose is to uncover the main socio-economic variables that explain fertility variation and to assess the fertility level of the non-religious European population. A similar analysis enables us also to asses the fertility level of the non-religious Asian-African population.

Data and Variables

The analysis covers Israel's Jewish *urban* population that forms some 90 percent of the total. The units of analysis are based on aggregated populations in geographical areas that are either localities or parts of localities when these are large.

Census coverage is not complete among the religious population. Most conspicuous in this respect are the extreme *Naturei Karta* and similar extreme factions (Bleich 1984). However birth registration is complete, for it is very difficult to evade the registration of a birth, and it would be very costly to do so, particularly for large families who receive significant welfare benefits. Hence, age-specific fertility rates for geographical units that contain relatively high proportions of these religious factions are biased. We have, therefore, estimated total fertility for these units by stable-population techniques. It has been shown that the stability assumption is reasonable.

In all, 215 urban units are used in our analyses. For each of these units, total fertility, as well as various socio-economic variables, have been estimated.

Beginning with the major dependent variable we have:

Total fertility 1983-85, for women born either in European countries or born in Israel to fathers born there (i.e. of European ethnicity).

Several explanatory variables are used in the analysis:

The economic-status variable is the proportion employed, whose income in 1983 was within the upper decile of Israel's income distribution. This variable will be referred to as the *high-income* variable.

The social-status variable is the proportion of women aged 25-34 who had received more than twelve years of formal education. This is referred to as the *high-education* variable.

The *religiosity* variable is based on the general election results of 1984. It is the aggregated percentage vote for religious parties.

Women's participation in the labor force at ages 25-34 is a proxy for women's extra-familial activities during the major childbearing ages. It is referred to as *women's employment.*

Metropolitan is a variable that indicates whether a unit belongs to the Tel Aviv or Haifa metropolitan areas. The meaning of metropolitan residence is complex, and is related to opportunities in general.

Is Israel's Population on the Route to Below-Replacement Fertility?

We show in this section that in spite of the current relatively high *overall* total fertility a major part of Israel's population is proceeding toward the new European low-fertility pattern.

An examination of the distribution of total fertility of the European ethnic group shows that even *with no control on religiosity*, total fertility in over 55 percent of the 215 population units are below 2.5, and in about half of these below 2.1. However, when we regress total fertility rate on socio-economic and religiosity explanatory variables (to be discussed in a following section), and compute predicted values of total fertility on the assumption of zero religiosity, the percentage of units with below-replacement fertility is 94 percent. Considering the Asian-African ethnic group, which is at an earlier stage of the process, their total fertility is below 2.5 in 21 percent of the population units. However, when the predicted total fertility values for this ethnic group of zero religiosity are used, the percentage of units in which total fertility is less than 2.5 comes to 56 percent. Hence, it appears that the respective total fertility of 2.60 and 2.84 of the European and the Asian-African ethnic groups disguise a process of fertility decline towards below-replacement levels. The European group has reached an advanced stage in this process, the Asian-African is just at its beginning.

The association of religiosity with total fertility is the strongest for the explanatory variables, as is shown in table 2.1. This table presents the proportions of units with above average values by various explanatory variables for three ranges of total fertility. Although the associations between fertility and each of these explanatory variables are not controlled by others, they provide some indication to the explanation of low fertility. For example, the high-education variable in the table shows that the overall percentage of women with more than twelve years of formal education was 36.4 among all units. However, 64.2 percent of geographical units in which total fertility was 2.1 or lower, contained an above-average proportion of women with high education. This percentage was 59.4 and 31.6, among units in the medium and high-fertility categories respectively. Hence, there is a strong negative association between educational levels and fertility. Similarly, income, women's employment, and metropolitan residence are negatively associated with fertility. Religiosity is positively related with fertility and appears to be the strongest among the associations shown in this table.

We conclude from this part of the analysis that fertility of Israel's population of European ethnicity is similar to the new European pattern, and that they can be explained in terms of social status and economic welfare levels, and women's extra familial activities; variables which have been regarded as important in the explanation of low fertility in European countries. However, Israel differs from these European countries in the effect of religiosity, which provides the most important explanation for Israel's *overall* high fertility. These relationships will be restated in terms of specific hypotheses, and tested through multivariate analyses.

Major Hypotheses

The hypotheses listed below are based on explanations proposed for below-replacement fertility patterns in various European countries, and on theoretical considerations of fertility processes.

Religiosity: The higher the proportion of the religious population in the unit, the higher its fertility level, other things being equal. This relationship has been analyzed mostly in micro-level studies, and found to be significant (Lawton 1988, Schmelz 1985, Finnäs 1991).

High Income. The relationship between income and fertility has been studied extensively since the 1940s. The leading hypothesis was that income and fertility are positively related when other variables are controlled, because the conflict between an additional child and alternative non-familial goals is weaker, given higher income. The relationship was described as "elusive," because in contrast to expectations, it was found to be negative in many studies (Freedman and Thornton 1982). A negative relation is also shown in table 2.1, but this is before controlling for other variables. Our hypothesis is that the effect of income on fertility in our multivariate analyses is positive.

Table 2.1
Percentages of units with above average values in various explanatory variables for three ranges of total fertility levels (for the population of European ethnicity

	Explanatory variables*			
Total fertility rate (1)	High education (2)	High income (3)	Women's employment (4)	Religiosity (5)
TF ≤2.1	64.2	67.9	62.3	7.5
2.1 < TF ≤2.5	59.4	54.7	59.4	19.9
TF > 2.5	31.6	22.1	36.8	56.8
Means	36.4	11.2	64.0	13.5

*See explanations in action on data and variables.

Women's Employment. A high proportion of women in the labor force is expected to be negatively related to fertility levels. For example, it has been shown that women who are employed are more likely to postpone childbearing (Jones 1981). Women's employment does not only tend to lengthen birth intervals, but may also lead many women to stop reproducing, at relatively low fertility levels. The relation between fertility and women's employment has been studied extensively (Hartman 1978).

Education. The higher the educational levels of the adult population in a community, the lower their expected fertility levels. This is assumed to be the result of two indirect effects. First, women who have received more years of education tend to marry at older ages, and this would affect total fertility negatively. Secondly, such women tend to participate more in extra-familial activities, (one of these is their participation in the labor force) which will again affect fertility negatively.

Metropolitan Residence. Fertility levels in metropolitan areas are thought to be lower, when other variables are controlled. In such areas childbearing is more costly, extra-familial alternative activities are more diverse, and the society is more competitive.

Testing the Hypotheses

The above hypotheses imply that two variables are likely to have positive effects on fertility: religiosity and income. The remaining variables: educational levels, women's employment, and metropolitan residence, should affect fertility negatively. We use multivariate regressions to test these hypotheses.

Some explanatory variables are obviously intercorrelated, and this could affect the estimation of the regression coefficients. Preliminary analysis suggested that due to multicollinearity, only one of the economic-status, social-status and women's-employment variables, can be included in a single regression. Hence, we consider three alternative models as specified in table 2.2.

In each of Models 1 to 3 only one of the education, income and women's employment variables is included, in addition to metropolitan residence and religiosity. The table shows that Models 1 and 3 are consistent with our hypotheses, while in Model 2 the income variable has a negative coefficient, contrary to expectation. Modifying the income variable, by removing the effect of education does not alter the sign of the income coefficient. Hence, as in many other studies, the coefficient of high income is negative, that is, higher income is not associated with higher fertility. These regressions explain nearly 80 percent of the variance, and confirm that religiosity is invariably the most important explanatory variable, making the largest contribution to the explained variance.[2] Hence, the findings, so far, show that the new low European fertility pattern is present in Israel's population, particularly in the European ethnic group. Low proportions of religiosity tend to reduce fertility very considerably, while

Table 2.2
Regressions of total fertility on various explanatory varaiables, population of European ethnicity

Explanatory variables*	Model I		Model 2		Model 3	
	t	ΔR^2	t	ΔR^2	t	ΔR^2
High education	−3.60	0.017	–	–	–	–
High income	–	–	−2.45	0.006	–	–
Women's employment	–	–	–	–	−3.18	0.011
Metropolitan residence	−3.07	0.01	−2.54	0.013	−3.40	0.013
Religiosity	26.17	0.759	24.69	0.759	25.13	0.759
R^2	0.785		0.778		0.783	

*See explanations in action on data and variables.

increased socio-economic status, or women's employment, as well as urban residence, further reduce fertility levels.

The Explanation of Fertility Levels through a Recursive Model

The above relationships can be expressed by a model of structural equations in a recursive system. It provides a useful way of explaining and interpreting fertility levels and their relationships with the explanatory variables. We first present a theoretical recursive model of fertility illustrated by Equations (1)-(3), and figure 2.1 which is justified by its assumed interrelationship structure as specified below:

$$W=a_w+b_{ws}S+b_{wr}R+b_{wm}M+\varepsilon_w \quad (1)$$

$$I=a_i+b_{is}S+b_{ir}R+b_{im}M+b_{iw}W+\varepsilon_i \quad (2)$$

$$F=a_f+b_{fs}S+b_{fr}R+b_{fm}M+b_{fw}W+b_{fi}I+\varepsilon_i \quad (3)$$

where W, S, R, M, I and F, represent women's employment, social status, religiosity, metropolitan residence, income, and total fertility, respectively. ε_w, ε_i, and ε_f are residual error terms.

It is assumed in such a model that all the explanatory variables, that is, social status, religiosity, metropolitan residence, women's employment, and income, could affect total fertility, while total fertility does not affect these variables. Similarly, social status, religiosity, metropolitan residence, and women's employment may affect income, but cannot be affected by it. Also, status, religiosity and metropolitan residence may affect women's employment, but this variable does not affect the former variables (see figure 2.1). If, in addition, it is also assumed that the error terms ε in the three equations are uncorrelated, the system becomes a recursive model and can be appropriately estimated by ordinary least square methods (Johnston 1987).

In this model, women's employment and income may be considered as "intervening" between the status, religiosity, and metropolitan residence variables

Figure 2.1
Recursive Model: The Theoretical System

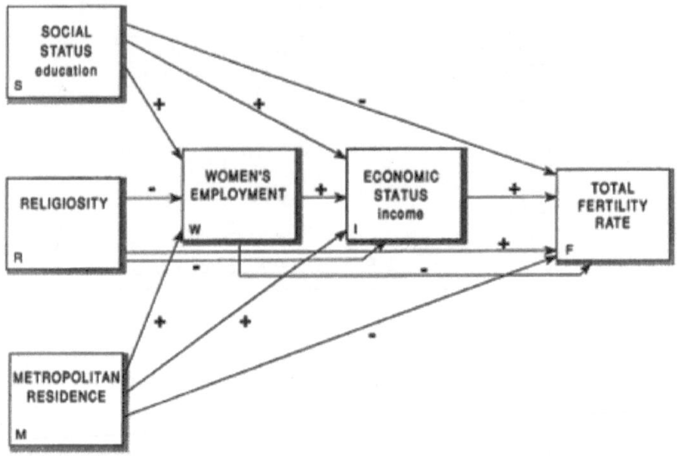

on one hand, and total fertility on the other. Therefore, the status, religiosity, and metropolitan residence variables may affect the total fertility directly, and/or indirectly, through the two intervening explanatory variables. Similarly, women's employment may have direct and/or indirect effects, while high income may only have a direct effect on total fertility.

An example of a general hypothesis within such a model is illustrated in the first panel of table 2.3, and by the signs above the arrows in figure 2.1. Accordingly, extensive extra-familial activities, such as women's employment, can be expected in high-status populations. Such activities conflict with high fertility. By implication, the high-status variable would have an indirect negative effect on fertility through such intervening 'conflict' variables. However, at least according to our initial hypothesis, the income variable should have a positive effect on fertility and is expected to reduce that conflict.

In addition to these potential indirect effects, a large proportion of high status might also have a negative direct effect on fertility because in such populations there is a high propensity for modern consumption patterns, and for raising "quality" children while limiting their numbers.

Religiosity may imply an idealistic approach to childbearing with a positive direct effect on fertility. But it also has potential indirect effects on fertility. Religiosity is likely to reduce women's employment, and they affect fertility positively. However, social organization within the religious community, certainly among the ultra-orthodox, is likely to reduce the conflict between women's employment and high fertility, as is argued in the next section. The role of income is similar to that stated above.

Similar considerations can be applied to the direct and indirect relationships between urban residence and fertility.

While such a general model of assumed relationships has merit in theory, it cannot be fully estimated in practice due to multicollinearity. Hence, we use three sub-models to avoid this difficulty. Table 2.3 shows the t-values of the regression coefficients for these sub-models. Their signs can be compared to those in the general relationships in the first panel of table 2.3.

Sub-model 1 in that table illustrates one specific empirical link. Women's employment has a negative effect on fertility, and is positively related with status. Hence, consistently with the assumed relationships, high status tends to reduce fertility indirectly by way of such' conflict' variables. However, its direct relationship with fertility is insignificant, whereas we expected it to be negative (see figure 2.2 and table 2.3).

Religiosity affects fertility positively both directly and indirectly, consistently with the general hypothetical system.

The direct relationship between metropolitan residence and fertility can be interpreted as being due to the higher costs of child rearing in metropolitan areas, which is consistent with the hypothetical system. However, there is no indirect significant relationship between metropolitan residence and fertility.

The comparison between the assumed, and the empirical relationships of sub-models 2 and 3 show reasonably good consistency (see table 2.3). Studies of the emergence of low total fertility in European countries have suggested that delayed marriage played a major role in the establishment of the new pattern of low fertility (Bourgeois-Pichat 1986). Hence, we propose another model to analyze the effects of social status, metropolitan residence, and religiosity on fertility by way of a nuptiality variable. This model is expressed by Equations (4) and (5).

Table 2.3
Structural Equations of a Recursive System: Values of t and R^2

	Dependent variables in structural equations†									
	General hypotheses			Sub Model 1		Sub Model 2		Sub model 3		
Explanatory variable*	W	I	F	W	RF	I	F	W	I	F
High education (S)	+	+	–	21.68	N.S.	20.13	– 3.60	‡	‡	‡
Religiosity (R)	–	–	+	–4.46	28.38	– 6.09	26.17	– 2.11	– 1.86	25.13
Metropolitan residence (M)	+	+	--	N.S.	–2.46	5.58	– 3.07	N. S.	5.33	–.3.40
Women's employment (W)	‡	+	–	‡	– 3.85	‡	‡	‡	9.53	–3.18
High Income (I)	‡	‡	+	‡	‡	‡	N.S.	‡	‡	N.S
R^2				0.701	0.82	0.71	0.785	0.021	0.405	0.783

* See explanation in section on data and variables.

† W = Women's employment; F = Total Fertility; I = High Income.

‡ Varaible not in the equation.

$$N = a_n + b_{ns}S + b_{nr}R + b_{nm}M + \varepsilon_n \quad (4)$$
$$F = a_f + b_{fs}S + b_{fr}R + b_{fm}M + b_{fn}N + \varepsilon_f \quad (5)$$

where S, R, M, N, and F, represent the status level, religiosity, metropolitan residence, nuptiality (the proportion of married women in the 20-24 age group) and total fertility respectively. These regressions, which are not specified in the tables, show that, as in European countries, social structure affects fertility levels, at least partly, through nuptiality.

Some Comments on the High Fertility of the Religious Population

The aim of this study was to show that when religiosity is controlled, each of the two major ethnic groups can be shown to have joined, or is about to join, the transition to below replacement fertility. However, the fertility levels of the religious and the nonreligious populations can only be estimated indirectly.

We use estimates from the regression equations discussed above to illustrate numerically the effect of religiosity on fertility for the European ethnic group. These are presented in table 2.4.

The dominant effect of religiosity on fertility is evident. The table shows quite clearly the descent from extremely high fertility levels in religious communities, to below replacement fertility in non-religious ones. For example, total fertility for a unit with 80 percent religiosity is over 7. Although this figure is an extrapolation, its comparison with alternative independent estimates shows consistency.

Stable population fertility levels for two religious sub-groups could be estimated by using their age distributions in school populations. Hence, we obtain

Figure 2.2
Recursive Model: Sub Model 1

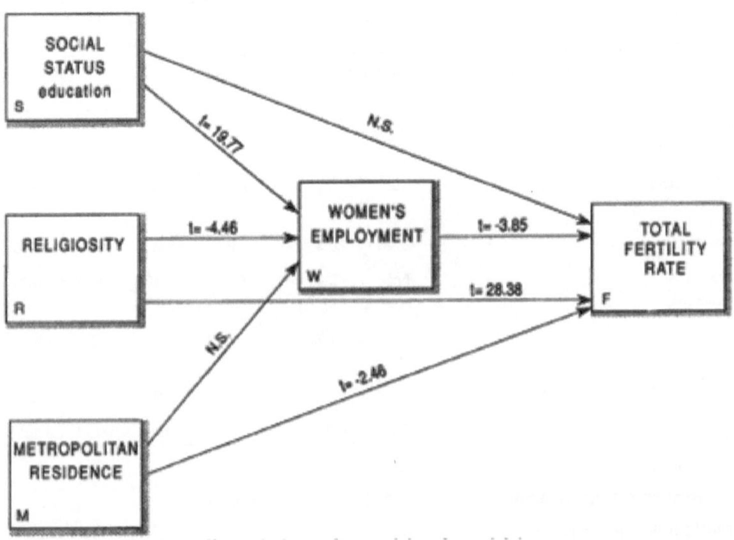

Table 2.4
Predicted Total Fertility Under Assumed Values for Major Explanatory Variables

Per cent religiosity	Per cent Women's High Education			
	36 Per cent		50 Per cent	
	Metropolitan residence			
	Yes	No	Yes	No
80	7.25	7.02	7.14	6.92
50	5.27	5.04	5.16	4.94
25	3.62	3.39	3.51	3.29
0	1.97	1.74	1.87	1.64

* The mean percentage for women's education is 36.

total fertility of 7.2 and 4.6 respectively for the ultra-orthodox and the national religious populations. These are consistent, in general, with the extrapolated regression estimate.

A third estimate based on indirect standardization (Schellekens 1991). According to this, total fertility in the ultra-orthodox population of Jerusalem is about 7.5, a figure which should, however, be considered an upper limit.

Is it possible to explain the very high fertility levels of the religious population, in view of its being part of a modern society? We argue that the socio-cultural structure of the religious population, particularly of the ultra-orthodox group, explains its high fertility. Heilman and Friedman have argued that the key instrument of the high fertility levels, the high growth rate, and the survival of this group, is its own independent educational system. Education begins at a very early age, and male students remain in the more advanced educational institutions until their mid-thirties, if not forties. Hence, the ultra-orthodox created a "society of scholars," of "persons who first and foremost saw themselves as people of the book" (Heilman and Friedman 1991: 9). At the same time, women are regarded as supports of scholars. Indeed, women are the main breadwinners in many ultra-orthodox families. They are engaged in various occupations such as teachers—in an ever growing young "closed" population—clerical and sales workers, particularly in employments which do not involve the necessity of mixing with people of the "outer" world.

Marriages in the ultra-orthodox community are "arranged" and take place at an early age. Couples are expected to have their first child within one year of marriage, while high fertility is an encouraged norm throughout marriage (Shilhav and Friedman 1985). Obviously, many years of education for men, early marriages and household formation, high fertility, and rapid population growth, are societal characteristics which require economic resources over and above those generated by this community. Where do such additional economic sources come from? One source consists of donations made by ultra-orthodox communities around the world. However, the major source comes from the larger society of Israel through generous child allowances, assistance in housing young couples, etc. A most important source is specific funds which are allocated to families by their own community institutions, and which are secured by various governmental authorities. These have been granted for years as part of coalition agreements between the ultra-orthodox parties and the main political parties either on the left or on the right. It has, therefore, been argued that the ultra-orthodox population "lives in an ambivalent relationship with the larger culture and society. It shuns the values of that larger world while depending on it ... " (Heilman and Friedman 1991: 22). Hence, at the individual level there is no conflict with high fertility, as long as women can work while children are either at school for the day, or with boarding arrangements, with no costs to parents. Younger children are looked after by relatives through family arrangements, when the mother is unable to do so. On the economic side, state allowances given directly to families, or funds secured through the community, which are at least partly allocated in relation to family size are clearly pro-natalist. Social norms and religious commands related to marriage and childbearing clearly encourage early marriage and high fertility. And in this respect the importance of internal community pressures on individuals to conform with its norms, should not be underestimated. Clearly, rapid population growth under such optimal conditions is a source of community power both internally and towards the larger society.

Conclusions and Implications

Fertility has declined to below replacement levels in many of the modern industrialized countries during the last three decades. This decline has been explained by various modern socio-economic characteristics, which are in conflict with high, even moderately high fertility levels. The change in women's status was associated with increased participation in non-familial activities such as employment. The increasing costs of raising "quality" children is another example of such a conflict. Such processes of change have affected fertility both through declines in nuptiality and delayed childbearing within marriage.

The Jewish population of Israel is a modern society with characteristics similar to those of European populations. Recent changes in the status of women, in women's employment, in consumption patterns and in many other characteristics are common to Israel and to European countries. Yet, total fertility in Israel during the early 1980s was well above replacement level and at least one child higher than in most European countries. We have shown that social heterogeneity makes this an oversimplified and misleading comparison. It has been shown that fertility in the European ethnic group is, indeed, at European levels, if religiosity is controlled at low levels. It has also been shown that the Asian-African ethnic group is proceeding towards low fertility, given its increasing educational levels and other modernization characteristics. Hence, it is the very high fertility of the orthodox population and the moderately high, but declining, fertility of the Asia-Africa ethnic group, combined with the low fertility of the non-orthodox European ethnic group, which produce the high average fertility of the population as a whole.

A review of the major patterns of fertility and their determinants since the 1950s suggests a very significant transformation. While in the 1950s and 1960s the major explanations of fertility variation were ethnicity and socio-economic status, these have been replaced by religiosity during the 1970s and the 1980s (Friedlander and Goldscheider 1978).

The high fertility of the ultra-orthodox has been explained by its way of life, its socioeconomic structure, and its political power. Only a radical change in the economic and political relationships between this group and the larger society can reduce motivations for very large families, a contingency which seems unlikely in the foreseeable future. Hence, given the very high fertility of the religious population combined with below-replacement fertility of the non-religious population, a continuous increase in the proportion of the religious population and its political power can be expected. Will this population, eventually, achieve majority status?

Acknowledgement

While Ron Freedman was Einstein Visiting Fellow at the Hebrew University in 1987, he often expressed astonishment at the high national fertility in Israel compared with Europe, despite its modernity. This article is dedicated to him with the hope that it clarifies the issue.

We are grateful to Jona Schellekens for his valuable comments on an earlier version.

Notes

1. Total fertility adopted and/or calculated from Central Bureau of Statistics (1949-1990).
2. Very similar relationship patterns are obtained when the dependent variable is the average number of births per married woman in the twenty-five to thirty-four age group.

References

Bleich, J. D. 1984. "The Halachic controversy concerning the Israeli census." *Journal of Halacha and Contemporary Society* 8: 62-86.

Bourgeois-Pichat, J. 1986. "The unprecedented shortage of births in Europe." In Kingsley Davis, Mikhail S. Bernstam and Rita Ricardo-Campbell (eds.), *Below Replacement Fertility in Industrial Societies: Causes, Consequences, Policies* (Supplement to Volume 12 of *Population and Development Review*), 3-25.

Central Bureau of Statistics. *Statistical Abstract of Israel*, Vol. 1-41. Jerusalem: Central Bureau of Statistics.

Davies, K. 1986. "Low fertility in evolutionary perspective." In Kingsley Davis, Mikhail S. Bernstam and Rita Ricardo-Campbell (eds.), *Below Replacement Fertility in Industrial Societies: Causes, Consequences, Policies* (Supplement to Volume 12 of *Population and Development Review*), 48-68.

Finnäs, F. 1991. "Fertility in Larsmo: the effect of Laestadianism." *Population Studies* 45: 339-351.
Friedlander, D.and C. Goldscheider. 1978. "Immigration, social change and cohort fertility in Israel." *Population Studies* 32: 299-317
Freedman, D. S. and A. Thornton. 1982. "Income and fertility: The elusive relationship." *Demography* 19: 65-78.
Hartman, M. 1978. "Number of children and work experience of married women in Israel." Unpublished manuscript.
Heilman, S. C. and M. Friedman. 1991. *The Haredim in Israel: Who Are They and What Do They Want?* New York: The Institute on American Jewish-Israeli Relations.
Johnston, J. 1987. *Econometric Methods*. Singapore: McGraw-Hill International Editions.
Jones, E. F. 1981. "The impact of women's employment on marital fertility in the U.S., 1970-1975." *Population Studies* 35: 161-173.
Lawton, L. 1988. "The impact of religious commitment on fertility among Israeli Jews." Paper presented at the annual meeting of the Population Association of America, New Orleans.
Shilhav, J. and M. Friedman. 1985. *Growth and Segregation: The Ultra Orthodox Community of Jerusalem*. Jerusalem: The Jerusalem Institute for Israel Studies (In Hebrew).
Schellekens, J. 1991. "Estimating the total fertility rate of the ultra orthodox population." Unpublished note.
Schmelz, U. O. 1985. "Religiosity and fertility among the Jews of Jerusalem." In *Papers in Jewish Demography*. Jerusalem: The Institute of Contemporary Jewry, The Hebrew University of Jerusalem.

3

Religiosity, Nationalism and Fertility in Israel

Jon Anson and Avinoam Meir

Israel has a consistently higher level of fertility than its European counterparts, despite having a comparable standard of living (Keysar et al. 1992). The present chapter seeks to re-evaluate explanations for this apparently unusual situation. We suggest that previous explanations, based on the ethnic origin and composition of the population, and on religiosity, are sociologically incomplete. Such explanations identify those segments of the population with high fertility and then argue, *post hoc, ergo propter hoc,* that because there is a clear empirical correlation between religiosity, ethnic origin and fertility, *therefore* the higher fertility is explained by religiosity and ethnic origin. To anticipate, we shall show that neither of these putative causes can explain Israeli high fertility:

1. High fertility is not the cultural residue of a population in transition to modernity (the ethnic origin argument), as even those sections of the population that have already made this transition show an inexplicably high level of fertility.
2. Neither can it be explained by a religious injunction to "be fruitful and multiply," as there are a large number of examples (including Jewish populations outside Israel) in which such an injunction is not associated with high fertility.

Instead, we argue that normative orientations, or cultural explanations of the value of children, are but *intervening variables* (Davis and Blake 1956). Along with the high fertility that they support, they are products (but also a part) of the social conditions under which Israelis live their lives. We shall argue that Israel's high fertility needs to be explained not in terms of the internal qualities of particular parts of the population, but rather in terms of Israel's special position in the Middle East and in the world-economy as a whole, and the nationalist sentiment which this engenders in the *conscience collective* (the set of symbols, meanings and ideas which are more or less common to all members of society, see Durkheim 1915; 1953). This nationalism, of course, is not a homogeneous sentiment, and its differentiation is reflected in support for the different political parties. Using census data and voting returns for Jewish urban statistical areas in the early 1980s, we shall present evidence that high fertility is directly associated with nationalism, rather than with religiosity, and will argue that the association of the latter with high fertility in Israel derives from the special circumstances which make it a reflection of nationalist consciousness.

Fertility in Israel

Figure 3.1 plots total fertility against a measure of real gross domestic product per person (Slottje et al. 1991), as a measure of standard of living, for Israel and 28 European states in the early 1980s. In general we can see that as the standard of living increases, fertility tends to decline, even if the association is not particularly strong. The outer lines represent a 99 percent confidence

Figure 3.1

Fertility by Domestic Product. European Countries, circa 1983

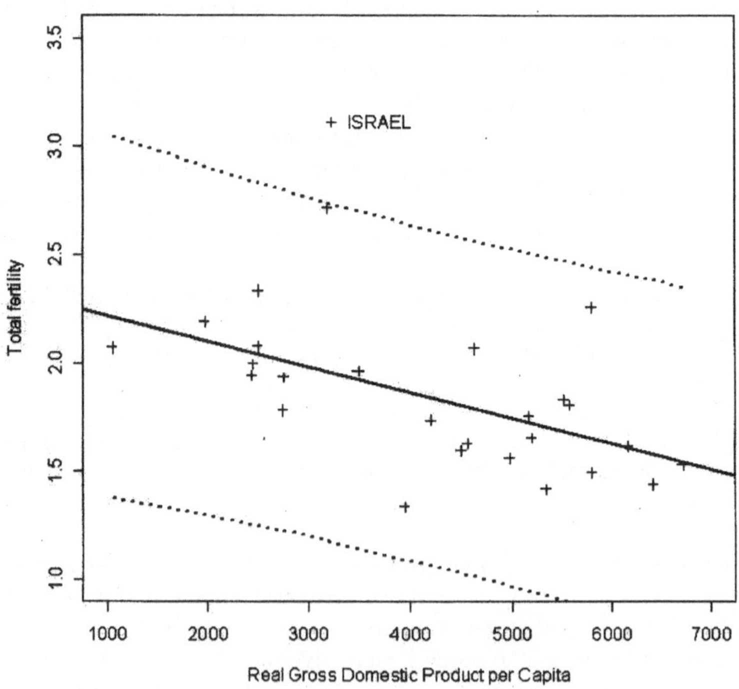

Note: Outer lines are 99% confidence bounds for indivdual prediction

interval for the prediction of individual cases (based on the European countries alone). Although Israel at the time was in the second quartile, in terms of its domestic product (standard of living), its fertility level was higher than that of any European country, and significantly greater than would be expected on the basis of the European experience of fertility as a declining function of living standards. It what ways, then, is Israel different?

Fertility and Ethnic Origin

Previous discussions of Israeli fertility have focused on two major explanatory frameworks, which we may label the cultural and the normative. The first argues that the reason for Israel's high fertility lies in the social origins of what is still, essentially, a population in the process of modernization. Approximately one sixth (17 percent) of the population in the early 1980s was Moslem or Druze Arab, and almost half (44 percent) of the Jewish population was of North African or West Asian origin (Central Bureau of Statistics 1984, tables 2, 3). Both these groups have a recent history of high fertility and high family size norms, so that even if their fertility has dropped dramatically since the early 1960s (Friedlander, Eisenbach, and Goldscheider 1979; 1980), they still show a higher level than do Jews of European or American origin; or than can be expected from a European population under similar circumstances. Implicitly, this argument suggests that as time passes, and modem, urban, Israeli-born women become the overwhelming majority of child-bearers, fertility will draw closer to the European standard. Thus, Peres and Brosch (1991), on the basis of a large scale interview survey of Jewish women, argued that while various income measures have no net effect on the number of children ever born, there are important differences by mother's education and individual modernity. In practice, this leads to more children in families of Asian and African, rather than European or American origin. Neuman and Ziderman (1986) reached similar conclusions.

The difference between fertility levels for the different groups is plotted in figure 3.2, which shows time trends in total fertility for Arab women (Moslems, Druze and Christians), and for Jewish women born in Israel, in Asia-Africa and in Europe-America (Central Bureau of Statistics 1993). The pattern of convergence can be clearly seen, as also the consistency of the fertility level of Israeli-born Jewish women (the sudden increase in Asian-African fertility and the decline in European-American fertility, since 1990, are almost certainly attributable to the recent wave of immigration from Ethiopia and Eastern Europe respectively). It is important to note, however, that even if we focus on the group with the *lowest* fertility, European-American women, we find that their fertility *rose* in the 1960s, and that in the early 1980s total fertility (2.75) was substantially higher than the mean European level to be expected, given the Israeli standard of living. In other words, even Israel's low fertility group (whose standard of living is *above* the mean level), is clearly over-reproducing in comparison with the European standard. The cultural traditions of the Arab

Figure 3.2
Total Fertility, Israel, by Population Group

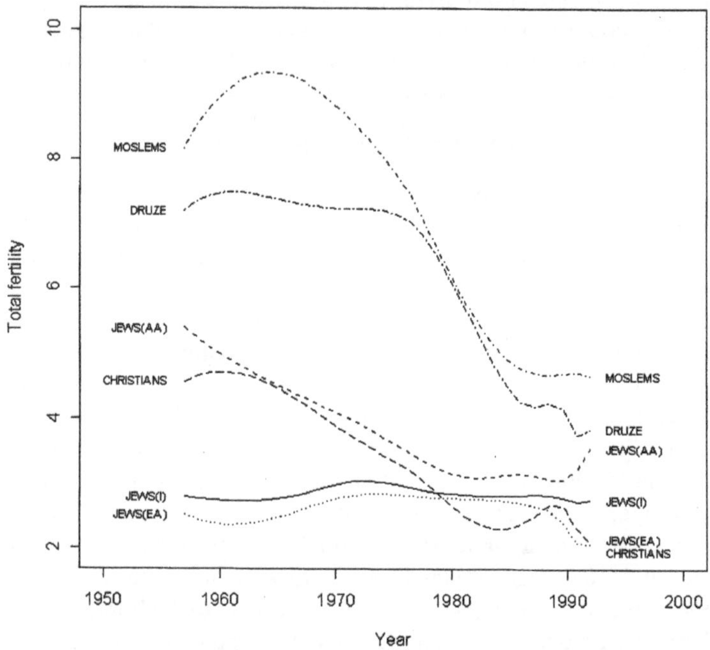

Note: I = Israeli born; AA = Asian, African born; EA = European, American born.

population, or of the Asian-African immigrants, cannot explain the high fertility of Israel as a whole, as even those women who are not heirs to this tradition show an inexplicably high level of fertility.

Fertility and Religiosity

A complementary explanation has focused on the religiosity of large segments of the Israeli population. Peritz (1992), summarizing the findings of a recent fertility survey in Israel, noted that "[t]he difference in fertility between religious and non-religious [Jewish] women pervades most of our other analyses" (p. 189), and Kupinsky (1992), using data from the same survey, found religiosity to be the variable with the greatest effect on fertility, net of all other variables examined. Indeed, Friedlander and Feldmann, chapter 2, have recently argued that were it not for this religious section, Israeli fertility would be at, or approaching, the level found in European countries. Their model argues that social status (education), religiosity and metropolitan residence all act as independent, exogenous variables and that, directly and indirectly, they affect the total fertility rate in urban statistical units through their effects on women's employment and economic status (income). In this, they reflect a large and consistent body of data showing that fertility is higher among religious segments of the population (Neuman and Ziderman 1986; Lazerwitz 1980), even if conclusions vary as to the relative importance of religiosity and of standard of living variables (income and mother's education).

This focus on religiosity is problematic, however. By claiming that were it not for the religious population, Israel's fertility would be at, or approaching, European levels, Friedlander and Feldman are comparing the lower end of the Israeli distribution with the whole of the European distribution. In effect, they are arguing that the Israeli distribution is bimodal, there being a lower distribution for the non-religious, and a higher distribution for the religious population. They then argue that the lower mode is comparable with European fertility patterns, and indicates Israel's level of fertility were it not for the effects of religiosity. Now, while there may be support for the first argument of a bimodal Israeli distribution (Peres and Brosch 1991), we have no evidence that ethnic and religious differences do not create similar bimodal distributions, at a far lower level, in European countries.

A Critique of Explanations Based on Religiosity

A statistical relationship, however well substantiated, is no proof of a causal relation. Statistical analysis, however competent, can only evaluate the match between the data and a particular model of relationships between variables. Statistical analyses, in and of themselves, can offer no indication of what processes lie behind the relationships uncovered (though they may offer insights leading to fruitful hypotheses). We have no argument with the claim that religious groups in Israel have higher fertility than do non-religious groups—we do argue that the religious injunctions to be fruitful and multiply, in and of themselves, are an insufficient explanation of this difference. On the contrary, we shall go so far as to argue that the religiosity-fertility relationship is spurious, that where religiosity is associated with augmented fertility this is because a common explanation can be found for both the religiosity and the high fertility, and that in the absence of this common cause religiosity is not necessarily associated with high fertility.

Jewish Fertility Outside Israel

If the specifically Jewish injunction to high fertility were a cause of high fertility, we would expect Jewish groups in Europe and North America to show a higher fertility than other groups in a comparable social situation. This however is not the case. Jews have had consistently lower fertility than have their Gentile neighbors in Europe and in North America for at least the past century (Goldscheider 1967), or even the past two centuries (DellaPergola 1968), and this difference remains even after controlling for race, urban or metropolitan residence, education, occupation, income, and other socio-economic variables (Goldscheider and Uhlenberg 1969). In more recent studies, DellaPergola (1993) has shown that this difference is maintained even under the very low fertility conditions prevailing in European countries today; and Goldscheider and Mosher (1988) compared different religious groups in a national U.S. sample, and showed that Jewish women have the highest proportion of contraceptive users, overall, and as a proportion of women at risk of an unwanted pregnancy (neither pregnant, infertile, postpartum, or actively seeking pregnancy). Jewish women also had the highest proportion in this at risk group, and the lowest proportion postpartum. Comparing different Jewish denominations in the United States, Cheskis (1980) showed that while denominationally affiliated Jews had higher fertility than the non-affiliated, this effect was stronger for Conservative than for Orthodox Jews. Thus, even if Jewish religiosity in the Diaspora is associated with higher fertility (relative to other Jews), this is more a function of Jewish affiliation and identification than of orthodoxy *per se.* An explanation of Israeli high fertility in terms of religiosity must therefore show why, in this particular case, norms are directly translated into practice.

Normative Injunctions

The injunction to "be fruitful and multiply" is a classic example of a pro-natalist norm. The religiosity-based explanation of Israeli higher fertility argues implicitly that this norm is *necessarily* translated into practice among Israel's religious population (or at least, serves to increase fertility levels above what they might otherwise be, given the particular social-economic conditions in which people live). Yet such an argument ignores the large and consistent body of evidence that argues that people do not necessarily act according to pro-natalist norms, and indeed, that populations with declared pro-natalist norms may often have no higher fertility than do their non pro-natalist neighbors:

1. S. Goldstein (1970) noted that though Moslems in pre-transition Thailand declared a greater preference for large families than did the majority Buddhists or the Confucians, they nonetheless had lower fertility, even after accounting for their higher standard of living and predominantly urban residence;
2. Jiobu and Marshall (1977) compared the fertility of three culturally coherent groups (Chinese, Filipino, and Japanese Americans in California) to that of the majority white Anglo population. They found that of the three groups, only the Filipinos had explicitly pro-natalist norms, yet they were precisely the group whose fertility (adjusted for background, socio-economic characteristics) was less than that of the whites.
3. Sabagh and Lopez (1980) compared the effects of religiosity on fertility among the (pro-natalist) Chicanos of Los Angeles. They found religiosity

to have a positive effect on the fertility of Chicanos reared in the United States, but not for those reared in Mexico, and this difference remained after allowing for a variety of socio-economic and other background variables.

On the basis of the above evidence, we argue that there is no necessary relationship between declared pro-natalist norms and fertility; and in particular, that there are ample indications that Jewish pro-natalism is not necessarily translated into childbearing practice. If Israeli fertility is higher than social conditions would lead us to expect, and if this higher fertility is to be found particularly among the religious groups in the population, we need to understand the specific conditions which generate such a high level of compliance with the pro-natalist norm.

Fertility and Nationalism

The religiosity-fertility connection is generally based on a simple, normative argument: people believe that having many children is the right thing to do, and therefore they have many children. Yet most measures of religiosity are based on religious *practice* (what people do), not on religious *beliefs* (what people think) (Marcum 1988). *Within* religious communities, a high commitment to doctrine is not necessarily associated with high fertility (Marcum 1986). Religion is essentially a group phenomenon, not a personal worldview (Durkheim 1915; Stark 1984; O. Anson et al. 1990), and religiosity is a commitment to the group—and only indirectly to its practices and its doctrine. These practices may well include a high fertility, but not necessarily. Only very rarely do they include the unrestricted fertility implied by a doctrine of "be fruitful and multiply" (even the Islamic government of Iran now directly supports lowering the fertility rate, by subsidizing family planning services, see Roudi 1993). Figure 3.2 indicates a growing degree of fertility control among all sectors of Israeli society, and a convergence to a common Israeli level considerably above the European. The critical question thus becomes, how do we explain a particular level of fertility control, even in a population that normatively disavows the practice?

Surprisingly, there has been little attempt to relate Israeli fertility to the country's special position in the Middle East, and the constant state of tension between the Jewish and Arab populations within Israel, and between Israel and its Arab neighbor states. Yet the minority group fertility hypothesis (Goldscheider and Uhlenberg 1969; Ritchey 1976) has long argued that group fertility should be analyzed in terms of a group's relations with other groups with which it interacts. There are two parts to this theory. The more common argument (as applied, for instance, to the Jews in the United States) states that if a minority group is well endowed financially and upwardly mobile, but this mobility is blocked by discrimination, then member families will reduce their fertility as part of a rational strategy for the concentration of individual and group effort to overcome discrimination (note, for instance, the relatively low fertility of the Christians in Israel). The second part of the argument, however, is that if the group is ill endowed, and its low social status is compounded by blatant discrimination, then it will resort to high fertility as a strategy to strengthen the group, and as a defense against the external threat. Lopez and Sabagh (1978), for instance, showed that among the Chicanos in Los Angeles (a group with pro-natalist norms), those with strong cultural and personalities to the ethnic group had *lower* fertility than those without these ties (controlling, of course, for education and income). In Israel, Meir and Ben-David (1995) compared fertility preferences between aboriginal and fellaheen Bedouin. The latter are more sedentary, better educated and have a higher standard of living, yet are viewed both by themselves and the aboriginal Bedouin as being of lower status within Bedouin society. When sedentarization, education, and standard of living were statistically controlled, the fellaheen were found to desire larger families (and in particular more sons) than the aboriginal Bedouin. We may interpret both these findings by arguing that fertility was higher in those populations that did not benefit from the enhanced security of the integrated ethnic and social group.

Looked at in this light, fertility becomes (consciously or unconsciously) a part of the group's survival strategy. As figure 3.2 shows, Palestinian (Arab) fertility is also high, but this is only partially explicable in terms of their lower standard of living. Furthermore, it is to be noted that the decline in Moslem fertility ceased, and Christian and Druze fertility both increased in the mid to late 1980s, at the time of the *intifada* uprising in the West Bank and Gaza. Now, although Israel's Jewish population is in no sense a minority, the particular nature of the conflict, as one over the establishment and maintenance of a specifically Jewish State, with its continual risk of war and of nationally motivated violence, is likely to bring about a similar response. It is also very likely that such a response will find expression in the articulation of specifically Jewish values in daily life, that is, in an enhanced religiosity. If this is the case, then both high fertility, and a high degree of religiosity, may be explained by reference to the radical nationalist response. Let us examine this possibility.

Nationalism and the Minority Group Hypothesis

Nationalism is a political principle by which a group of people recognize each other as belonging to the same culture, with consequent rights and duties (Gellner 1983, chapter 1), an assertion by the group-for-itself that it must "assert or extend [its] rights in the political arena in order to defend possibilities for [its] continued existence as a group . . . " (Wallerstein 1979: 184). By definition, then, this is a competitive sentiment, as it necessarily defines the group in terms of its struggle for resources *against* another group with a putative claim to the same territory. This very process of political mobilization, however, also makes nationalism into a powerful source of group integration (Coser 1956). Within the context of modern democratic states, this is then reinforced through the public dialogue between political parties, which assumes and reasserts the existence of the homogeneous *national* community united in struggle, and the ritual process of group definition leading up to the election comes to focus on the shaping of the specific *subgroup* identities (Gellner 1983, chapter 9; Herzog 1987; Sinnot and Davis 1981).

The strength of nationalist sentiment cannot be understood, however, strictly within the context of a particular nation-state. The nationalist struggle has its origins not in group subjectivity *sui generis,* but in the uneven development of the modern world-economy, in which there is a constant struggle for preferential access to resources, and in which a strong state has always been the principal mechanism by which the local bourgeoisie has been able to control its own fortunes (Wallerstein 1974; Delacroix and Ragin 1981; Cochrane 1986). Nationalism thus takes many forms. It is the revolt of the weak, resisting the predations of this uneven development whereby material progress has come to mean domination of the less by the more (materially) advanced nations, the break-up of traditional communities and the generation of expectations far exceeding the material benefits; it is the demand by successful semi-peripheral states, who are seeking to transform their structural role in the world-economy, to enjoy the fruits of their new progress; and it is the rearguard action of one-time central economies seeking to preserve their advantage over the encroachments of new centers (Nairn 1977; Gellner 1983; Wallerstein 1984). As Nairn points out (1977: 188-9), the nationalist tension is liable to be particularly intractable in those semi-peripheral outposts of the center in which settler implantation has led to the growth, in the periphery, of a genuine, self sustaining middle class society. Because it is a settler initiative, this relative over-development occurs in the "wrong place," from the point of view of the prevailing geopolitical order, thus pitting the settler community, Janus-like, against two contradictory adversaries: the displaced indigenous, peripheral population on the one hand, and the center of the international world-economy on the other. On both fronts it must defend both the legitimacy of the settler enterprise; and its rights to the fruits of the new development. This double-structuring of the nationalist tension, on two fronts, will ensure that it maintains a consistently high level of vitality, for a decrease in tension on one front will only ensure an increase on the other.

Nationalism, particularly that of the settler nation, thus expresses, at the level of the nation-state, precisely those pressures and tensions which the minority group fertility hypothesis attributes to the ethnic group at the intra-state level. Whether this nationalist consciousness leads to a higher or lower fertility will depend, as with the minority group, on the specific nature of the salient conflict. If the conflict is economic, directed at the position of the semi-peripheral formation in the global world-economy, we may expect fertility to be reduced, as in the case of Hong Kong, Japan, Singapore and Taiwan, all of which had reduced their total fertility by 1985 to below 2.00. If on the other hand the conflict is a local one, between the settler and the indigenous population, then the effect is likely to be one of an enhanced fertility by both parties to the conflict, as in Northern Ireland, with a total fertility of 2.45 in 1985; or South Africa, with a total fertility of 4.48 for total population in 1985, and 2.57 for the non-black population (Keyfitz and Flieger, 1990).

Fertility as a Social Fact

Fertility is generally measured as a construct at the group level, either as a group mean (crude birth rate; general fertility rate; child-woman ratio); as the realization of a nominal group potential (I_f, I_g); or as a strictly synthetic measure (total fertility; intrinsic birth rate) representing a cohort or period average which would be attained under certain highly improbable conditions. This is true even when individual measures (children-ever-born) are analyzed by least squares regression procedures. This form of analysis seeks to predict, or reproduce, the number of children born to date (fertility), as a function of the woman's age, and other group and individual characteristics (ethnic group, urban-rural residence, education, income, occupation, etc.) Although the measurement is individual, the analysis actually focuses on variations in group means (often confounding, along the way, individual and group level variability) (H. Goldstein 1988).

Now the implications of the above discussion of nationalism and its relation to the minority group hypothesis is precisely that we should forego the temptation to interpret this social phenomenon in terms of an *individual* propensity of women to bear children (subject to biological age constraints). Such an individual-level interpretation would argue, for instance, that *because* the group is defined in terms of a common religious belief, its high fertility is *necessarily* a function of that belief. This argument is problematic on a number of grounds. It is logically fallacious, in that it imputes causality to what may be no more than a correlative association; it is ecologically fallacious in that it imputes directly from group to individual level associations (Robinson 1950), without accounting for in-group variability; and by treating religious belief as primordial it gives up on any attempt to explain why some people are more religiously observant than others, treating religiosity itself as an individual quirk, rather than a social phenomenon. Our point is not to deny the validity of individual level analysis, only to argue that it must be performed by appropriate methods at an individual level (see, e.g., Courgeau 1994), not by analysis of group means.

Our approach, by contrast, is explicitly macro-sociological. We treat fertility as a supra-individual phenomenon, indeed a socially sanctioned way of acting which imposes itself on individuals, and which can be interpreted only through theoretically based analysis of its relations with other such socially defined ways of acting and thinking (Durkheim 1964; Gane 1988). We have argued above that Israeli high fertility may be a function of Israel's special position at the semi-periphery of the world-system. This special position expresses itself, politically, in an activist nationalism; and practically, in an enhanced propensity to bear children. The particular self-definition of group identity, and its claim to legitimacy, may be a religious one, but not necessarily. We may hypothesize, therefore, that:

1. Those subgroups of the population which show a strong nationalist response will be the subgroups of the population which also have a particularly high level of fertility.

Furthermore, if religiosity is another expression of this special situation, then:

2. Once the nationalist response is controlled, there will be no special effect of religiosity on the fertility of the population.

Method

We analyzed fertility in urban statistical areas, as a function of mean material resources, religiosity, and nationalism. These urban areas (census enumeration districts) are the basic units by which census results are reported, and in which population accounting is managed between censuses. At the time of the 1983 census of population and housing, when they were last updated, they averaged about 3,500 inhabitants. These areas are not strictly homogeneous, of course, but given the natural process of residential segregation and regional inequalities (Lipshitz 1986), the variation between them should be sufficient to render their internal heterogeneity negligible. Fertility and resource levels were measured using data from the 1983 census; and religiosity and nationalism from voting patterns in the national elections that took place approximately a year after the census.

The Israeli national political system is one of proportional representation, so that all voters vote for the same party lists, which are then represented in the Knesset (Parliament) in direct proportion to their showing at the polls. Voting returns are thus directly comparable between districts as all voters are responding to the same "question," and the voting districts themselves have no political significance (as they do in a constituency system). Furthermore, to ease the work of the analyst, the boundaries of all polling districts are subsumed within the statistical areas used for the presentation of census data, so votes from Knesset elections can be aggregated over geographical units exactly matching those for which data are available from the census. As the population is mostly residentially segregated by national group (of the 1,010 urban statistical areas with a population of over 1,000, 94 percent were homogeneously Jewish or Arab) it is possible to restrict this analysis to the Jewish population, thus recognizing that the two groups make different readings of the party programs and messages.

Religiosity and Nationalism

We obtained distributions of votes cast, by statistical area, for each party in the 1984 Knesset elections. The resulting matrix of area by votes cast was then analyzed by Correspondence Analysis (Greenacre 1984; Weller and Romney 1990; Anson and Slonim-Nevo 1995) to identify the voting patterns of the different areas. Correspondence Analysis (CA) is a graphic technique for representing the data from a two- or multi-way contingency table in a manner that enables simple and concise interpretation of the relations between the column and row variables. This it does by locating the categories of each variable in geometric space along a common set of axes. Row categories (statistical areas) with similar distributions of the columns (that is, with similar voting patterns) will be located close to each other, whereas those with dissimilar patterns will be distant from each other. At the same time, column categories with similar row distributions (that is, parties with support from the same statistical areas) will be close to each other, and those with dissimilar distributions will be distant. The row categories are thus ranked in terms of the columns, and the column categories are ranked in terms of the rows. By examining the location of the parties, for instance, in terms of the content of their appeal to the voters, it is possible to give meaning to the axes (in a manner akin to the labeling of factors), and then interpret the statistical areas in terms of their locations along these axes. (Similarly, it would be possible to give meaning to the axes by examining relevant properties of the statistical areas, and then interpreting the parties in terms of their locations along these axes. The axes themselves are unchanged, only their meaning changes, depending on whether they are labeled by reference to the parties (columns) or to the statistical areas (rows). In this way, it becomes possible to see the relationship between the categories of the row and column variables, and thus to obtain a fuller interpretation of the table than may be obtained by examination of just one distribution (e.g., percent votes for a religious party); or salient cells (e.g., classifying each district by modal party, or the modal standardized residual from a simple chi-square analysis).

The analysis was restricted to urban statistical areas with an homogeneous Jewish population (95 percent of the population Jewish in the 1983 census), and with a total population of 1,000 or more. Parties analyzed were restricted to those parties that polled at least 1 percent of the total vote in this population. A total of 792 areas were available for analysis. Figure 3.3 presents results of the CA in two dimensions, which between them account for 80 percent of the variation among the cells (in the sense of their deviation from a random distribution of the votes).

Figure 3.3a shows the distribution of the parties within this two-dimensional space. As we move down the Y-axis, we move from the radical religious party (AGUDA) which does not recognize the legitimacy of Israel as a Jewish State, pending the revelation of the Messiah, and demands that the secular authorities

Figure 3.3
Correspondence Analysis of Voting Patterns Israel, Jews, General Elections 1984

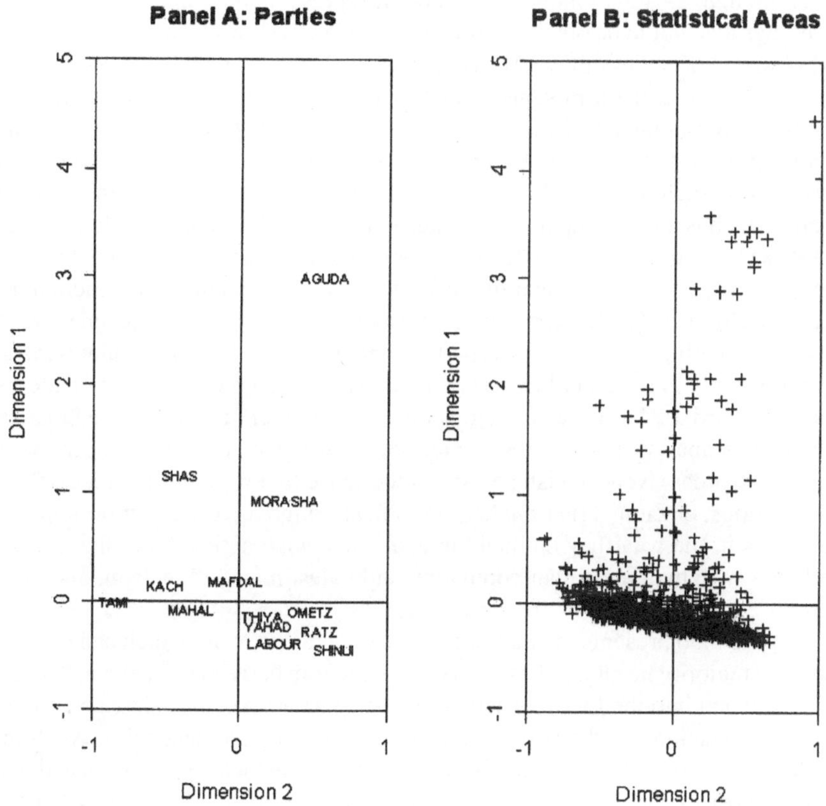

operate strictly in accordance with Jewish Law; through the National Religious Party (MAFDAL) which views the establishment of the State, and its military achievements, as an act of Revelation, and demands that Jewish Law and the Rabbinate (the established religious authority) be accorded a privileged position within the secular state; to the radically secular parties, RATZ and SHINUI, which argue that religion is a strictly private affair, and that neither Jewish Law, nor the Rabbinate, are entitled to a position of privilege. Clearly, then, the first dimension represents the religiosity of the party, its doctrine, and its supporters. The second dimension presents a double distinction. On the one hand, it distinguishes between the radically nationalist parties (KACH, MAHAL, MAFDAL) and the more pragmatic (LABOUR) and liberal, conciliatory parties (RATZ, SHINUI). At the same time, the axis also distinguishes parties with an emotional appeal (TAMI and SHAS on the basis of ethnic identity, MAHAL on the basis of Jewish activism) from those with a more rational appeal to the electorate. In essence, then, this axis represents the nationalist commitment of the population, even though, as a nationalist dimension, it represents only approximately the rankings that would be obtained from a content analysis of the party manifestos. This would doubtless move MORASHA, TEHIYA, and OMETZ over to the right of MAHAL in the plot, and TAMI closer to the center. However, combined with the emotional nature of the appeal, and the fact that these locations on the plot represent the voting patterns and affiliation of the voters (which do not necessarily match exactly the intentions of party leaders), we feel that radical nationalism is the most appropriate interpretation of this axis. The relative sizes of these axes indicate a high degree of geographical segregation on the basis of religiosity, and a far less clear distinction between nationalist and conciliatory areas. Religiosity is thus represented here as a fairly unambiguous distinction, in that areas voting for the religious parties tend not to vote for the secular parties. Nationalism, on the other hand, is more a matter of degree, and voting patterns in this regard are far more heterogeneous. In particular, it is to be noted that all the parties analyzed here (those which received 1 percent or more of the vote in Jewish areas) were Jewish parties, in the sense that they defined themselves as religious, or Zionist (nationalist) or both, although there were important differences in the way they defined the goals of Jewish nationalism; the desired relation with the Palestinian population and Palestinian nationalism; and their proposed policies (tactics) for achieving these goals.

Figure 3.3b presents the plot of the statistical areas, from which can be seen that the majority lie along a broad curve running from the second quadrant, through the third and into the fourth quadrant. For these areas there is a clear correlation between locations on the two axes, a movement along the nationalist axis from radical nationalist to conciliatory being, in general, matched by a movement down the religiosity scale. However, there is also a second, minor trend, moving from this broad curve in the second quadrant, across into the first. For these areas, a decrease in nationalism is associated with a large *increase* in religiosity. We may thus suggest two different patterns of religiosity, the one associated with a radically nationalist political response, the other disassociated from such a response.

On the bases of these plots we can divide the statistical areas into four main groups:

Quadrant 1: Religious, conciliatory (71 areas);
Quadrant 2: Religious, nationalist (142 areas);
Quadrant 3: Non-religious, nationalist (240 areas);
Quadrant 4: Non-religious, conciliatory (339 areas).

It should be emphasized that these areas are not homogeneous, and the labels are used to typify the ambient social current, or *conscience collective* in the different areas. These differences are reflected, for instance, in the distribution of votes to the major parties in each of the four quadrants (table 3.1). In quadrants 2 and 3 MAHAL (nationalist) has almost half the votes, whereas in quadrants 1 and 4 it has less than a third. AGUDA (ultra-orthodox) has a high showing in quadrant 1, SHAS (a radically religious party with a strong appeal to African and Asian Jewish ethnicity) has a high showing in quadrant 2 and some support in quadrant 3, and neither are supported in quadrant 4. RATZ (social democrat) and SHINUI (liberal), by contrast, both of which were secular, conciliatory parties with a rationalist appeal, have most of their support in quadrant 4, and little to none elsewhere. Typifying the area as nationalist or conciliatory, religious or non-religious thus represents the relative strengths of the nationalist and religious sentiments that are to be found in all parts of the Jewish population of Israel.

Fertility and Standard of Living

Published fertility data, at the local level, is restricted to the number of births in each local authority. We thus have no direct measure of fertility by statistical area. We therefore measured fertility using the Child/Women Ratio (CWR) in each statistical area, taking the number of children aged 0-5 divided by the number of women aged 18-49, these being the women at risk of giving birth in the past five years. To reflect the decreasing fecundity of women, with age, we have weighted the age groups according to the relative probability of birth to married women under a regime of natural fertility (Chernichovsky and Anson 1993), according to the following table (the weights were calculated from a summary of research in natural fertility, given in Wilson, Oeppen and Pardoe 1988):

Age	18–24	25–29	30–34	35–39	40–44	45–49
Weight	1.00	0.95	0.86	0.72	0.41	0.08

Table 3.1
Party Support in the Four Quadrants

First Quadrant Religious Conciliatory		Second Quadrant Religious Nationalist		Third Quadrant Non-religious Nationalist		Fourth Quadrant Non-religious Conciliatory	
LABOUR	24.0	MAHAL	48.5	MAHAL	46.3	LABOUR	44.7
MAHAL	22.5	LABOUR	19.2	LABOUR	30.5	MAHAL	27.8
AGUDA	15.5	SHAS	8.4	TEHIYA	3.7	TEHIYA	5.1
SHAS	10.0	MAFDAL	4.0	SHAS	3.0	SHINUI	4.2
MORASHA	7.3	TEHIYA	3.4	MAFDAL	2.6	RATZ	3.7
MAFDAL	6.0	TAMI	2.9	TAMI	2.2	MAFDAL	2.7
TEHIYA	4.0	AGUDA	2.7	YAHAD	1.8	YAHAD	2.5
RATZ	2.1	KACH	2.3	KACH	1.6	OMETZ	1.9
SHINUI	2.0	MORASHA	1.8	RATZ	1.5	MORASHA	1.2
KACH	1.3	YAHAD	1.3	SHINUI	1.3	SHAS	1.1
YAHAD	1.2						
OMETZ	1.1						

As a measure of the standard of living in the population, we used the published data from the census on mean household income per standardized individual in salaried (employed, but not self-employed) households. The standardization allows for the greater costs per head of maintaining a smaller household, and the measure is thus a useful proxy for average real material resources in the statistical area (Ben Tuvia, 1987).

Results

Table 3.2 presents ordinary least-squares analyses of the co-variation between fertility on the one hand, and religion, nationalism, and income on the other.

Table 3.2
Religiosity, Nationalism, Income and Fertility Regression Results

Panel 1: Single effects of religiosity and nationalism (t-values in parentheses)

Variable	Religiosity	Religiosity & Income	Nationalism	Nationalism & Income
Constant	– 0.285	0.943	– 0.325	1.52
Religiosity	0.0846* (5.72)	– 0.717* (4.71)		
Nationalism			0.131* (10.4)	–1.57* (8.58)
Log Incone		– 1.06* (14.9)		– 1.52* (14.3)
Religiosity * Log(Income)		0.659* (4.76)		
Nationalism * Log(Income)				1.38* (8.57)
R^2	0.0398	0.259	0.121	0.303

Notes:
1. * indicates slope coefficient at $p < 0.05$
2. The regressions indicate logarithmic relatioships, thus column 1 (religiosity) should be read as:

$$\log(CWR) = -0.285 + 0.0846(\text{religiosity})$$

or

$$CWR = 10^{(-0.285 + 0.0846(\text{religiosity}))}$$

indicating a mean CWR of 0.519 ($=10^{-0.285}$) for non-religious areas, and 0.630 in religious areas. Religiosity thus increases fertility by a factor of 21.5% ($10^{0.0846} = 1.215$).

Table 3.2 (cont.)

Panel 2: joint effects of nationalism and religiosity

	Regression Coefficients	Mean Effects	Regression Coefficients (t-values)
Quadrant 1 (religious conciliatory)	– 0.211	0.616	1.52
Quadrant 1* log(income)			–1.49¤ (6.04)
Quadrant 2 (religious nationalist)	– 0.195	0.638	– 0.125
Quadrant 2* log(income)			-0.0685 (0.34)
Quadrant 3 (non-religious nationalist)	– 0.194	0.640	0.0613
Quadrant 3* log(income)			– 0.237 (1.37)
Quadrant 4 (non-religious conciliatory)	– 0.349	0.447	1.39
Quadrant 4* log(income)			– 1.42¤ (11.36)
R^2	0.161		0.309

Note:
¤ indicates slope coefficient significant at $p < 0.05$
Column 1 is equivalent to the regression equation:
log(CWR) = constant + religiosity + nationalism + religiosity*nationalism, where:
Quadrant 1 = constant + religiosity
Quadrant 2 = constant + religiosity + nationalism + religiosity*nationalism
etc.
Column 2 is $10^{coefficient}$ of column 1
Column 3 is equivalent to the equation:
log(CWR) = constant + religiosity + nationalism + religiosity*nationalism + log(income) + log(income)*religiosity + log(income)*nationalism + log(income)*religiosity*nationalism

Both fertility and income are transformed to their logarithms, to obtain the most parsimonious form of the relation between them (see figure 3.4 below). The first column considers the religiosity effect, showing clearly that religious areas have, on the average, 21.5 percent more children in the five years prior to the census than did women in non-religious areas. The interaction between religiosity and income level in the second column indicates that this difference derives from a muting of the negative effect of income on fertility in religious populations. Column 3 shows that the baseline effect of nationalism is far greater than that of religion, and that women in nationalist areas had 35 percent ($10^{0.131}$) more children than did women in conciliatory areas. Column 4 shows a strong positive interaction between the effects of radical nationalism and of income, so that in the nationalist areas the income slope is effectively annulled. Taken by themselves, religiosity and nationalism both correlate positively with higher fertility, although a comparison of the R^2 values of column 1 with column 3, and column 2 with column 4, also indicates that when each is considered separately, the nationalist commitment of a population (as expressed in its voting pattern) is a better predictor of fertility than is its religiosity.

When we combine nationalism and religion we obtain the separate analyses for each quadrant, given in the second panel of table 3.2 and displayed in figure 3.4. The first 2 columns give the regression coefficients for the constant effect (income excluded), and their translation into mean CWR values (coefficients raised to the power 10). Mean fertility is highest in the 2 nationalist quadrants (2 and 3), lowest in the conciliatory, non-religious quadrant 4. The religious, conciliatory quadrant 1 is close to, but lower than, the nationalist quadrants. The third column gives the regression of 1og (CWR) on log (income) in each of the four quadrants. In the two nationalist quadrants (2 and 3) the slopes are non-significant, indicating that there is *no effect* of mean income on fertility in these areas. The intercepts do not differ significantly either, showing that if an area is nationalist, religiosity adds nothing to its *level* of fertility. Comparing the two conciliatory quadrants (1 and 4), we can see that both slopes are significant, but they do not differ significantly, so that in conciliatory areas, the effect of material resources (income) on fertility is significantly negative, but unaffected by the religiosity of the area. The constant terms do not differ either. Thus the resources-fertility relationship is very different in nationalist and conciliatory areas, but once nationalism is controlled, is unaffected by religiosity. We can see this by comparing this final regression with the fourth column of Panel 1 (CWR as a function of nationalism and income). The R^2 difference, after adding 4 extra terms for the religiosity effect, is 0.006, which is not significant ($F_{4,784} = 1.71$, $_{P} > 0.05$). "Adding" nationalism to a devoutly religious district, therefore (quadrant 2 vs. quadrant 1), dramatically alters the pattern of fertility, and effaces the effects of local standard of living on fertility. On the other hand, "adding" religiosity to a non-nationalist area (quadrant 1 vs. quadrant 4) has no real effect either on the baseline level of fertility *or* on the effects of local standard of living on fertility.

As can be seen in figure 3.4, the religious areas are poorer, as a group, than the non-religious areas, and as figure 3.3 indicated, there is a positive relationship between religiosity and nationalism. Taken by itself, then, it appears as if there is a consistent relationship between religiosity and higher fertility, even when standards of living are controlled (table 3.2, Panel 1, column 2). However, when religiosity, nationalism and material resources are considered together, we find that there is no independent, significant effect of religiosity on fertility.

Figure 3.4
Fertility by Mean Household Income in Statistical Areas by Religosity and Nationalism

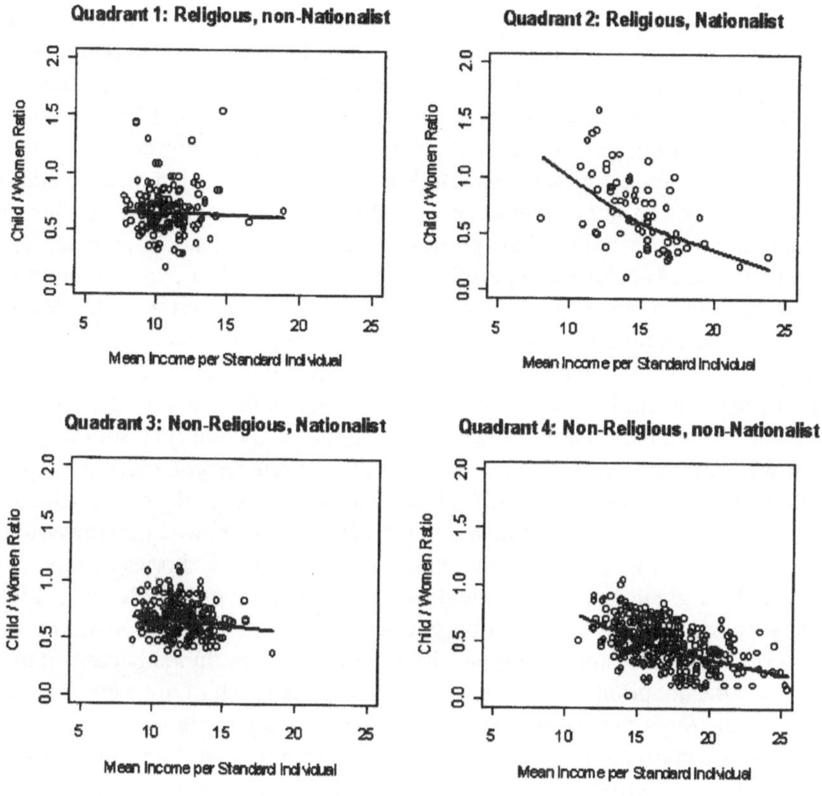

Conclusions

Explanations of Israel's high level of fertility have often focused on the salience of nonnative religious injunctions. In doing so, they have taken at face value a particular statistical association, without considering the theoretically problematic aspects of such an explanation: that Jews outside Israel do not have the same high level of fertility; and that there is much evidence to indicate that verbalized nonnative injunctions are not necessarily a good guide to what people actually do. The roots of Israel's high fertility need to be sought in Israel's singular position in the world-system, and in the specific conditions in which Israelis live their lives, and we are arguing that these conditions give rise both to a high degree of religious identification, and a high level of fertility.

One of the major themes in Israeli life, and in Israeli consciousness, is the ongoing struggle over the establishment of the State and the form that the

State is to take. The conditions of this struggle, including periodic wars and an endemic and salient threat of random violence, are conditions that highlight the importance of group strength, and yet at the same time maintain a constant situation of personal insecurity. At points in the social structure in which this threat is felt most it is also expressed in support for political parties that are nationally activist, and which make an emotional appeal to group pride, and it is here that the personal response of enhanced fertility is most noticeable.

However, we are not arguing that Israel's fertility is high because there is a large group of radical nationalists in the population. Nor are we arguing that the Israeli-Palestinian (or Israeli-Arab) conflict can be interpreted simply as the result of an intransigence or unwillingness to compromise on the part of one or other (or both) of the parties. Israel is an outstanding example of a semi-peripheral enclave in a peripheral region, engaged in two contradictory struggles. On the one hand it must maintain its autonomy vis-à-vis the center, and at the same time it must maintain its advantage vis-à-vis the surrounding periphery. On both fronts it is threatened with a loss of its semi-peripheral status, and absorption into the periphery, though in the early 1980s (perhaps even more than today) it was the struggle on the peripheral (Palestinian) front that was salient. As a result, the whole of the *conscience collective* is imbued with nationalism, mostly focused on Israel's special role in the region (Shamir 1986, notes that surveys conducted in the early 1980s showed that fewer than 20 percent of Israeli Jews favored withdrawal from the territories occupied in 1967). To a greater or lesser extent this nationalist ethos affects all Israelis, invoking a high degree of sensitivity to nationalist and religious symbols and rhetoric, and increasing the propensity to have children. In many cases it also involves the adoption of a traditional, religious approach to life, certainly to a far greater extent than would be expected under comparable social conditions without the constant external threat. We are arguing, therefore, for a macro-perspective on fertility analysis, seeing fertility as a social phenomenon, a reflection of what Durkheim might have termed a "fertilogenic force," and something which needs to be explained by reference to other such social facts, We have not attempted, here, to tackle the micro-question, of how nationalism, as ideology, translates into a particular propensity to have children, nor the effects of this high fertility on the nationalist *conscience collective.* Clearly, these questions deserve further attention in future studies. For the moment, we are merely suggesting that much of the religiosity recorded in fertility surveys is an expression, in consciousness and in the mode of daily living, of a strongly felt nationalist sentiment, and that once this nationalist sentiment is controlled for, there is no direct effect of religiosity on fertility. Among those sections of the population in which the nationalist spirit is strongly felt, it is powerful enough to annul even the general relationship between living standards and fertility. The peace process currently under way, in which Israel is gradually disengaging from its control of the territories occupied in 1967 and is moving towards an accommodation with its Arab neighbors, is being accompanied by growing tensions within Israeli (Jewish) society focusing not only on the desired extent of Israeli physical hegemony, but also on the role of religion in public life. This process may also be indicative of a relative change in the salience of the two fronts: the central and the peripheral. Implicitly, our analysis suggests that if and when this occurs, and Israel's struggle moves from one of establishing its position in the region to one of establishing its autonomy in the world-economy, there will also be a decline in the level of fertility, although expressions of religiosity may yet remain high.

Acknowledgements

We wish to express our gratitude to the Social Science Data Archive at the Hebrew University in Jerusalem, for providing the data required for this analysis in machine-readable form. Previous versions of this chapter were presented at the annual meeting of the British Society for Population Studies, Durham, 1994, and the Israel Sociological Society, Eliat, 1995. The authors wish to acknowledge the helpful and constructive criticisms offered in Durham and by colleagues in Israel, as well as those of the editor and reviewers for the European Journal of Population, but insist that all errors of omission and commission are strictly their own!

References

Anson J. and V. Slonim-Nevo. 1995. "Correspondence analysis, a graphical tool for the presentation and interpretation of cross-classified data: An illustration using contraceptive behavior of male adolescents." *Journal of Applied Social Sciences* 19: 61-71.

Anson, O., S. Carmel, D. Y. Bonneh, Arieh Levenson, and Benjamin Maoz. 1990. "Recent life events, religiosity and health: An individual or collective effect." *Human Relations* 43: 1051-1067.

Ben Tuvia, S. 1987. *Classification of Geographic Units According to Socio-economic Characteristics of the Population.* 1983 Census of Population and Housing Publications, No. 15. Jerusalem: Central Bureau of Statistics.

Central Bureau of Statistics. 1993. *Statistical Abstract of Israel.* Jerusalem: Central Bureau of Statistics.

Central Bureau of Statistics. 1984. *Localities, Populations and Households: Demographic Characteristics from the Complete Enumeration, By locality.* 1983 Census of Population and Housing Publications, No.3. Jerusalem: Central Bureau of Statistics.

Chemichovsky, D. and J. Anson. 1993. "Cost recovery and the true cost-effectiveness of contraceptive provision." *International Family Planning Perspectives* 19: 129-133.

Cheskis, R. 1980. "Jewish identification and fertility: An analysis of subgroup fertility and differentials." Paper presented at the annual meeting of the Population Association of America, Denver, CO.

Cochrane, A. 1986. "Industrialisation and nineteenth century states." In J. Anderson (ed), *The Rise of the Modern State*, 64-90. Brighton: Harvester.

Coser, L. 1956. *The Functions of Social Conflict.* Glencoe, IL: Free Press.

Courgeau, D. 1994. "Du groupe à l'individu: l'Exemple des comportements migratoires." *Population* 49: 7-26.

Davis, K. and J. Blake. 1956. "Social structure and fertility: An analytic framework." *Economic Development and Cultural Change* 4: 211-235.

Delacroix, J. and C. C. Ragin. 1981. "Structural blockage: A cross sectional study of economic dependency, state efficacy, and underdevelopment." *American Journal of Sociology* 86: 1311-1347.

DellaPergola, S. 1968. "La popolazione Ebraica d'ltalia: Caratteristiche demografiche, economiche e sociali." *Genus* 24: 135-175.

DellaPergola, S. 1993. "Jews in the European community: Sociodemographic trends and challenges." *American Jewish Year Book* 93: 25-82.

Durkheim, E. [1895] 1964. *The Rules of Sociological Method.* New York: Free Press.

Durkheim, E. 1915. *The Elementary Forms of the Religious Life.* London: George Allen and Unwin.

Durkheim, E. [1924] 1953. *Sociology and Philosophy.* London: Cohen & West.

Friedlander, D., Z. Eisenbach and C. Goldscheider. 1979. "Modernization patterns and fertility change: The Arab populations of Israel and the Israel-Administered territories." *Population Studies* 33: 239-254.

Friedlander, D., Z. Eisenbach and C. Goldscheider. 1980. "Family size limitation and birth spacing: The fertility transition of African and Asian immigrants in Israel." *Population and Development Review* 6: 581-593.

Friedlander, D. and C. Feldmann 1992. "The modern shift to below-replacement fertility: Has Israel's population joined the process?" *Population Studies* 47: 295-306.

Gane, M. 1988. *On Durkheim's Rules of Sociological Method.* London: Routledge.

Gellner, E. 1983. *Nations and Nationalism.* New York: Cornell University Press.

Goldscheider, C. 1967. "Fertility of the Jews." *Demography* 4: 196-209.

Goldscheider, C. and W. D. Mosher. 1988. "Religious affiliation and contraceptive use: Changing American patterns." *Studies in Family Planning* 19: 48-57.

Goldscheider, C. and P. Uhlenberg. 1969. "Minority group status and fertility." *American Journal of Sociology* 74: 361-372.

Goldstein, H. 1987. *Multilevel Models in Education and Social Research.* London: Charles Griffin.

Goldstein, S. 1970. "Religious fertility differentials in Thailand, 1960." *Population Studies* 24: 325-337.

Greenacre, M. 1984. *Theory and Applications of Correspondence Analysis.* London: Academic Press.

Herzog, H. 1984. "The election campaign as a liminal stage: Negotiations and meanings." *Sociological Review* 35: 559-579.

Jiobu, R. and H. Marshall. 1977. "Minority status and family size: A comparison of explanations." *Population Studies* 31: 509-517.

Keyfitz, N. and W. Flieger. 1990. *World Population Growth and Aging: Demographic Trends in the Late Twentieth Century.* Chicago, IL: Chicago University Press.

Keysar, A., E. Sabatello, I. Ziegler, R. A. Shtarkshall, S. Kupinsky, R. Zur, and E. Peritz. 1992. "Fertility patterns in the Jewish population of Israel." In E. Peritz and M. Baras (eds), *Studies in the Fertility of Israel:* 21-57. Jerusalem: The Institute of Contemporary Jewry, Hebrew University.

Kupinsky, S. 1992. "Jewish fertility patterns: Norms, differentials, and policy implications." In C. Goldscheider (ed.), *Population and Social Change in Israel*, 149-175. Boulder: Westview.

Lazerwitz, B. 1980. "Religiosity and fertility: How strong a connection?" *Contemporary Jewry* 5: 56-63.

Lipshitz, G. 1986. "The stability of spatial patterns of welfare - the Israeli case." *Geoforum* 17: 353-366.

Lopez, D. E. and G. Sabagh. 1978. "Untangling structural and nonnative aspects of the minority status—fertility hypothesis." *American Journal of Sociology* 83: 1491-1497.
Marcum, J. P. 1986. "Religious affiliation, participation and fertility: A cautionary note." *Journal for the Scientific Study of Religion* 27: 621-629.
Marcum, J. P. 1988. "Explaining Protestant fertility: Belief, commitment and homogamy." *Sociological Quarterly* 27: 547-558.
Meir, A. and Y. Ben-David. 1995. "From latent surplus to changing norms: Fertility behavior of the Israeli Bedouin along the nomadism-sedentarism continuum." *Journal of Comparative Family Studies* 26: 389-409.
Nairn, T. 1977. *The Break-Up of Britain: Crisis and Neo-Nationalism.* London: New Left Books.
Neuman S. and A. Ziderman. 1986. "How does fertility relate to religiosity: Survey evidence from Israel." *Sociology and Social Research* 70: 178-180.
Peres Y. and I. Brosch. 1991. "The impact of social and economic factors on the size of Israeli Jewish families." *Journal of Comparative Family Studies* 22: 367-378.
Peritz, E. 1992. "Overview of the findings." In E. Peritz and M. Baras (eds), *Studies in the Fertility of* Israel, 187-199. Jerusalem: The Institute of Contemporary Jewry, Hebrew University.
Ritchey, P. N. 1976. "The effects of minority group status on fertility: A re-examination of concepts." *Population Studies* 29: 249-257.
Robinson, W. 1950. "Ecological correlations and the behavior of individuals." *American Sociological Review* 15: 351-357.
Roudi, N. 1993. "Population policies vary in Middle East." *Population Today* 21: 3-10.
Sabagh, D. and D. E. Lopez. 1980. "Religiosity and fertility: The case of Chicanos." *Social Forces* 59: 431-439.
Shamir, M. 1986. "Realignment in the Israeli party system." In A. Arian and M. Shamir (eds.), *The Elections in Israel – 1984*, 267-296. Tel Aviv: Ramot.
Sinnott, R. and E. E. Davis. 1981. "Political mobilization, political institutionalization and the maintenance of ethnic conflict." *Ethnic and Racial Studies* 4: 398-414.
Slottje, D. J., G. W. Scully, J. G. Hirschberg and K. Hayes. 1991. *Measuring the Quality of Life Across Countries: A Multidimensional Analysis.* Boulder, CO: Westview Press.
Stark, R. 1984. "Religion and conformity: Reaffirming a *Sociology* of Religion." *Sociological Analysis* 45: 273-282.
Wallerstein, I. M. 1974. *The Modern World System.* New York: Academic Press.
Wallerstein, I. M. 1979. *The Capitalist World-Economy: Essays.* Cambridge: Cambridge University Press.
Wallerstein, I. M. 1984. *The Politics of the World Economy: The States, the Movements, and the Civilizations.* Cambridge: Cambridge University Press.
Weller, S. C. and A. K. Romney. 1990. *Metric Scaling: Correspondence Analysis.* Newsbury Park, CA: Sage Publications.
Wilson, C., J. Oeppen and M. Pardoe. 1988. "What is natural fertility: The modelling of a concept." *Population Index* 54: 4-20.

4

Innovation and Adaptation in Fertility Transition: Jewish Immigrants to Israel from Muslim North Africa and the Middle East

Barbara S. Okun

Introduction

Beginning with Carlsson's (1966) alternative characterizations of fertility transition—one in terms of innovation and diffusion, the other in terms of adjustment or adaptation—there has been a major controversy over which model better describes the process of marital fertility decline. While it is likely that both innovative and adaptive behavior play roles in fertility transition, the literature has been largely polarized around these two views. In their discussion of the policy implications for developing countries of the European historical record, Knodel and van de Walle (1986) stress an innovation in family limitation by a vanguard followed by diffusion to the many. In summarizing the results of the European Fertility Project, Watkins (1986) echoes this view, and emphasizes the importance of cultural boundaries to the spread of the innovative behavior. The innovation and diffusion of stopping behavior—fertility control exercised once women have already attained their desired family size—are seen as the driving force behind the European fertility transition.

The adaptation hypothesis maintains that fertility transition is accompanied by increases in the extent or amount of fertility control that is already practiced by a more limited proportion of the population, rather than by the innovation of a new behavior. Fertility control is thought to reflect couples' adaptation to changes in the socioeconomic environment that affect the costs and benefits of children. Classical demographic transition theory, for example, highlights economic development as a major influence on declining fertility (e.g., Coale and Hoover 1958). Also, most economic demographers and economic historians see reduced demand for children as the fundamental driving force behind fertility transitions. Essentially, economic development transforms a society, in which large families are assets to parents, to an industrialized, market-oriented economy that increases the economic advantages of small families. Modernization reduces children's role as security for parents, and the trend toward mass education decreases their availability for work.

Empirical support for the adaptation view is presented, for example, in the context of the decline of Mormon fertility in the nineteenth century United States, where fertility transition is thought to have reflected adaptation to the decreasing ability of the Church of Jesus Christ of Latter-day Saints to maintain an economic, political, educational, and religious separation from the national system (Bean, Mineau, and Anderton 1990). This adaptive fertility control behavior took the form of larger proportions of women practicing spacing behavior, that is, lengthening birth intervals, even at low parities, in order to reduce completed family size.

The innovation hypothesis, as generally discussed in the literature, maintains that the diffusion of innovations in knowledge of, attitudes towards, and behavioral changes in fertility control is impeded by the existence of cultural and linguistic boundaries. For example, diffusion is thought to be slowed when populations are less culturally homogeneous. Diffusion of knowledge, attitudes, and behaviors takes place through social networks, and may be aided by mass media and family planning programs. Because it may emphasize informational and contraceptive constraints as major obstacles to lower fertility levels, the innovation/diffusion hypothesis can be viewed as a justification for government and institutional expenditures on family planning programs. On the other hand, the adaptation hypothesis maintains that fertility falls in response to changing economic conditions that affect the costs and benefits of children. Thus, its adherents suggest that economic development is the path to lower fertility and controlled population growth.

The literature has generally assumed that the origins of an innovation-diffusion process were either new knowledge about contraception, the availability of a new method, or changes in social and cultural conditions that, for the first time, make fertility control acceptable on moral grounds. We suggest here, however, that the innovation may also take the form of interpretations of, or responses to, changes in socio-economic and mortality conditions that, for the first time, make the practice of fertility control advantageous. This occurs for example, when fertility decision-makers interpret changes in the socio-economic environment that affect the costs and benefits of having children. An understanding of the implications of these socioeconomic changes, or the new behaviors that are responses to these changes, may spread through the population via the process of interpersonal diffusion, just as the information concerning new types of fertility control techniques may diffuse through the population. In any case, the diffusion process affects the speed of the fertility decline, while the innovation refers to the initial change that triggers the decline. Thus, the distinction between innovation and adaptation as triggers of fertility transition is artificial. In this paper, we discuss the distinction between innovative and adaptive fertility control behavior only in the sense that the former is a *new* behavior while the latter is not. These issues are further discussed in Friedlander, Okun, and Segal (1997) and Friedlander and Okun (1996).

Below, we explore the roles of new, as well as old, fertility control behaviors in the fertility transition of a population of Jewish immigrants to Israel from Muslim countries of North Africa and the Middle East. We investigate the roles played by socio-economic factors and cultural boundaries in the spread of fertility control. We also explore the ways in which contact with the broader Israeli society affected contraceptive use among Asian-African women, after controlling for socio-economic factors.

The Setting

Following the foundation of the state of Israel in 1948, massive Jewish immigration created an extremely diverse society, marked by different cultures, languages, levels of socio-economic status, and demographic regimes. Differences were especially dramatic between Jews of European origin and those of North African and Middle Eastern origin (referred to here as of Asian-African origin). Most European immigrants to Israel were born in Poland, the former U.S.S.R., Romania, Germany, and Austria, and arrived between the 1930s and 1970s. Most immigrants of Asian-African origin arrived in Israel during the late 1940s and 1950s from Morocco, Iraq, Tunisia, Egypt, Yemen, Turkey, and Iran. After arriving in Israel, women of Asian-African origin began a fertility transition. Census data from 1983 (the latest census available for public use at this time) indicate that Jews of Asian-African origin reduced their cohort total fertility by about 33 percent, from a predecline level of approximately 6.5 children per woman in cohorts married in the early 1930s, to approximately 4.3 children per woman in cohorts married during the early 1960s. A large proportion of the decline in total fertility—approximately 75 percent—is attributable to reductions in fertility within marriage, while approximately 25 percent is due to increases in age at marriage. Thus, one of the important responses of immigrants to the dramatic cultural and socio-economic transformations they experienced was an increase in their use of fertility control, resulting in rapid fertility reduction (Schmelz, DellaPergola, and Avner 1991). The proportions of Asian-African women who ever married were very high and varied little over time during the period in question. Thus, changes in the proportion ever-married contributed little to changes over time in the total fertility of birth cohorts.

Since, in most cases, the mass migration comprised virtually all the Jews living in the Arab countries of origin, these immigrants were not selected on the basis of socio-economic characteristics, as is true of most migrant groups (Kahn 1988; Ford 1990). This non-selectivity of migrants substantially simplifies the study of immigrant fertility since the migrants were not especially likely to adapt quickly to Israeli society, nor were they similar to the Europeans before their arrival in Israel.

Israeli society in the early 1950s was dominated by Eastern European Jews. Some of these Jews were the first to immigrate to Palestine, and were the founders of almost all political, economic, and cultural institutions, including the trade unions, the kibbutz movement, the first Jewish cities, the premiliary organizations, and the national theatre. In general, immigrants from Muslim countries were characterized by low levels of economic development and educational attainment. Asian-African immigrants had usually lived in urban slums or primitive rural areas in their countries of origin (Roumani 1979).

Immigrant groups from Asia and Africa were confronted with severe economic pressures. During the 1950s, these immigrants suffered from high illiteracy rates and faced unemployment rates that were twice as high as the rest of the population (Sicron 1967; Patinkin 1967). They came from countries where they had worked in family businesses or as independent craftsmen, and were confronted with the need to search for hourly jobs as unskilled laborers or as employees in large industrial enterprises. The large family, beneficial in a traditional society in which children, especially sons, were economic assets, was ill-suited to the market economy in which children's education was compulsory and their economic costs outweighed their economic benefit. In addition, a remarkable reduction in infant and child mortality left immigrant women in Israel with larger proportions of their children surviving than they had experienced in their countries of origin (Friedlander and Goldscheider 1984). Thus, in contrast with the controversy concerning conditions surrounding other fertility transitions (e.g., Costa Rica, Sri Lanka, and Thailand), there can be little doubt that changes in socio-economic and mortality conditions played very important roles in the reduction in fertility among Asian-African Jews in Israel.

In addition to the substantial differences in the economic structure of their new country, the immigrants from Asia and Africa faced a radically different culture. The Asian-African family was the centre of religious and social life. The influence of Islam and local cultures in their countries of origin made Asian-African Jewish families resemble their Muslim neighbours in patterns of relationships and way of life (Eickelman 1981). The Asian-African Jewish family had come to possess, to a greater extent than their European counterparts, many social characteristics of families in traditional societies: veneration accorded to the father as head of the family; low status and minimized role of women; importance of sons; and absorption of the bride into her husband's family (Bernstein 1979; Okun 1996).

Moreover, the Asian-African Jews were generally less secular and less individualistic in outlook than their Eastern European counterparts. As Bernstein (1979) explains, "The (Asian-African Jew) ordered his world according to the social units he belonged to—his kinship group and his religious-communal group. He accepted both religious and secular authority as something taken for granted, as the will of God. He himself was not an autonomous entity striving to assert itself and to control its fate independently of these larger social frameworks" (p. 39).

After arrival in Israel, a process of cultural integration began. Over time the Asian-African ethnic groups have adapted themselves to the norms and values of mainstream Israeli society. While Asian-African norms and attitudes have left their marks on Israeli culture, the Asian-Africans have yielded more toward European-American behavior than vice versa (Peres 1989).

With regard to reproductive behavior, the Asian-African immigrants entered a society in which the use of fertility control within marriage was already well accepted and widespread. With cohort total fertility less than three, women of European descent had already been experiencing low fertility for decades. Thus, exposure of the Asian-African immigrants to this relatively secular culture, in addition to the more modern economy, may have also played an important role in reducing fertility (Lesthaege and Surkyn 1988).

There were few other changes that could have affected fertility. In particular, there were no large-scale (or even small-scale) government or private family planning programs aimed at reducing family size among the Asian-African population. Indeed, family planning policies in Israel have often been described as pronatalist, since the strengthening and growth of the Jewish population in Israel was a national, Zionist goal. As just one example of this pronatalist stance in the Israeli government, we note Prime Minister David Ben Gurion's prize payment incentive scheme, offered between 1949 and 1959, of approximately $300 (a substantial sum at the time) to every woman who bore a tenth child (Friedlander and Goldscheider 1979).

The pronatalist stance contrasts sharply with the situation in other countries that experienced socio-economic development and rapid fertility declines, in conjunction with large-scale family planning programs (e.g., Korea, Taiwan, Indonesia, Singapore, and Mexico). The experience of Asian-African Jews in Israel provides us with an unusual example of a modern fertility transition that occurred in the absence of the effects of a family planning program.

As will be discussed below, two important changes occurred in contraceptive use among the Asian-African population: increases in the use of the birth control pill, and increases in the use of any type of deliberate fertility control (contraception or abortion) before parity two. Since the birth control pill became available in Israel only in the late 1960s, we view the spread of its use as the diffusion of an innovation. In contrast, fertility control for spacing purposes (at parities zero or one) was practiced to a significant extent even among very early, pre-transitional cohorts of Asian-African women. Thus, we view the increase in the extent of spacing behavior as adaptive behavior. Below, we investigate the development of these innovative as well as adaptive behaviors in the fertility transition, and explore the roles played by socioeconomic factors and cultural boundaries in the spread of fertility control.

Theoretical Considerations

Socio-economic status

Socio-economic status variables are presumed to be related to both motivation to use birth control and accessibility or affordability of modern methods. In terms of motivation, we hypothesize that more highly educated women in higher status families are more motivated to use effective birth control. The empirical inverse relationships between fertility and economic and educational attainment have long been noted (e.g., Cochrane 1979). Economic explanations of these relationships point to the greater direct and indirect costs of children in higher status households. Presumably, higher status women and their husbands have higher expectations for their children, and thus want to invest in their quality. Also, the value of time for more educated women is greater because their wage is higher.

In terms of accessibility and affordability of modern fertility control methods, birth control pills and IUDs could be obtained, from the late 1960s and onward, primarily through visits to private doctors who would provide prescriptions. The fees for the doctors' visits and the costs of the contraceptives were paid by the patient. Unlike most medical services, which were provided by the socialized system of Kupot Cholim (the Sick Funds), contraceptive services were not provided by the Kupot. In addition, the publicly funded infant and child healthcare stations (Tipot Chalav) did not generally provide family planning services. Thus, both for reasons of motivation and accessibility, we expect higher status women, married to more educated men and living in households with a higher standard of living, to make more extensive and intensive use of fertility control. It is worth noting, however, that unlike the pill and other modern methods, abortion was provided free of charge by the State, if women were "approved" by committees that were set up to decide when abortion was acceptable. Of course, women who were rejected by these communities, or who did not want to go through them, could resort to illegal (but generally very safe) abortion by paying for an abortion by a private doctor. As of 1952, doctors who provided private illegal abortions were not prosecuted.

Religiosity

Religiosity is a particularly important explanatory variable, given the wide variation in religiosity within the Jewish population, and the generally pronatalist stance of the Jewish religion, which holds that it is a duty to "be fruitful and multiply, and replenish the earth." Although there is no single source that absolutely determines whether the use of birth control is permissible within the Jewish religion, most scholars agree that the use of birth control is not condoned (Feldman 1974). Therefore, we expect that more religious women are less likely to feel comfortable with the use of fertility control. Religiosity has been shown to be an important determinant of fertility in the Israeli context (Friedlander and Feldmann, see chapter 2), and is a widely discussed ideational variable (Lesthaeghe and Surkyn 1988).

Social integration

Next we consider military service as a measure of social integration or assimilation. Army service can be thought of as a vehicle of socialization or as a vehicle of departure from traditional culture (Bloom and Bar-Yosef 1985). Although service is in theory mandatory, exemptions for girls could be easily obtained by those who claimed to be religious.[1] It is widely known that many girls who were exempted on the basis of religiosity were actually secular Jews. Asian-African women were much less likely to have served in the military than their counterparts of European descent.

The Israeli military's role in the integration of new immigrants has often been presented as a prime example of what is known as "nation building." The Israeli Defense Forces (IDF) act as a channel for acculturation, education, and absorption in the new society (Azarya and Kimmerling 1980: 471). The *de facto* residential and educational segregation of Asian-African Jews from Jews of European origin often made the integrated military service the first life-cycle experience in which Asian-Africans and Europeans mixed together in an organized social environment. The socialization and educational processes of the IDF changed Asian-African soldiers who left the family milieu and spent two or three years in a Western and modern social organization (Roumani 1979). Military service can thus also be understood from the perspective of the diffusion of ideas, if we assume that activities away from home decrease the influence of the family (particularly the male family members) on decision-making, and increase the influence of new contacts (Axinn 1992).

Evidence that the military may serve as a vehicle for departure from traditional culture is presented by Bloom and Bar-Yosef (1985), who report the results of a panel study of girls interviewed at age seventeen in 1974, and reinterviewed four years later in 1978. The study shows that women who served in the IDF became more achievement-oriented, as well as more interested in mastering and controlling their environment over the four-year interim. In addition, they became more open about their sexual feelings. In contrast, the non-servers became more compliant and more deferent, thus leading the authors to conclude that not serving reinforces the traditional role and self-concept of young women.

Military service on the part of girls is probably also an indication of how conservative or traditional her family is. Serving in the IDF shows a willingness, on the part of the girl's male relatives, to allow the girl to leave the parents' home, and to have more exposure to the wider society. The social norm in the Asian-African subpopulation during the 1950s and 1960s—that "the army is not for girls"—was probably motivated by fear on the part of male relatives of girls' greater exposure to non-familial forces (Bloom and Bar-Yosef 1985). Thus, a girl's service in the military may be an indicator of weakening resistance to a changing society on the part of her family.

Other effects of military service may include enhancement of a girl's ability to manage her way around a large, bureaucratic system in a way that may aid her in overcoming administrative obstacles in other life situations, including those entailed in obtaining contraception or abortion services. Previous research has also shown that, in some contexts, military service can have important effects on post-service economic opportunities of veterans. However, this research has focused primarily on the U.S. context for male servicemen (Angrist 1990; Angrist and Krueger 1994). There has been no research that has examined the economic consequences of military service for Israeli women. While we do not dismiss the possibility that military service may increase economic opportunities for women, for example, by providing them with various forms of work experience, it is widely believed that the primary influence of military service on girls in Israel is via socialization and acculturation.

Additional measures of exposure to Israeli society or social integration are whether an immigrant married before or after her arrival in Israel, and if after, how many years she lived in Israel before getting married. Friedlander, Eisenbach and Goldscheider (1980) found important effects on fertility outcomes of the timing of marriage relative to immigration among older cohorts of Asian-African immigrants. Following this previous research, we hypothesize that women who married before immigration, or shortly thereafter, spent more of their formative years in their countries of origin, and were thus less exposed to new socio-economic conditions in Israel, and less likely to adopt Israeli patterns of behavior, including contraceptive use.

Finally, we consider the response of women to questions concerning their desired family size and future childbearing intentions. As discussed in Coale (1973), motivation to use birth control depends first on the consideration of fertility control as within "the calculus of conscious choice," that is, within the realm of human control. As discussed by van de Walle (1992) the calculus of conscious control is often absent from populations where desired family size is not a numeric concept—that is, when couples do not have a target towards which they progress as they live out their reproductive lives.

Motivation to use birth control may also depend on the strength of the desire to prevent or postpone the next birth. Previous research has suggested (Watkins 1986) that in historical Europe, the attempts to stop childbearing were the driving force behind the fertility transition. In contrast, Friedlander, Eisenbach, and Goldscheider (1980) suggest that increasing early birth intervals (spacing) as well as early termination of childbearing (stopping) were important components of the fertility transition of Asian-African women in Israel. We will test whether women who desire to stop childbearing are more likely to use effective means of birth control than women who want more children in the future.

Data and Methods

The data come from a fertility survey conducted in 1974 and 1975 on a random sample of married, urban Jewish women aged 18-54. Since approximately 90 percent of the Jewish population in Israel resides in urban areas, the exclusion of rural women from the survey is largely immaterial. Indeed, given the great differences between Israel's rural and urban populations (for example, special kibbutz populations are included as rural), an analysis of the urban population separately is probably desirable. Also, given the very different fertility patterns of the minority non-Jewish (primarily Muslim) women in Israel, we focus here on Jewish women only.

The sampling frame was based on complete lists of dwelling units, and the response rate of the surveys was 99 percent. In the survey, 2,974 currently-married women who had married once only were asked detailed questions about their fertility and contraceptive histories. The contraceptive histories include information on types of methods used, and when use of each method was initiated. The timing of the retrospective survey is ideal for capturing the experience of Asian-African women in the process of demographic transition.

The fertility survey analyzed here was carried out as part of a larger project that also included another survey with a larger sample size (approximately 10,000 women), but no information on contraceptive use. The larger survey, which contained fertility data, has been analyzed extensively in numerous publications (see Friedlander and Goldscheider 1978; Friedlander, Eisenbach, and Goldscheider 1980). This previous research focused on changes in fertility outcomes (birth intervals and completed family size), rather than on contraceptive use, which is an important proximate determinant of fertility, and the primary mechanism driving the fertility transition.

Table 4.1 presents characteristics of the sample women, by ethnicity (place of birth) and age at survey. After eliminating women who had missing information on at least one variable of interest, we are left with a total sample size of 2,601. Place of birth was either Asia-Africa, Europe, or Israel. The older birth cohort of women were aged 36-54 at the time of the survey; the younger women were aged thirty-five and under at survey date. By analyzing women by age at survey, we can compare the behavior of earlier and later birth cohorts, and thus note changes in behavior over time. Israeli-born respondents were generally the children of very early Jewish immigrants from Europe, and were similar, in terms of socio-economic status and cultural factors, to women born in Europe. In general, women born in Asia or Africa differed from the other two groups in terms of most of the important variables under consideration.

First, we note that women in the earlier birth cohorts of all three ethnicity groups were unlikely to have ever used the birth control pill (first row of table 4.1). This result follows from the timing of the introduction of the pill in Israel, during the late 1960s. By the time of the survey in 1974-1975, women aged 36-54 were unlikely to have ever used the pill, since it was introduced so late in their reproductive lives. Women in the later birth cohorts were more likely to have used it. Among women in the later birth cohorts, Asian-African women were much less likely than European women or Israeli-born women to have ever used the birth control pill. That is, the Asian-African women adopted innovative behavior at a slower rate than the other women. This will be discussed further below.

The second row in table 4.1 reports the probability of having used any means of contraception or abortion before parity two (that is, at parities zero or one). Fertility control exercised before parity two is an indicator of spacing behavior. Note that this form of spacing behavior was practiced fairly widely by all women in all ethnicity groups, although women of Asian-African origin practiced the behavior to a smaller extent than other women. Also note that there were increases in spacing behavior between the two birth cohorts, for women of all three ethnicities, and especially for women of Asian-African origin. This will be discussed further below.

In terms of socio-economic status variables, table 4.1 indicates that women of Asian-African origin were much less likely to be highly educated (at least twelve years of school) and to be married to highly educated men. These women were also much less likely to have at least three of the following four consumer durables in their households: telephone, washing machine, air conditioner, and television. In addition, we see that women of Asian-African origin lived in households with substantially lower monthly incomes than women of European-American or Israeli origin. We note important gains in educational attainment between the two birth cohorts, for all ethnicity groups. Since ownership of consumer durables and household income variables refer to the time of the survey, it is not surprising that the younger women often lived in households with fewer consumer durables and lower household incomes than their older counterparts.

Next we consider religiosity. We define a woman as religious if she responded that she did not travel on the Sabbath, that she adhered to kosher rules by separating milk from meat, and that she attended monthly ritual baths (the *mikvah*). Attending the monthly bath is meant to purify the woman following menstruation and is a prerequisite for entering into sexual relations. We defined a woman as secular if she did not meet any of these three criteria. Women who met one or two of these criteria were defined as traditional. As can be seen from table 4.1, Asian-African women were more likely to be traditional or religious than European or Israeli-born women. Among all ethnicity groups, we note a trend toward secularization between the two birth cohorts.

Table 4.1
Characteristics of sample women by continent of birth (reported members are proportions unless otherwise stated)

	Place of birth/Birth cohort[a]					
	Asia - Africa		Europe		Israel	
	Earlier cohort	Later cohort	Earlier cohort	Later cohort	Earlier cohort	Later cohort
Dependent variables						
Ever-use of pill (%)	11.0	21.4	9.0	44.9	19.5	39.6
Use before parity 2 (%)[b]	33.3	53.2	55.0	73.6	58.9	69.5
Exposure (years)						
Mean marital duration	22.8	8.4	23.3	6.7	20.0	5.9
Status						
12+ years education (%)	10.3	20.1	38.7	59.1	47.3	57.7
Husband 12+ years education (%)	21.9	27.1	44.7	64.6	52.0	57.5
Consumer durables (%)[c]	43.4	30.0	60.4	58.3	73.8	54.6
Mean lolg of household income	6.66	7.01	7.04	7.38	7.15	7.27
Religiosity						
Traditional (%)	42.9	45.5	29.2	21.3	32.8	28.7
Religious (%)	28.2	16.4	10.1	10.2	11.3	9.9
Social integration						
Served in Israeli army (%)	4.4	6.6	17.2	33.1	46.5	45.0
Married before immigration (%)	50.5	7.0	42.9	15.9	N/A[d]	N/A
Married 0 – 3 years after immigration	23.3	14.0	20.0	14.6	N/A	N/A
Married 4 or more years after immigration (%)	26.1	79.0	37.3	70.5	N/A	N/A
N	476	457	644	254	256	515

[a] The earlier birth cohort of women were aged 36 and over at the time of the survey. The later birth cohort were aged 35 and under at the survey date
[b] Use before parity two includes fertility control initiated at parities zero or one. Fertility control includes all methods of contraception as well as abortion.
[c] The percentage of women living in households with a selection of durables. See text for details
[d] N/A not applicable

Matras and Auerbach (1962) make an interesting point that religiosity may take on different meanings for European and Asian-African women. The religious women of European origin had rejected secular culture, while those of Asian-African origin had not (yet) been fully integrated into it. Matras and Auerbach also note that many Asian-African women who say they are religious and go to the mikvah actually have little understanding of why they do so. Attendance at the mikvah is more of a social norm than a religious duty (*mitzvah*). Thus, the Asian-African religious women may be less religious than the European religious women, since the former may not connect the mikvah with the timing of sexual relations, whereas the latter do.

Next we consider social integration variables. In terms of military service, women of Asian-African origin were much less likely than all other women to have served in the IDF. Among the immigrant groups, approximately half of women in the earlier birth cohort were married before immigration, while among women in the later birth cohort the great majority were married in Israel. Thus, immigrants in the later cohort were much more exposed to Israeli society during their youth than were their counterparts born in the earlier cohort. We note also that the vast majority of immigrants in the later cohorts had lived in Israel at least four years before getting married.

Women aged forty-five and under were asked "How many children do you want all together?" Slightly more than 8 percent of the Asian-African respondents answered non-numerically; that is, their responses were typically, "As many as God gives" or "As many as possible" (not reported in table 4.1). This proportion is similar to, but slightly higher than the proportions of European-American and Israeli-born women providing non-numerical answers (5 percent and 6 percent respectively). We hypothesize that the provision of a non-numerical response by the interviewed woman is negatively related to use of birth control (van de Walle 1992).

We view non-numerical responses as intermediate outcomes of other explanatory variables. For example, it is quite likely that religiosity is an important determinant of the tendency to provide non-numerical responses. Thus, we estimate the effect of the non-numerical response variable on various measures of contraceptive use, net of other effects.

For those women who did provide a numerical response to the question concerning desired family size, we were able to determine which women had already attained that size by the time of the survey, and wanted to stop childbearing. That is, for women who already had at least as many children as they stated that they desired, we assigned a value of one to a dummy variable for "wanting no more." For those women who wanted more children than they currently had, or provided a non-numerical response to desired family size, that dummy variable takes on the value zero. Women of European origin and Asian-African origin were somewhat more likely to want to stop childbearing than women who were Israeli-born (not reported in table 4.1).

The dummy variable for "wanting no more" is problematic in that it measures fertility desires at the time of the survey, whereas we are examining use of fertility control prior to the survey. Nevertheless, we will attempt to see whether this variable has an effect in a multivariate framework, with and without other control variables, because this motivation variable is probably also a function of the other explanatory variables.

Trends in Contraceptive Use among Cohorts Married between 1940 and 1970

As can be seen in figure 4.1, early marriage cohorts of Asian-African women contained smaller proportions of ever-users of contraception or abortion than did European women who married during the same periods. However, even among

Figure 4.1
Proportions who have ever used fertility control, by ethnicity and marriage cohort. Fertility control includes all methods of contraception as well as abortion.

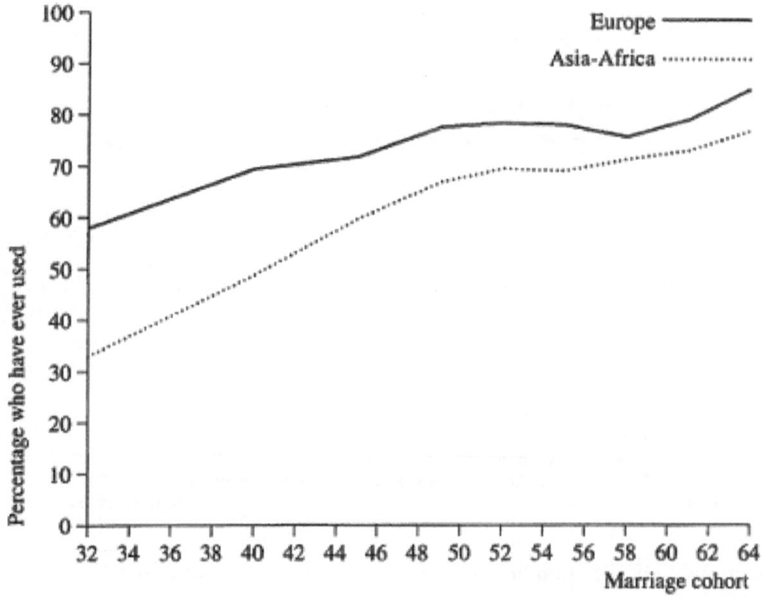

early Asian-African cohorts who married between 1948 and 1951, more than 70 percent had ever used fertility control, despite completed fertility of five to six children per woman. Ever-use did not increase much as cohort fertility fell among Asian-African women married after 1948. Overall, ever-use among Asian-African women increased by only about 8 percentage points between the cohorts of 1948-1951 and 1964-1967.

So how did marital fertility fall dramatically, if ever-use hardly changed over the marriage cohorts? Fertility must have fallen as a result of more intensive, earlier, and more effective use of fertility control. In terms of earlier use of fertility control, figure 4.2 shows that among Asian-African women, there were large increases in use of fertility control before parity two (control initiated at parity zero or parity one). The increases in use before parity two after the 1948-1951 cohort were much larger (almost 40 percentage points) than the increases in ever-use after the 1948-1951 cohort. More modest increases before parity one (at parity zero) are seen among women of Asian-African origin, but, even in the latest cohorts, use before parity one among Asian-African women lags far behind that of European women. Thus, one important factor in the fertility decline is the large increase in fertility control at early parities among Asian-

Figure 4.2
Proportions who practised spacing behaviour at early parties, by ethnicity and marriage cohort. Note that contraceptive use before parity two includes use at parities zero or one. Use before parity one includes only use at parity zero. Fertility control includes all methods of contraception as well as abortion.

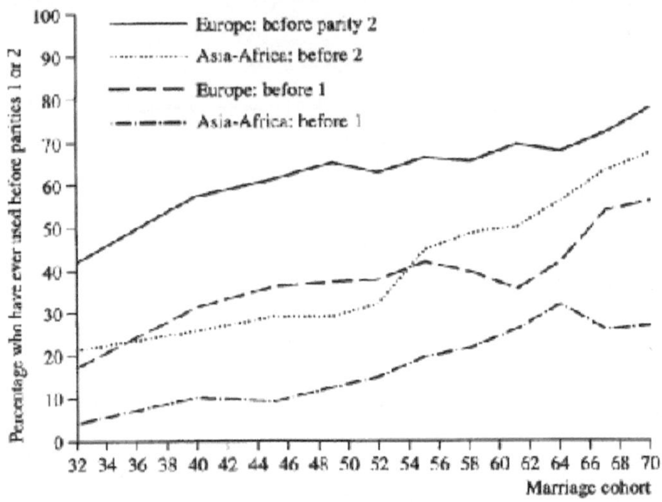

African women who married after the founding of the state in 1948.

Note, however, that this spacing behavior is practiced by a significant minority of women, even in the earliest marriage cohorts available (1930s). Traditional methods—primarily withdrawal—were the major forms of fertility control used by Asian-African women for spacing at low parities. We conclude that the increase in spacing behavior which accompanied the fertility transition of the 1950s and 1960s marriage cohorts represented adaptation to new conditions through increased use of a behavior already practiced in pretransition populations.

We see a very rapid increase in pill use among European marriage cohorts after 1958 (figure 4.3). This rise in ever-use of the pill is not matched by Asian-African women, even though overall ever use among Asian-African women rises together with that of European women. The difference is explained by absolute and relative increases in the use of withdrawal among Asian-African women (figure 4.4). Starting with the 1948-1951marriage cohort, ever-use of withdrawal drops steadily among European women, while it rises among Asian-African women, at least until the explosion in pill use in the early 1960s cohorts. Once ever-use of the pill starts rising, withdrawal levels off among Asian-African women, but does not decline. A cross-over thus occurs, so that by the mid-1950s cohorts, Asian-African women have higher ever-use rates of withdrawal than do corresponding European women.

Figure 3
Proportions who have ever used the birth control pill, by ethnicity and marriage cohort.

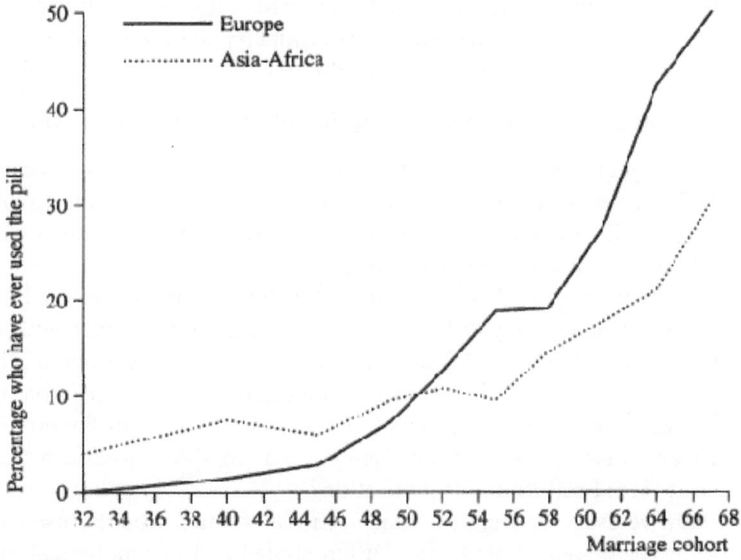

Figure 4.4
Proportions who ever used withdrawal, by ethnicity and marraige cohort

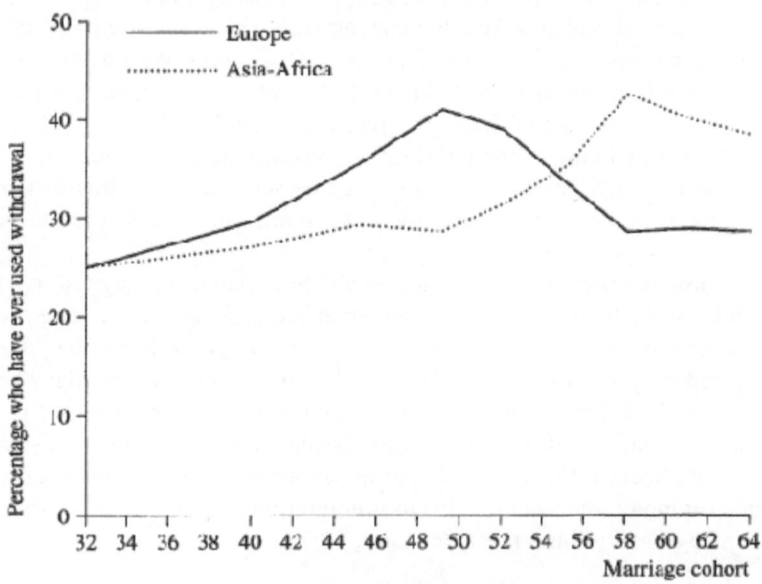

Thus, European women were adopting the pill and abandoning withdrawal, but Asian-African women were slower to do so, and continued to use withdrawal, while adopting the pill at a lower rate. The Asian-African women continued using the more traditional, male method longer.[2] Still, the Asian-African women did adopt the pill as well, which may help to explain part of the fertility decline. Below, we explore the ethnic gap in the adoption of the birth control pill.

Explaining the Ethic Gap in Adoption of Modern Contraception

Among women aged thirty-five and under at the time of the survey, nearly 45 percent of women born in Europe and 40 percent of women born in Israel had ever used the pill, while only 21 percent of the corresponding group of women born in Asia or Africa had ever used the pill.

We first consider why this innovation—the new technology offered by the pill, with its greater efficacy and greater convenience—was adopted with lower frequency among the Asian-African population. Are the obstacles to pill use grounded in socio-economic factors that are related to the motivation to use effective birth control and the accessibility and affordability of the pill? Were there also cultural barriers, entrenched among women of Asian-African descent, which held them back from this innovation?

Second, we ask who were the Asian-African women who did use the pill when it first came out. What factors differentiated them from the majority of the Asian-African subpopulation? Again, are the factors mostly socio-economic in nature, or are they related to culture, or to the extent that these women were integrated into Israeli society? We attempt to address these questions through multivariate analyses of pill use in a logistic regression framework.

Table 4.2 reports results from logistic regression analyses of pill use among women aged thirty-five and under at the time of the survey. We did not consider older women because, as indicated in table 4.1, very few women over the age of thirty-five at the time of the survey had ever used the pill. The pill became available in Israel only in the late 1960s. Thus, immigrant women who were more than thirty-five years old in 1974 were exposed to the pill primarily during the latter part of their reproductive lives, when pill use was not recommended by most Israeli physicians.

As is also indicated in table 4.1, almost all immigrant women aged thirty-five and under at the time of the survey were married in Israel, after a long period of exposure to Israeli society during their formative years. Since the pill was introduced only several years before the date of the survey, and many years after most of the immigrants arrived in Israel, it is not surprising that in our preliminary analyses of pill use, we did not find any important or statistically significant effects of the timing of marriage relative to immigration. We do not include timing of marriage relative to immigration as an explanatory variable in the analyses of pill use presented here.

Table 4.2
Logistic regression model of ever-use of birth control pill among all women aged < 35 at survey date

Explanatory variables	(1) Odds ratio	(2) Odds ratio	(3) Odds ratio	(4) Odds ratio
Ethnicity				
Asian-African	0.045*** (0.0001)	0.74* (0.08)	0.80 (0.20)	0.79 (0.17)
European	1.18 (0.32)	1.12 (0.50)	1.16 (0.39)	1.12 (0.54)
Marital duration				
< 2 years	0.63* (0.07)	0.73 (0.23)	0.72 (0.23)	0.80 (0.41)
2 – 4 years	0.98 (0.90)	0.98 (0.90)	0.98 (0.93)	1.01 (0.96)
> 10 years	0.51*** (0.0001)	0.51*** (0.0001)	0.52*** (0.0002)	0.49*** (0.0001)
Socio-economic status				
12+ years education	–	1.66*** (0.002)	1.60** (0.004)	1.63*** (0.003)
Husband 12 + years education	–	1.25 (0.17)	1.23 (0.20)	1.24 (0.18)
Consumer durables in household	–	1.62*** (0.001)	1.59*** (0.002)	1.57*** (0.002)
Log of household income	–	1.16** (0.02)	1.16** (0.02)	1.16** (0.03)
Religiosity				
Traditional	–	0.77* (0.09)	0.79 (0.13)	0.81 (0.18)
Religious	–	0.52*** (0.006)	0.56** (0.02)	0.65** (0.08)
Integration				
Military service	–	–	1.30 (0.11)	1.29 (0.12)
Response to desired family size				
Non-numerical response	–	–	–	0.48*** (0.04)
Wants no more	–	–	–	1.25 (0.19)
N	1,093	1,093	1,093	1,093
– 2 Log likelihood	1,346.0	1,285.0	1,282.5	1,275.1

Figures in parentheses are *p*-values of Wald χ^2 statistics (with one degree of freedom), computed as squares of the parameter estimates divided by their estimated standard errors. *** $p < 0.01$; ** $p < 0.05$; * $p < 0.10$; – indicates that the variable is not included in the model.

In table 4.2, we explore various explanations for the large ethnic gap in ever-use of the birth control pill noted above. The table reports odds ratios; odds ratios that are greater than one are associated with variables that raise the odds of having used the pill, relative to the omitted category, or relative to a lower value of the listed variable. Conversely, odds ratios that are less than one are associated with variables that lower the odds of pill use relative to the omitted category, or relative to a smaller value of the listed variable. The larger the deviation of the odds ratio from one, the larger the magnitude of the effect. The table also includes *p* values of Wald χ^2 statistics (with one degree of freedom), computed as squares of the parameter estimates divided by their estimated standard errors.

In model (1), which controls only for marital duration, we see that women of Asian and African origin have 55 percent lower odds of pill use than women who were Israeli-born (the omitted category). Model (1) indicates that women who were born in Europe were not significantly more or less likely to have used the pill than the Israeli-born. The lower odds of pill use among Asian-African women accords with our earlier descriptive findings.

In model (2), we introduce educational attainment variables, economic status variables, and religiosity variables. As expected, women with at least twelve years of education have significantly higher odds than less educated women of ever having used the pill. The effect for husbands' education is in the same direction, but is not statistically significant. Thus, we see that women's education is a more critical determinant of pill use than is husbands' education. This is consistent with much research suggesting the greater importance of women's educational attainment for contraceptive adoption. We also note that, as expected, women living in households with a greater variety of consumer durables and higher monthly incomes have significantly higher odds than other women of having used the pill. Also as expected, women who are traditional or religious are significantly less likely to have used the pill than are secular women (the omitted category). As seems reasonable, the effect of being religious is more sizeable than that of being traditional. In all, we see that, while a combination of socio-economic status and religiosity variables explains a large part of the ethnic gap in pill use, there still remains a statistically significant and important effect of place of origin.

In model (3), presented in table 4.2, we examine the effects of the military service variable, net of all other previously mentioned explanatory variables. Women who served in the Israeli military are more likely than other women to have ever used the pill. Although this effect is not statistically significant at conventional levels ($p = 0.11$), the importance of the military service variable will be illustrated in more in-depth analyses below. We note that, once we control for military service, the ethnicity effect associated with Asian-African origin is no longer statistically significant. The effects of the other explanatory variables remain largely unchanged.

In model (4), we examine the effects of the non-numeracy and want-no-more dummy variables on the likelihood of pill use, controlling for all other previous variables. The omitted category is women whose desired family sizes (numerical responses) were larger than their total number of children ever born at the time of the survey. We see that providing non-numerical responses to questions concerning desired family size is, as expected, negatively associated with pill use. Desire to stop childbearing is positively associated with pill use, but the effect is not statistically significant. Thus, we find support for van de Walle's (1992) argument concerning the importance of numeracy. On the other hand, we find little support for the importance of stopping behavior in motivating pill use; although our variables are not ideally suited to this type of analysis, we do find some support for the notion that the desire to space births was as important a motivation for pill use as the desire to stop childbearing altogether. The effects of most of the rest of the explanatory variables in model (4) are similar to those in model (3). We see some reduction in the size of the effect of religiosity in model (4), relative to model (3); this reflects the positive association between religiosity and the non-numeracy dummy variable. In all, we conclude from table 4.2 that while socio-economic status and religiosity variables are critical to explaining the slower adoption of modern contraception among immigrant women from Muslim North Africa and the Middle East, they do not explain the entire ethnic gap. Military service and numeracy variables explain some of what remains of this gap. The next section explores these factors in greater depth.

Who are the Innovators in Pill Use?

Who were the innovators in pill use among the Asian-African subpopulation? What factors differentiate the innovators from the majority of Asian-African women who did not adopt the pill when it first became available to them? Also, are the factors that differentiate the Asian-African innovators the same factors that identify the innovators among the European and Israeli-born population? We focus our attention primarily on the differential importance of military service for the various ethnic groups.

We estimate different models of pill adoption for the different origin groups. Because of the relatively small size of our subsample of women aged thirty-five and under who were born in Europe, and because separate analyses indicate that these women behave in a similar fashion to young women born in Israel, we combine the subsamples of young women of European origin with those of Israeli origin. Below, we contrast the behavior of these women with that of the women of Asian-African origin.

Table 4.3 reports the results of logistic regression analyses of pill use among the two origin groups. The left-hand panel reports the results for the subsample of women of Asian-African origin, and the right-hand panel reports the results for all other women. Within each panel, model (1) includes marital exposure, socio-economic status, religiosity, and military service as explanatory variables. Within each panel, model (2) includes the explanatory variables related to desired family size (the non-numerical response and want-no-more dummy variables) in addition to all those variables included in model (1). It is instructive to compare the results across panels in order to see ethnic differences in

Table 4.3
Logistic regression model of ever-use of birth control pill among all women aged < 35 at survey date, by orgin group

	Origin Group			
	Asian - African		Europe or Israel	
Explanatory variables	(1) Odds ratio	(2) Odds ratio	(1) Odds ratio	(2) Odds ratio
Marital duration				
< 2 years	0.46 (0.25)	0.58 (0.42)	0.81 (0.49)	0.86 (0.64)
2 – 4 years	0.71 (0.30)	0.72 (0.34)	1.10 (0.65)	1.12 (0.59)
> 10 years	0.53*** (0.03)	0.45*** (0.008)	0.50*** (0.002)	0.48*** (0.001)
Socio-economic status				
12+ years education	1.63 (0.12)	1.68* (0.10)	1.67*** (0.01)	1.68*** (0.01)
Husband 12 + years education	1.25 (0.43)	1.26 (0.41)	1.22 (0.31)	1.23 (0.30)
Consumer durables in household	1.23 (0.44)	1.17 (0.56)	1.82*** (0.001)	1.81*** (0.001)
Log of household income	1.13 (0.32)	1.10 (0.44)	1.16** (0.05)	1.16** (0.05)
Religiosity				
Traditional	0.80 (0.41)	0.89 (0.65)	0.76 (0.16)	0.76 (0.17)
Religious	0.71 (0.36)	0.79 (0.53)	0.43*** (0.008)	0.47** (0.03)
Integration				
Military service	3.11*** (0.007)	3.08*** (0.008)	1.06 (0.74)	1.07 (0.71)
Response to desired family size				
Non-numerical response	–	0.25* (0.06)	–	0.70 (0.41)
Wants no more	–	1.55 (0.12)	–	1.14 (0.52)
N	418	418	675	675
– 2 Log likelihood	422.3	413.5	851.9	850.7

Figures in parentheses are *p*-values of Wald χ^2 statistics (with one degree of freedom), computed as squares of the parameter estimates divided by their estimated standard errors. *** $p < 0.01$; ** $p < 0.05$; * $p < 0.10$; – indicates that the variable is not included in the model.

the determinants of innovative behavior. It important to keep in mind that, since the subsample of Asian-African women is smaller than that of the other women ($N = 418$ *v.* $N = 675$), it is not appropriate to compare statistical significance across ethnic groups. Rather, we focus on the relative magnitudes of the odds ratios across the subsamples.

First we compare the results of model (1) in the two different subgroups. With respect to status variables, the positive link between socio-economic status and pill use is present among women of Asian-African origin, as well as among other women, although the odds ratio associated with the dummy variable concerning number of household consumer durables in the Asian-African subsample is smaller in magnitude than the corresponding figure in the other subsample. In neither of the two subsamples is the effect of husband's education sizeable or significant.

Second, we note that the negative effects of religiosity on pill adoption are smaller in magnitude for the Asian-African subsample. For example in model (1), women categorized as religious in the Asian-African subsample have 29 percent lower odds of pill use than other Asian-African women, while in the subsample of European or Israeli women, the corresponding figure for women categorized as religious is a much more extreme 57 percent lower odds. This finding is consistent with Matras and Auerbach's (1962) suggestion that the meaning of religiosity may differ in the two subgroups.

Most striking is the powerful, positive effect of military service on the likelihood of pill adoption among the Asian-African women. The odds ratio is 3.11. There is no similar effect for the other women. We interpret this finding as evidence that military service is an important vehicle of socialization for immigrants from Muslim countries, and a reflection of lessening resistance to a different culture and tradition. Thus, we find that this ideational variable plays an important role among the more disadvantaged population group. In contrast, for women of European and Israeli origin who are members of the dominant cultural, economic, and political group in Israel, this variable has no significance at all. This finding may shed some light on the possible importance of cultural effects. Culture may be a more important factor in explaining the behavior of population subgroups that are not fully integrated into the dominant society.

Results reported in table 4.3 require the estimation of models that include both religiosity and military service variables. Chi-square tests indicate that there is a negative association between these variables, as can be expected since one of the acceptable reasons for military exemption was a claim of religiosity. However, as mentioned above, it is well known that many secular women were exempted from military duty on the basis of false claims of religiosity. The inclusion of both religiosity and military service variables in the same model poses a problem of multicollinearity, since it may not be possible for both these effects to be statistically significant. Perhaps differing effects of multicollinearity in the two subsamples led to the contrasting results concerning the association between military service and pill use. To address this issue, we estimated models that included either religiosity variables or the military service variable (in addition to the other socio-economic and marital duration variables). The results of these models, not reported here, indicate that, even when religiosity variables are not included in the model, the effect of military service is small and not statistically significant among women of European or Israeli origin, while the effect is very large and significant for Asian-African women. Also, when military service is not included in the model, the effect of religiosity is important and statistically significant for the European and Israeli origin group, but small and insignificant for women of Asian-African origin. Thus, we conclude that the differential importance of military service and religiosity between the two ethnic groups is not a consequence of multicollinearity, but rather a reflection of differing cultural meanings associated with these explanatory factors. Moreover, the differential importance of military service between the two ethnic subpopulations was obscured in the analyses reported in table 4.2, where women of different ethnicities were analyzed altogether, and where the military service variable was not found to have a statistically significant effect on pill use.

Turning to model (2) in table 4.3, we see additional differences between the two subsamples. After controlling for other factors, the effect of a non-numerical response to the question on desired family size is important for Asian-African women, but not for the other women. The explanation for this difference may lie in the fact that the European and Israeli-born women who want "as many as God gives" are likely to be religious, but still aware of the fact that fertility control is practiced by others. They personally reject the concept of fertility control, in theory, if not in practice. On the other hand, the Asian-African women who report "as many as God gives" or "as many as possible" may be willing to accept Israeli society and the use of fertility control, but have not yet been fully integrated into that society. Thus, the non-numerical response may be some indicator of a shortfall in cultural integration for the Asian-African woman, while for the European and Israeli-born woman, it is not.

Our analysis of innovators in pill use suggests that there were different factors of importance in the Asian-African subpopulation as opposed to the European and Israeli-born women. Both models (1) and (2) indicate that the relative importance of some of the ideational variables (military service and non-numerical response to questions on desired family size) compared to the socio-economic, structural variables may depend on the status of the subpopulation in the overall population.[3]

Increases in Fertility Control at Early Parities

In this section, we consider the determinants of early use of contraception or abortion, that is, use of fertility control before parity two (at parities zero or one). As seen in figure 4.2 above, there were significant increases in use of birth control at these early parities among the Asian-African cohorts. We are interested in the socio-economic and cultural determinants of birth-spacing behavior. This issue is particularly interesting in this context, since, in the absence of an official family planning program, women's adoption of spacing and stopping behavior is unaffected by targeting of specific demographic groups by family planning proponents.

Table 4.4
Logistic regression model of ever-use of fertility control before parity 2 among women, by age at survey

	Birth Cohort					
	Earlier			Later		
Explanatory variables	(1) Odds ratio	(2) Odds ratio	(3) Odds ratio	(1) Odds ratio	(2) Odds ratio	(3) Odds ratio
Ethnicity/exposure to Israeli society						
Asian-African married outside Israel	0.24*** (0.0001)	0.41*** (0.0001)	0.43*** (0.0001)	0.36*** (0.004)	0.76 (0.48)	0.79 (0.55)
Asian-African married in Israel	0.47*** (0.0001)	0.64*** (0.007)	0.65*** (0.01)	0.51*** (0.0001)	0.92 (0.65)	0.96 (0.80)
Socio-economic status						
12+ years education	–	1.28* (0.10)	1.25 (0.14)	–	1.92*** (0.001)	1.89*** (0.002)
Husband 12 + years education	–	1.14 (0.34)	1.14 (0.34)	–	0.95 (0.77)	0.94 (0.76)
Consumer durables in household	–	1.45*** (0.002)	1.42*** (0.004)	–	1.76*** (0.0006	1.73*** (0.0009)
Log of household income	–	1.18*** (0.0003)	1.17*** (0.0005)	–	1.12 (0.11)	1.12 (0.11)
Religiosity						
Traditional	–	0.73* (0.01)	0.74*** (0.13)	–	0.59*** (0.002	0.60*** (0.003)
Religious	–	0.22*** (0.0001)	0.23*** (0.0001)	–	0.22*** (0.0001)	0.23*** (0.0001)
Integration						
Military service	–	–	0.31* (0.10)	–	–	1.18 (0.42)
N	1,405	1,405	1,405	849	849	849
– 2 Log likelihood	1,838.6	1,712.4	1,709.8	1,080.0	997.0	996.2

The earlier birth cohort of women were aged 36 and over at the time of the survey. The later birth cohort were aged 35 and under at the survey date. Women who married less than five years before the survey are excluded from this analysis. Fertility control includes all forms of contraception as well as abortion.
Figures in parentheses are p-values of Wald χ^2 statistics (with one degree of freedom), computed as squares of the parameter estimates divided by their estimated standard errors. *** $p < 0.01$; ** $p < 0.05$; * $p < 0.10$; – indicates that the variable is not included in the model.

Do we see the same influence of cultural integration variables (e.g., military service) on spacing behavior as we saw in the context of pill adoption? It may be that the process of increasing birth spacing at earlier parities differs from the process of pill adoption since the latter is certainly a new, innovative form of behavior, while the former is not. Figure 4.2 indicates that at least 20 percent of even the earliest cohorts of Asia-African women practiced spacing behavior before parity two.

Since spacing behavior was practiced even in the earliest marriage cohorts, our analysis of fertility control before parity two is not limited to women aged thirty-five and under, as in the analysis of pill use. In order to examine how the determinants of spacing behavior differed across time, we classify women into two groups—those aged thirty-five and under at the time of the survey, and those aged 36-54. We exclude from this part of the analysis women who married less than five years before the survey, since it is likely that many of these women had not yet attained parity two, so that their experience would have been censored.

Table 4.4 presents the results of logistic regression analyses of the use of contraception or abortion before parity two, among women of all ethnicities. The left-hand panel of the table presents the results for the earlier birth cohort (the older group of women), and the right-hand panel presents the results for the later birth cohort (the younger group of women). The later birth cohort (aged thirty-five and under) are a subsample of the women included in the pill analysis above, since women who married less than five years before the survey are excluded.

As mentioned above, Friedlander, Eisenbach, and Goldscheider (1980) found important effects of the timing of marriage relative to immigration on the fertility behavior of the earlier cohort of Asian-African women, because of the importance of exposure to Israeli socio-economic structure and culture during adolescence and early childhood. We consider this effect by specifying interaction terms between ethnicity and exposure to Israeli society. Women of Asian-African origin who married before immigration (outside Israel) are compared with the reference group (women born in Europe or Israel), separately from women of Asian-African origin who married subsequent to immigration (in Israel).

First, consider women in the earlier cohort (left-hand panel). In model (1), the odds of Asian-African women who married outside Israel of having used fertility control at the early parities are approximately 75 percent lower than those of women of European and Israeli origin (the omitted category). Women of Asian-African origin who married in Israel also have significantly lower odds of having used fertility control before parity two than do women in the reference group (53 percent lower odds). However, odds for Asian-African women married in Israel are much higher than those of their Asian-African counterparts who married outside Israel. Thus, the findings of Friedlander, Eisenbach, and Goldscheider (1980) concerning the significance of exposure to Israeli society in the elongation of early birth intervals are confirmed here in an analysis of contraceptive use at early parities.

In the left-hand panel, models (2) and (3), which control for socio-economic status and religiosity, and socio-economic status, religiosity, and military service, respectively, suggest smaller effects of Asian-African ethnicity, both for women married outside and inside Israel, but the ethnicity effects remain large and statistically significant. Further, in models (2) and (3), there are positive

Table 4.5
Logistic regression model of ever-use of fertility control before parity 2 among women aged 35 and under, by ethnicity

Explanatory variables	Asia–Africa	Europe/Israel
Socio-economic status		
12+ years education	2.15**	1.87**
	(0.03)	(0.02)
Husband 12 + years education	1.00	0.89
	(1.00)	(0.65)
Consumer durables in household	1.52*	1.93***
	(0.09)	(0.003)
Log of household income	1.09	1.13
	(0.44)	(0.17)
Religiosity		
Traditional	0.48***	0.75
	(0.004)	(0.24)
Religious	0.24***	0.21***
	(0.0001)	(0.0001)
Integration		
Military service	1.09	1.18
	(0.86)	(0.48)
N	357	492
– 2 Log likelihood	456.8	536.5

Women who married less than five years before the survey are excluded from this analysis. Fertility control includes all forms of contraception and abortion.
Figures in parentheses are *p*-values of Wald χ^2 statistics (with one degree of freedom), computed as squares of the parameter estimates divided by their estimated standard errors. *** $p < 0.01$; ** $p < 0.05$; * $p < 0.10$; – indicates that the variable is not included in the model.

effects of high socio-economic status, negative effects of religiosity, and in model (3), positive effects of military service. Overall, among the earlier birth cohort of women, an important ethnicity effect remains after controlling for other variables. We do not consider the desired family size variables (non-numeracy and want-no-more) in the analysis of ever-use before parity two because these variables are not relevant to the decision to space births.

Turning now to the later birth cohort (the right-hand panel of table 4.4), we see much more modest effects of ethnicity in all the models. In models (2) and (3), the ethnicity effects are small and not statistically significant. That is, unlike the case concerning the older women, once we control for socio-economic and religiosity effects among the younger women, there is no longer any sizeable effect of ethnicity on the probability of exercising fertility control before parity two. This finding accords with Figure 4.2 that shows a distinct narrowing of the ethnic gap in spacing behavior at early parities among more recent marriage cohorts. The disappearance of the effect of ethnicity on spacing behavior among the later birth cohorts of Asian-African women contrasts with the greater persistence of the ethnicity effect on pill use, even after controls for other important factors are implemented (table 4.2, model (2)).

We turn now to table 4.5 that presents the results of an analysis of the determinants of spacing behavior among the younger birth cohort of women, by ethnicity. Again, we exclude women who were married less than five years before the survey. Preliminary analyses indicated that there was no significant role for the timing of marriage relative to immigration among this later birth cohort, so this variable was not included in the model presented in table 4.5.

Recall that in the analysis of ever-use of the birth control pill among Asian-African women aged thirty-five and under, we saw an important positive effect of military service (table 4.3). In contrast, table 4.5 indicates that the military service variable has no significant effect on the use of fertility control at low parities among the younger Asian-African women (nor among European or Israeli-born women). These contrasting results are interesting because they suggest that an ideational variable (military service) is much less important in explaining the determinants of a behavior (birth spacing) that is already accepted and practiced by the subpopulation undergoing the fertility transition.

Summary and Discussion

In this chapter, we begin by identifying two distinctive changes in fertility control behavior associated with the rapid fertility decline experienced by Asian-African immigrants to Israel. These changes are increases in the use of the birth control pill, and increases in the use of any type of fertility control at very early parities (zero or one). We note that use of the birth control pill is an innovative form of behavior, since the pill became available in Israel only in the late 1960s. In contrast, use of fertility control at early parities is an adaptive behavior because it was practiced by a substantial minority of women even in the earliest marriage cohorts under consideration.

We analyze each of these changes in behavior in turn, first focusing on the innovative behavior of pill use. We note the persistent negative effect of Asian-African ethnicity, relative to European or Israeli ethnicity, on pill adoption, even after controlling for socio-economic and religiosity variables. This finding suggests the existence of important cultural effects in the adoption of innovative behavior, and prompts us to look more closely at the select group of women of Asian-African origin who took up pill use within the first few years of its availability. We find that beyond important socio-economic status effects that are also apparent in the analysis of European and Israeli-born women, there is a powerful positive effect of female respondents' military service on pill use among the Asian-African women. We interpret the military service variable as a factor in reduced conformity to traditional Asian-African culture, since service in the Israeli Defense Forces is an important non-familial experience during late adolescence and early adulthood. Service in the IDF is a vehicle of socialization and departure from traditional culture, as well as a reflection of the extent of integration in the larger Israeli society.

In addition to the effects of military service on pill use among Asian-African women, we also find an effect of non-numerical response to a question on desired family size. Even after controlling for religiosity and educational attainment, non-numerical response is associated with a reduced likelihood of Asian-African women ever having used the pill. The non-numerical response dummy variable provides another example of the importance of ideational variables to the adoption of innovative behavior.

We note that among the relatively high-status, European and Israeli-born group, two of the ideational factors (military service and non-numerical response) are not important in determining pill use; only socio-economic and religiosity factors are found to be consistently important. In contrast, among the low-status, disadvantaged and marginalized group, the Asian-Africans, the military service and non-numeracy factors are important. Thus, these two ideational factors matter less within the elite group where norms of fertility control and small families are already accepted. The relative importance of structural and ideational variables in identifying the innovators of a new behavior depends on the status of the subpopulation of interest relative to the wider society.

With regard to use of fertility control at early parities, we first confirm earlier results, based on a study of birth intervals (Friedlander, Eisenbach, and Goldscheider 1980), concerning the importance of increases in spacing behavior in the fertility decline of Asian-African Jews. Thus, we note the importance of spacing behavior in the context of a modern fertility transition in the absence of a family planning program. Further, we analyze the determinants of spacing behavior among Asian-African Jews, and find that, after controlling for socio-economic and religiosity variables, the negative ethnicity effect completely disappears among women aged thirty-five and under at the time of the survey. Thus, while the effect of culture is evident in models of the adoption of innovative behavior (pill use), it is absent from models of spacing behavior, a reproductive behavior that was already firmly entrenched among the Asian-African subpopulation. Moreover, the important effect of military service noted in the models of pill use does not exist in the models of spacing behavior. We take this as further evidence of the diminishing importance of ideational variables in explaining behaviors that are already widely accepted and practiced.

We note the consistent evidence of the importance of socio-economic status variables in explaining use of fertility control in all models, and the importance of religiosity in many of the models. These findings are not new, and have been established in much previous research on fertility transition. Our major findings are the differential effects of certain ideational variables on innovative and adaptive behaviors. For example, we find important effects of military service on the adoption of innovative behavior by a socio-economically disadvantaged and culturally marginalized subpopulation undergoing rapid fertility decline in the absence of a family planning program. In contrast, military service plays no important role in explaining the spread of a type of reproductive control, spacing behavior, which was already practiced by a substantial minority of women in the earliest marriage cohorts of this same population subgroup. Nor was this ideational variable important in explaining innovative or adaptive fertility control behavior by the culturally and economically dominant population subgroup. These findings thus identify the existence of cultural barriers to the adoption of new behavior by a disadvantaged subgroup.

Acknowledgements

This research was supported by Grant 0321212 from the Israel Academy of Sciences and Humanities. The author thanks Zvi Eisenbach, Dov Friedlander, Moshe Lissak, Jona Schellekens, and seminar participants at the Hebrew University of Jerusalem for useful comments.

Notes

1. The Defense Law of 1959 states that all men and women must report for conscription into national service at the age of eighteen. Exemptions for men are much more difficult to obtain than exemptions for women. The army has never had as much need for women because women do not serve as fighters; most women serve as support staff. Among recent cohorts of Jewish youths, only about 67 percent of women serve in the IDF. In contrast, nearly 85 percent of men serve (National Council of Child Welfare (1995: 64).
2. See Santow (1993) for a discussion of the use of withdrawal among other twentieth-century populations.
3. While religiosity is a widely-discussed ideational variable (Lesthaeghe and Surkyn 1988), an examination of the effects of religiosity on contraceptive use is not the primary focus of this paper. The bulk of our analysis focuses on effects of other ideational variables—military service and non-numerical response to a question on desired family size.

References

Angrist, J. D. 1990. "Lifetime earnings and the Vietnam era draft lottery—evidence from Social Security administrative records." *American Economic Review* 80: 313-336.

Angrist, J. D. and A. B. Krueger. 1994. "Why do World-War-II veterans earn more than nonveterans?" *Journal of Labor Economics* 12: 74-97.

Axinn, W. G. 1992. "Family organization and fertility limitation." *Demography* 29: 503-521.

Azarya, V. 1983. "The Israeli armed forces". In M. Janowitz, and S. D. Westbood (eds.), *Civic Education in the Military*, vol. 2. Beverly Hills, CA: Sage Publications.

Azarya, V. and B. Kimmerling 1980. "New immigrants in the Israeli armed forces." *Armed Forces and Society* 6: 455-484.

Bacchi, R. and J. Matras. 1962. "Contraception and induced abortions among Jewish maternity cases in Israel." *Milbank Memorial Fund Quarterly* 40: 207-229.

Bacchi, R. and J. Matras. 1964. "Family size preferences of Jewish maternity cases in Israel." *Milbank Memorial Fund Quarterly* 42: 38-56.

Bean, L., G. Mineau and G. Anderton. 1990. *Fertility Change on the American Frontier: Adaptation and Innovation.* Berkeley, CA: University of California Press.

Bernstein, D. 1976. "The Black Panthers of Israel." Doctoral dissertation, University of Sussex.

Bloom, A. and R. Bar-Yosef. 1985. "Israeli women and military service: A socialization experience." Unpublished manuscript.

Carlsson, G. 1966. "The decline of fertility: innovation or adjustment process." *Population Studies* 20: 149-174.

Cleland, J. and C. Wilson. 1987. "Demand theories of the fertility transition: an iconoclastic view." *Population Studies* 41: 5-30.

Coale, A. 1973. "The demographic transition." *International Population Conference 1973*, 52-73. Liège, Belgium: IUSSP.

Coale, A. and E. Hoover. 1958. *Population Growth and Economic Development in Low-Income Countries.* Princeton, NJ: Princeton University Press.

Coale, A. J., and S. C. Watkins (eds.). 1986. *The Decline of Fertility in Europe.* Princeton, NJ: Princeton University Press.

Cochrane, S. 1979. *Fertility and Education: What Do We Really Know?* Baltimore, MD: Johns Hopkins University Press.

Eickelman, D. F. 1981. *The Middle East: An Anthropological Approach.* Englewood Cliffs, NJ: Prentice-Hall.

Feldman, D. M. 1974. *Marital Relations, Birth Control and Abortion in Jewish Law.* New York: Schocken Books.

Ford, K. 1990. "Duration of residence in the United States and the fertility of U.S. immigrants." *International Migration Review* 24: 34-68.

Freedman, R. 1990. "Family planning programs in the Third World." *Annals of the American Academy of Political and Social Sciences* 510: 33-43.

Friedlander, D., Z. Eisenbach and C. Goldscheider. 1980. "Family-size limitation and birth spacing: the fertility transition of African and Asian immigrants in Israel." *Population and Development Review* 6: 581-593.

Friedlander, D. and C. Feldmann. 1993. "The modern shift to below replacement fertility: has Israel's population joined the process?" *Population Studies* 47: 295-306.

Friedlander, D. and C. Goldscheider. 1978. "Immigration, social change, and cohort fertility in Israel." *Population Studies*: 32: 299-317.

Friedlander, D. and C. Goldscheider. 1979. *The Population of Israel.* New York: Columbia University Press.

Friedlander, D. and C. Goldscheider. 1984. "Israel's population: the challenge of pluralism." *Population Bulletin* 39: 1-39.

Friedlander, D. and B. S. Okun. 1996. "Fertility transition in England and Wales: Continuity and change." *Health Transition Review* (Supplement to Volume 6): 1-18.

Friedlander, D., B. S. Okun and S. Segal. 1997. "Demographic transition then and now: processes, perspectives and analyses." *Journal of Family History* 24: 493-533.

Kahn, J. 1988. "Immigrant selectivity and fertility adaptation in the United States." *Social Forces* 67: 108-128.

Knodel, J. and E. van de Walle. 1986. "Lessons from the past: policy implications of historical fertility studies." In Ansley J. Coale, and S. C. Watkins (eds.), *The Decline of Fertility in Europe.* Princeton, NJ: Princeton University Press.

Lesthaeghe, R. 1977. *The Decline of Belgian Fertility, 1800-1970.* Princeton, NJ: Princeton University Press.
Lesthaeghe, R. and J. Surkyn. 1988. "Cultural dynamics and economic theories of fertility change." *Population and Development Review* 14: 1-45.
Lesthaeghe, R. and C. Wilson. 1986. "Modes of production, secularization, and the pace of fertility decline in Western Europe, 1870-1930." In Ansley J. Coale, and S. C. Watkins (eds.), *The Decline of Fertility in Europe.* Princeton, NJ: Princeton University Press.
Matras, J. and C. Auerbach. 1962. "On rationalization of family formation in Israel." *Milbank Memorial Fund Quarterly* 40: 453-480.
National Council for Child Welfare. 1995. *Children in Israel Statistical Abstract.* Jerusalem: Ofek and Joint Israel (in Hebrew).
Okun, B. S. 1996. "Sex preferences, family planning and fertility: an Israeli subpopulation in transition." *Journal of Marriage and the Family* 58: 469-475.
Peres, Y. 1989. "Horizontal integration and vertical differentiation among Jewish ethnicities in Israel." In M. Lissak (ed.). *Stratification in Israeli Society: Ethnic, National and Class Cleavages,* vol. 2. Tel Aviv: The Open University of Israel.
Roumani, M. 1979. *From Immigrant to Citizen: The Contribution of the Army to National Integration in Israel.* The Hague, Foundation of Plural Societies.
Santow, G. 1993. "Coitus interruptus in the twentieth century." *Population and Development Review* 19: 767-792.
Schmelz, U. O., S. DellaPergola and U. Avner. 1991. *Ethnic Differences among Jews: A New Look.* Jerusalem: Institute for Contemporary Jewry, Hebrew University.
Sicron, M. 1967. "The economics of immigration to Israel: 1948-1963." *Proceedings of the World Population Conference, 1965*, Vol. 4, 230-234. New York: UN.
van de Walle, E. 1992. "Fertility transition, conscious choice, and numeracy." *Demography* 29: 487-502.
Watkins, S. C. 1986. "Conclusions". In Ansley J. Coale and S. C. Watkins (eds.), *The Decline of Fertility in Europe.* Princeton, NJ: Princeton University Press.

5

Fertility Behavior of Recent Immigrants to Israel: A Comparative Analysis of Immigrants from Ethiopia and the Former Soviet Union

Petra Nahmias

Introduction

Fertility changes of migrants have long provided fertile ground for demographers. The sharp transition from one society to another, with the accompanying changes in individual status as well as the more obvious contextual differences, are of great interest to those studying fertility dynamics. Societies usually change at a slower rate than the changes experienced by migrants, so migrants provide a picture of fertility changes in a rapidly changing context. Israel, as a largely immigrant society, provides a perfect case study of the fertility changes experienced by migrants. In addition to the large numbers of migrants, the registration of vital events is of a high quality, including migration that is notoriously difficult to track. Israel has the added advantage of having received migration waves from countries with vastly differing fertility regimes, both from one another and from that in Israel.

During the last twenty years Israel has absorbed large immigrant waves from both the former Soviet Union (the FSU) and Ethiopia. The immigrant wave from the FSU began at the end of 1989 and carried on throughout the 1990s (about 50,000 from the Asian republics and 770,000 from European republics). The vast majority of immigrants were from urban areas, with nearly half of the immigrants from 1989-1993 coming from Moscow and St. Petersburg alone (Tolts 1997). Immigrants from Ethiopia are less numerous than those from the FSU but nonetheless have had a significant impact on Israeli society. They have arrived in Israel in two main waves—one in the mid-1980s and the other in the early 1990s although immigrants have been arriving, albeit in fewer numbers, throughout the last twenty years. The immigrants from Ethiopia from each immigration wave also differ from one another, due to the differences in their absorption, the length of the exposure to Israeli society and also the routes used to arrive in Israel. Many of the immigrants in the 1990s have spent considerable amounts of time in transit in Addis Ababa, with its very different fertility regime, as opposed to earlier immigrants who had had little exposure to a modem lifestyle.

These immigrants arrived from countries with widely differing fertility regimes to those prevalent amongst the Israeli Jewish population. The chapter seeks to document the demographic data available, and to that end presents results on the main trends in fertility of immigrants to Israel from the FSU since 1989 and from Ethiopia since the 1980s, and also on their fertility in the country of origin. The chapter hypothesizes, based upon established fertility theories and also the experiences of immigrants to other countries, that the fertility behavior of immigrants will converge towards the norms prevalent amongst the Israeli Jewish population. It also aims to provide a contextual framework for the fertility behavior of immigrants based on previous experience and empirical theories developed thereof. It then goes on to discuss these changes in terms of

Table 5.1
Migration to Israel by Country of Birth, 1980-2000

Year	FSU	Ethiopia
1980-89	29,574	16,971
1990	184,602	4,137
1991	147,292	20,014
1992	64,921	3,650
1993	65,996	864
1994	67,956	1,193
1995	64,771	1,319
1996	58,970	1,414
1997	54,586	1,659
1998	45,963	3,109
1999	66,706	2,292
2000	50,776	2,205

Source: Central Bureau of Statistics [Israel], 2001

the fertility policy prevalent in Israel and the effect of the absorption process of the immigrants on fertility patterns and to predict future changes. The chapter ends with a brief set of conclusions.

Fertility Changes of Migrants

Research has been conducted on the changes in migrant reproductive behavior, particularly in terms of fertility changes towards the norm. One example is that of ethnic Germans in the Ukraine migrating to Germany in the 1990s (Dinkel and Lebok 1997). Prior to migration, the population had higher fertility levels than both the average for the German and USSR populations. It is suggested that an assimilatory process may be at work with a subsequent decrease in fertility to below the prevailing German levels.

Schoenmaeckers, Lodewijckx, and Gadeyne (1999) in their research on first and second generation immigrants to Belgium from Morocco and Turkey found that young women clearly preferred smaller families to older women and that this difference was more pronounced with Moroccan immigrants, who have higher fertility, than with Turkish. Migration to Belgium had a serious impact on contraceptive use with modem methods replacing traditional and overall usage increasing.

Abbasi-Shavazi and MacDonald (2000) gave precedence to cultural factors and the idea of "cultural maintenance" in their analysis of the changing fertility practices of immigrant women in Australia. Amongst their findings was the increased fertility of immigrants from the Netherlands, both first and second generation, in Australia, which is pertinent for the FSU immigrants to Israel.

Immigrant women to Israel in the 1950s from North African and Asian countries experienced fertility decreases towards the veteran population whereas immigrant women from European countries in the same period experienced an increase in fertility towards the norm. Friedlander and Goldscheider (1978) attribute the changes in the fertility of immigrants mainly to economic conditions and furthermore, Friedlander et al. (1980) found that socio-economic status, rather than cultural differences, is the determining factor of fertility decline amongst immigrants from Asia and Africa. Immigrants who were more exposed to elements of socioeconomic change in Israel, those who married after immigration or the more educated controlled their fertility through both spacing and stopping. However, the less educated and those married prior to immigration employed only stopping. In another study, it was found that immigrant women from Asia and Africa desired smaller families than their husbands. However, due to the prevalent gender power relations amongst such immigrants, women are not usually the reproductive decision makers. Thus fertility may be higher than desired or clandestine abortions may be sought (Okun, see chapter 4). Okun, in chapter 4, asserts that socioeconomic factors, or the adaptation approach, alone did not account for the fertility decline of Asia-Africa immigrants but acted in tandem with cultural factors, that is, the innovation-diffusion approach. It is likely that the absorption of Ethiopian immigrants will resemble the patterns of absorption of these non-European groups (Weinstein 1985) given the similarities in their original fertility regimes.

Sabatello (1992,1995) examined the fertility and abortion patterns of immigrants from the FSU who immigrated to Israel in the 1970s. The immigrants in their initial phase of immigration did not experience any significant change in their fertility but by the early 1990s their fertility was only 10 percent lower than that of Israeli Jewish women yet 50 percent higher than that of Jews in the USSR. Despite this, he found that even after ten to fifteen years exposure to Israeli family planning patterns, immigrants continued to use abortion as a means to control their fertility. However, although their abortion application rates were 26 percent higher than the average Israeli Jewish woman, the rates were significantly lower than those prevailing in the Soviet Union at the time. Interestingly, these immigrants preserved the pattern of early childbearing, followed by stopping rather than delaying childbearing. This immigrant group may provide less of a pre-cursor to the behavior of the current immigration wave due to the heterogeneity of fertility behavior within the FSU since a large majority of the immigrants of the 1990s, unlike the immigrants of the 1970s, came from the relatively developed European Soviet republics and especially from the large urban centers.

Fertility Changes in Country of Origin

Fertility Rates in the FSU

The fertility rates in the FSU are relatively low, even when compared with European countries. Although the fertility in some of the Asian republics is above replacement level, all other republics have fertility levels well below those of replacement level. That being said, childbearing is concentrated at younger ages, with high age specific fertility rates. Together with the low overall fertility rates, the fertility rates of older women will correspondingly be very low. Accordingly, the fertility control of FSU women has been achieved mainly through stopping rather than delaying childbearing.

The concentration of childbearing in younger ages has been increasing in recent years with rates at younger ages increasing along with decreasing overall levels. The decrease in fertility is accounted for by larger decreases in the older age groups, which decreased by more than 50 percent in the thirty-five and older age groups between the 1950s and the 1980s (Imbrogno and Imbrogno 1989). By 1991, the fertility rates of the 15-19 age group exceeded the rates in all age groups above thirty (Zakharov and Ivanova 1996).

Jewish women, in both the Ukraine and Russia have even lower fertility rates than those prevalent in the general population—in 1979 the Jewish fertility rate was about half that of the general population (Kostantinov 1991). Between 1988-

1989 and 1993-1994, the TFR of Russian Jewish women fell by 46 percent from 1.5 to 0.8 (lower than the overall urban TFR and lower even than overall TFR of Moscow and St. Petersburg) (Tolts 1997). The situation is further complicated by the fact that the fertility of the FSU population is in a state of flux, with the FSU experiencing a substantial decline in fertility since the onset of the socio-economic transition in 1989, which of course coincides with the beginning of the mass emigration to Israel (Kohler and Kohler 2002).

There are probably significant differences in fertility, as with other variables, between the various republics of the former USSR. It can be expected that immigrants from European republics will have lower fertility than immigrants from Asian republics, in accordance with the prevailing fertility regimes in those countries. Nonetheless, the overall fertility of the FSU is still significantly lower than the Jewish Israeli norm of about 2.5, with the mostly Jewish immigrants from the FSU to Israel having even lower fertility than the general population. Additionally, fertility has decreased in the FSU during the 1990s (although has been showing signs of recovery in recent years), and thus new immigrants to Israel can also be expected to reflect these trends (at least in terms of tempo).

The Proximate Determinants of Fertility in the FSU

The low fertility rate of the FSU is surprising given the high marriage rate. Prior to the 1990s, the prevalence of marriage was high and the mean age of marriage was low. During the 1990s, the marriage rates have decreased although the mean age of marriage has remained stable, indicating that people are not simply postponing marriage (Micevska 2002). However, marriage may no longer play such an important role in childbearing as in the past. In 1993, nearly one in five babies were born out of wedlock (Kingkade 1997), reaching nearly one in three by the end of the 1990s (Zbarskaya 2001). Thus the governing proximate determinant is now the age of entry into sexual union, which unfortunately is not registered in vital statistics.

Abortion is of particular importance when discussing the fertility behavior of FSU immigrants, as the abortion rate in the FSU is particularly high (Paltiel et al. 1997; Popov 1991). The FSU is the only country to have achieved low fertility with the use of abortion as the main form of birth control, with no analogous developed country (Popov 1991), apart from those Eastern European countries in the Soviet sphere of influence. The only easily accessible method was induced abortion, the principal means of fertility regulation (Scherbov and van Vianen, 2002). Reliable imported contraceptives were limited and expensive and other contraceptives, Soviet made or imported from East European countries, were unreliable and of poor quality (Amir et al. 1997). On the other hand, abortion was available using local equipment and personnel with no need for imported goods and available without charge (Popov 1991). Abortion was devoid of the values and the controversy present in other countries (Remmenick 1993; Amir et al. 1997), being regarded simply as an unpleasant medical procedure and found acceptable by the vast majority of Russian women (Bystydzienski 1989). Therefore, traditional methods such as withdrawal and rhythm were utilized, with abortion a back up for failure (Amir et al. 1997). Unlike the situation in developed countries, a high proportion of women in the FSU utilized abortion in order to stop childbearing, and not to postpone births or to space births. Young women have been more likely to marry and bring their first pregnancy to term in Eastern European countries than in other developed countries (Kulczychi 1999:9). Abortions are thus often obtained by older, married women who want to end childbirth but who use less efficient, traditional contraceptive methods (Kulczychi 1999:9).

Contraceptive use is much harder to measure. In general, the method mix of FSU women is different to women in developed countries, with a heavy reliance on traditional methods. Amongst modem methods, the IUD was the main method employed, with the Pill and condoms featuring very low (Popov 1991). Russian women (and presumably women from other Republics of the FSU) are increasingly using modem contraceptives to limit their fertility, with two-thirds of married women using some form of family planning in 1994 compared with 60 percent in 1990 (Kingkade 1997). The decline in fertility since 1988 has not been matched with an increasing abortion rate—in fact, the abortion rate has been decreasing (Zakharov and Ivanova 1996). Although the registration of induced abortions has deteriorated, evidence suggests that Russian women are indeed moving from abortion to efficient methods of contraception (Zakharov and Ivanova 1996; Kingkade 1997). Since these changes have been taking place while immigration from the FSU to Israel has been occurring, it is assumed that the fertility patterns of earlier immigrants will differ from those of later immigrants, and we can expect immigrants to arrive with higher levels of contraceptive use.

Fertility Rates in Ethiopia

Ethiopian immigrants arrived from a country with traditionally high fertility rates and low rates of abortion and contraceptive use. Data on Ethiopian fertility rates in general, and that of Ethiopian Jews in particular, is hard to come by. Ethiopia, like many less developed countries, has poor registration of vital events. As many Jewish communities in Ethiopia were in remote areas (most Jews immigrated originally from rural areas, with many coming from the northern and isolated region of Gonder),[1] there is no official data on Jewish fertility in Ethiopia. In less developed countries it is usual for the fertility of the urban and educated elite to be lower with higher contraception use. Therefore, given the rural and isolated nature of the Jewish community in Ethiopia, it can be expected that the fertility rates of Jewish Ethiopians are even higher. The DHS surveys provide more recent information.

Table 5.2
Fertility Rates by Age and Place of Residence, Ethiopia, 2000

	Age Specific Fertility Rates							TTotal Fertility Rate
Place of Residence	15-19	20-24	25-29	30-34	35-39	40-44	45-49	
Urban	50.2	139.3	142	154.7	91.6	17.3	4.8	3.0
Rural	114.4	256.4	277.5	258.7	182.8	98.7	20.8	6.0
Total	100.5	234.8	250.6	243.3	167.8	88.6	18.8	5.5

Source: DHS, 2002

It can be seen that the differences between urban and rural localities are marked. Furthermore, Addis Ababa has particularly low fertility. In 1990, reported fertility in Addis Ababa was 2.6 and in the mid-1990s it had declined further to 1.8 - below replacement level fertility (Ashagrea 2002).

The Proximate Determinants of Fertility in Ethiopia

Marriage in Ethiopia is nearly universal and occurs at young ages, with a median age of 16.4 and less than 0.5 percent of women aged forty and over never married. (Demographic and Health Surveys 2002). The median age of marriage is the same age as the median age of entry into sexual union, indicating that there is little sexual activity and resulting childbirth outside of marriage, with only approximately 1 percent of Ethiopian women cohabiting. This is in stark contrast to the situation in many other countries of sub-Saharan Africa that are characterized by an informal polygamous mating system.

Fertility in Ethiopia may be lower due to pathological sterility. Mammo and Morgan (1986) state that childlessness in Ethiopia is high due to sexually transmitted diseases, particularly gonorrhea. It is known that the prevalence of venereal disease resulted in remarkable levels of childlessness in Central Africa. The introduction of antibiotics reduced this phenomenon but fertility levels still remain depressed (Jones 1992:138). Although it is difficult to gauge how much this affected the Jewish community, it is feasible that the improved health conditions and increased awareness in Israel may lead to a decrease in infertility and possibly a rise in the natural fertility of the population. Additionally there are parts of Ethiopia where malaria is endemic that would lead to higher rates of spontaneous abortion and thus depress fertility.

Breastfeeding is an important proximate determinant in a traditional society, and is often employed in sub-Saharan Africa as a means of child spacing. It can be seen that in urban areas breastfeeding is shortened, leading to a shorter period of postpartum insusceptibility. In this case, urban women use contraceptives instead of breastfeeding to space their births so there is no overall rise in fertility.

DHS data show that contraceptive use in Ethiopia varies widely between urban and rural localities, and the use of contraceptives by urban women is more than eight times that of rural women. Amongst rural women, contraceptive use in 2000 is low, but still higher than the negligible 2.6 percent contraceptive use reported in 1990 (Ashagrea 2002). The low level of urban fertility was achieved with one of the weakest family planning programs in the world (Ashagrea 2002) and even resistance by medical personnel to the introduction of contraceptives (Kebede 2001).

Abortion data is hard to access since Ethiopia, has poor registration of vital events, let alone abortion, which is subject to restrictive laws and operates clandestinely. Given the remote nature of the Jewish communities in Ethiopia and the concentration of the few medical facilities in cities, the greater part of abortions would be performed using traditional methods. It is assumed that the abortion rate is low due to the high fertility rates and lack of access to safe medical procedures. However, in Ethiopia there is an interesting situation whereby Addis Ababa has very different fertility practices to those prevalent in other areas of the country. Ashagrea (2002) examined the prevalence of induced abortion amongst women in Addis Ababa and found a high level of awareness of the use of abortion. He further found a decreasing use of abortion amongst the youngest cohorts between 1990 and 1995, whereas older cohorts show increased use. This indicated that the youngest age groups are increasingly using contraception to limit their fertility as opposed to abortion. Nonetheless, unsafe illegal

Table 5.3
Selected Demographic Indicators, Demographic and Health Survey, Ethiopia, 2000

	Desire to limit childbearing (percent of currently married women)	Age at 1st marriage (women aged	Mean duration of postpartum insusceptibility 20-49)	Current use of contraceptives (% of currently married women)	
				Any	Modern
UUrban	40.3	17.8	10.5	35.6	28.3
RRural	30.9	16.2	20.1	4.3	3.3
TTotal	32	16.4	19.6	5.9	4.7

Source: Demographic and Health Surveys (2002)

abortion is the second killer of young women in Ethiopia, after tuberculosis (Kebede 2001), indicating that it may have wider prevalence. Abortion rates are likely to be much higher in urban areas, particularly in Addis Ababa due to lower fertility desires and superior access to health services.

Fertility Rates in Israel

Israel is a heterogeneous country in many respects, including the realm of fertility. The various population groups exhibit diverse fertility behavior. For example, the population group "Jews and others" had a TFR of 2.59 in 1999 as opposed to a TFR of 4.33 amongst the Arab population.[2] Since the immigrants are absorbed into Israeli Jewish society, it is assumed that their fertility will become more like the society into which they are absorbed. It is important to note that fertility in Israel, even Jewish fertility, is still significantly higher than that of other developed countries.

However, even amongst "Jews and others" fertility behavior is not homogeneous. Friedlander and Feldman (see chapter 2) point out that religiosity and fertility are correlated in Israel. Rough estimates of the TFR of the ultra orthodox are around seven children per women and those of the national orthodox about 4.5. FSU immigrants are, on the whole, non-religious and therefore it is to be expected that while there is an increase in the fertility rate it will not exceed the fertility rate of secular Jewish Israelis, which although higher than the FSU rate is about replacement level fertility. Many of the Ethiopian immigrants identify with more religious and traditional groups within Israeli society. Thus, although their fertility is expected to decrease, they may be more likely to adopt the fertility practices of the religious population rather than the secular population.

Israeli Jewish society is also relatively conservative regarding extra-marital childbearing. In 2000 only 2.8 percent of all births were to never-married women. Although many Jewish women cohabit prior to marriage, marriage is still the dominant framework within which childbearing occurs. Abortion behavior amongst Jewish women is similar to Western Europe in terms of the rates (the total abortion rate in 1999 was 0.45 abortions per woman). However, the marital status makeup is more similar to Eastern European countries (Amir and Benjamin 1997) and the percentage of births aborted is less than other developed countries due to the higher fertility rates. Data on contraceptive use in Israel is very hard to come by. The prevailing fertility rates, along with the abortion and marriage rates, indicate widespread use of contraception, particularly amongst secular Jews. However, it is very hard to quantify the extent and also to estimate the current method-mix being employed.[3]

Hypotheses

As has been demonstrated, immigrants tend to adopt the fertility practices prevalent in the absorbing society. As such, it is expected that the immigrants from the FSU will increase their total fertility rate to the level of secular Israelis, about replacement level. However, they will do so by increasing the fertility rates at older ages and there may even be a decrease in rates at younger ages. Ethiopian immigrants will also converge to the levels of Israeli society, although the society in to which they are absorbed may also include national-religious society. As a result, I expect the fertility of Ethiopian immigrants to decrease to a level slightly higher than secular Israelis—around 2.5 children per women. In both cases, it is hypothesized that the average age of first birth will increase, along with the overall average age of birth amongst FSU immigrants due to the delaying of childbearing amongst both groups, and the increase in fertility in older age groups amongst FSU immigrants.

The methods used to achieve the changes are not necessarily the same as those of the general population. It is known that the methods used by immigrants are not always the same as the receiving society, particularly during times of change. However, I do expect a number of changes to occur. Firstly, the age of first marriage of both Ethiopian and FSU women will increase. In other words, women will delay entering marriage and as a result (or perhaps a result of) delay childbearing. FSU immigrants will replace the use of abortions with the use of modern contraceptives and as a result, abortion rates will decrease. On the other hand, Ethiopian immigrants will increasingly use abortion to control fertility in conjunction with increasing contraceptive use.

Data

The data used in this study is mainly based upon the birth files of the Israel Central Bureau of Statistics (ICBS) from 1980 to 2000. Other data has been calculated from ICBS abortion and marriage files. In some cases it has been possible to further supplement the data with data from various publications of the ICBS, with the aim of constructing a time series of changes in rates during the 1990s.

Births

Birth data is provided from the population register when the birth is registered. By law, births have to be registered by the institution in which the birth took place or by the parents if the birth took place outside of an institution within ten days of the birth of a child. Variables recorded include identification details of mother, place of birth, religion, place of birth of parents, year of *aliya* (immigration), birth history of mother. Since the registration of a birth is necessary in order to obtain various benefits, it is assumed that coverage is nearly complete. The registration of a birth is controlled by the Ministry of the Interior, who, once a month, transfer the file of all births registered in that month to the ICBS. Most of the data is of high quality following record linkage with the national population register to fill in unknown variables, apart from variables that cannot be linked such as schooling and occupation that are of such poor quality that they cannot be reliably used.

Abortions

The abortion data is supplied by means of a form that applicants fill out when applying to the pregnancy termination board. Some of the variables on the form, particularly those of direct relevance to the outcome of the application such as age and marital status are statistically reliable. Others, such as contraceptive use are unreliable. A problem with estimating abortion rates is illegal abortions. Sabatello (1995) estimated that there are an additional 5,000-6,000 illegal abortions each year in Israel, which represent about a quarter of all legal abortion applications. From conversations conducted with social workers attached to the boards, it is suspected that many FSU immigrants seek an immigrant doctor from the FSU, often those not yet authorized to practice medicine in Israel, to conduct the abortion. This opinion is backed up by Remennick et al. (1995). Since the illegal abortion is most often performed under relatively safe and hygienic conditions, it is not possible to estimate the extent of this phenomenon from hospital emergency room admission records. Therefore we use data from applications to the board, but with the knowledge that it is an underestimation.

Marriage

Marriage in Israel is conducted by the relevant religious authorities. In the case of Jews, this is the Rabbinical authority, which fills out the marriage certificate. Due to the lack of civil marriage in Israel, there are no facilities to allow mixed religion marriages or the marriage of those whose Judaism is in doubt (according to the strict Orthodox definition). However, Israel is committed to recognize such marriages if performed abroad, although they are barred in Israel itself. As a result, in the last few years, many couples, particularly new immigrants from the FSU who are not able to, or prefer not to, marry in Israel are marrying abroad. On their return to Israel, they register their marriage with the Ministry of the Interior and this data also reaches the ICBS.

Fertility of New Immigrants

Fertility Changes in Israel

As expected, an increasing fertility rate is seen amongst immigrants from the FSU and a decreasing fertility rate is seen amongst immigrants from Ethiopia. Figure 5.1 shows the TFR of immigrants from the FSU and from Ethiopia compared with that of the Jewish Israeli population.

Figure 5.1
Total Fertility Rate by Country of Birth, 1986-2001

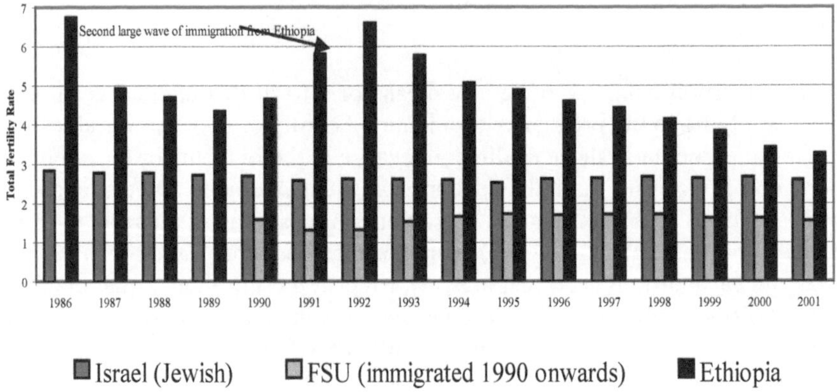

While the Israeli Jewish TFR has remained constant at slightly above 2.5 children, the TFR of immigrants from Ethiopia has decreased from 4.60 in 1996 to 3.85 in 1999—a decline of over 16 percent in four years. With immigrants from the FSU the picture is less clear and the TFR fluctuates from a low of 1.31 in 1991 to a high of 1.72 in 1995. However, due to the ongoing immigration both from the FSU during the 1990s and from Ethiopia during the 1980s and 1990s, these rates are obviously influenced by the continuous addition of new immigrants. Thus, the picture may be clearer if the population is divided according to immigration cohorts, as shown in table 5.4.

The cohort analysis is important, not only because it enables the amount of time since migration to be analyzed, but also because each cohort has a different socio-demographic make-up. Since some of the numbers are relatively small, particularly in the older age groups, the results were standardized using Jewish Israeli age specific fertility rates. However, the results were not significantly different from those in table 5.4, indicating that the results are not due to random factors caused by small population groups. Although there is an overall trend of increasing TFR with time in Israel, the immigrants arrive with varying TFR in different years. This may be attributable to the varying composition of the immigrants, such as age, marital status and republic of origin. The years 1992-1994 are unusual in that immigrants arrived with relatively high fertility that peaked four to six years after immigration and then dropped. As table 5.1 shows, the immigration to Israel in those years, although less than in 1990-1991, was still substantial. In no case does the number of annual births to the 1992-1994 immigration cohort fall below 700. Despite the slightly anomalous behavior by these cohorts, overall each additional year in Israel adds 0.076 to the TFR, if other intervening factors are assumed to be negligible.

Table 5.4
TFR by Year of Immigration, Immigrants from FSU, 1990-2000

	Years Since Migration										
Year of immigration	1	2	3	4	5	6	7	8	9	10	11
1990	1.39	1.38	1.59	1.75	1.84	1.79	1.83	1.78	1.8	1.8	1.7
1991	1.42	1.51	1.62	1.77	1.81	1.87	1.84	1.74	1.7	1.6	
1992	1.86	1.7	1.77	1.88	1.83	1.9	1.68	1.66	1.7		
1993	1.79	1.63	1.77	1.8	1.91	1.71	1.78	1.71			
1994	1.61	1.44	1.68	1.74	1.73	1.74	1.6				
1995	1.5	1.62	1.81	1.75	1.75	1.83					
1996	1.2	1.3	1.42	1.48	1.53						
1997	1.17	1.24	1.31	1.32							
1998	1.03	1.22	1.28								
1999	1.07	1.1									
2000	1.22										

With Ethiopian immigrants it is not possible to analyze their behavior by single year of immigration because their population size is much smaller. They are therefore grouped into two distinct groups by period of immigration—those who immigrated until 1989 and those who immigrated from 1989 and onwards.[4] Figure 5.2 shows their TFR according to this division between 1996 and 2001.

The data quite clearly show a significant decline in the TFR with time for both groups of immigrants. Although the TFR of both groups is still higher than that of Jewish Israelis, the 2001 TFR of immigrants who immigrated until 1989 is close to the Jewish TFR. The rate of decline of the TFR of new immigrants who immigrated since 1990 is greater and the gap between them and earlier immigrants is narrowing. Each additional year in Israel leads to a drop of 0.37 in TFR for newer immigrants and 0.21 for older immigrants.

Although the age specific fertility rates (ASFR) are the constituents of the TFR, they are also an important indicator of reproductive behavior in their own right and changes in TFR are not necessarily caused by proportional changes in the ASFRs. Amongst immigrants from the FSU the obvious trend is one of decrease amongst younger women, especially those in the 15-19 age group. This would seem to be contrary to the trend of increasing TFR, but the decrease amongst younger women is compensated for by increased fertility rates at older ages. These changes are in accordance with those expected since the age-fertility function is becoming comparable to that of the Jewish Israeli population.

These fertility changes hold true when a cohort analysis is conducted. The changes are greatest amongst the 15-19 age group which is presented in table 5.5. The 1992 immigration cohort stands out as having arrived with extremely

Figure 5.2
TFR of Immigrants from Ethiopia by Period of Immigration, 1996-2001

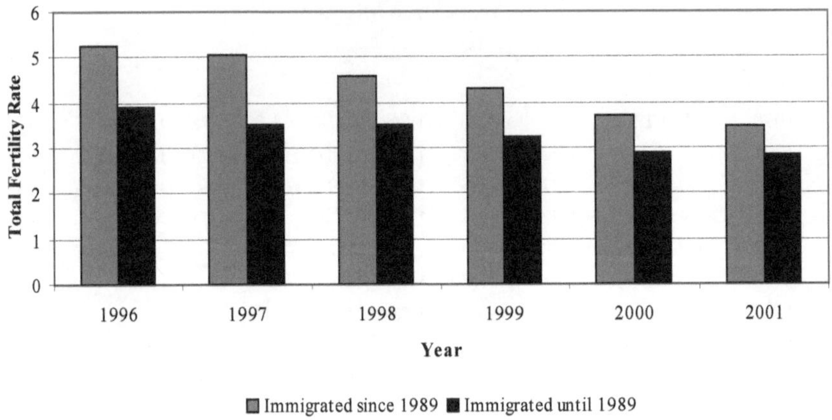

Figure 5.3
ASFR Selected Years, FSU immigrants

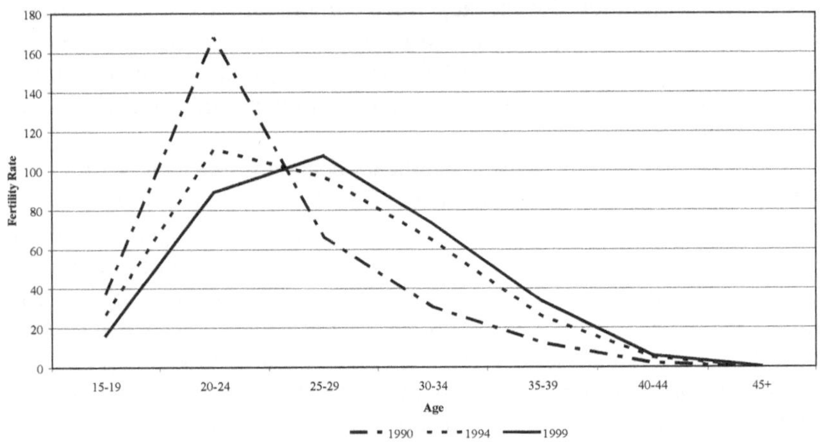

high fertility rates for the 15-19 age group. Within six years this rate was more than halved.

Immigrants from Ethiopia are also undergoing a decrease in the ASFR of young women. However, in this case it is accompanied by a decrease in the fertility of older women, leading to an overall decrease in TFR. The overall age-fertility function remains much the same, with the majority of childbearing concentrated in the 25-29 age group, apart from the 15-19 age group which shows a more marked decline. By 2001 the rates of young women are similar

Table 5.5
15-19 ASFR Immigrants from FSU by Years since Migration, 1991-2001

Year of immigration	Years since migration: 1	2	3	4	5	6	7	8	9	10	11
1990	24.7	18.79	18.48	14.55	15.15	13.33	12.43	12.42	8.79	8.79	8.95
1991	25.53	21.91	18.51	16.6	17.87	15.32	14.47	12.34	10.64	7.87	
1992	57.37	30 30	27.37	27.89	20	12.11	14.23	10			
1993	49.13	38.26	34.78	30.87	27.83	20.43	22.25	19.13			
1994	43.04	29.13	30 2	5.22	26.52	19.57	14.78				
1995	38.5	36	23.5	17	20.02	18.5					
1996	37.37	27.89	15.81	17.92	11.58						
1997	36.47	27.06	17.06	14.71							
1998	28.13	18.75	17.5								
1999	18.28	12.78									
2000	19.58										

to those of veteran Jewish Israelis (including ultra-orthodox with their elevated fertility levels) but diverge amongst women aged thirty-five and over who still have higher fertility.

As with immigrants from the FSU, the amount of time in Israel is an indicator of fertility behavior. When the immigrants are divided into two groups according to their period of immigration, their behavior can be seen to be different.

For both groups of immigrants the age-fertility functions are fairly similar to one another, although the fertility of the new immigrants is higher. Both groups show elevated fertility amongst older women. The fertility of women aged 40-44 is almost the same as that of women aged 35-39, which results in an odd age-fertility function. This does raise suspicions of the misreporting of age but since the function is similar in both groups it is possible that this is an accurate reporting of fertility patterns. Further work needs to be carried out in order to determine the cause of the age-fertility function, which deviates from that usually witnessed in populations.

Amongst younger women the process of convergence is apparent. The rates of women aged 15-19 are shown separately in figure 5.6. In 1996, the 15-19 ASFR amongst women who immigrated after 1990 was over fifty per thousand, whereas that of veteran immigrants was slightly less than ten. In 2001 the ASFR of immigrants before 1990 had risen slightly to 11.7 and that of new immigrants had dropped dramatically to 16.1. However, this rate was still much higher than the Jewish Israeli rate in 2001 of 6.9 (which includes in it also the ultra-orthodox population with elevated fertility levels). Thus it can be seen that the immigrant groups are converging with each other in terms of the fertility behavior of young women and not with secular Jewish Israeli society.

Figure 5.4
ASFR Immigrants from Ethiopia, Selected Years, 1986-2001

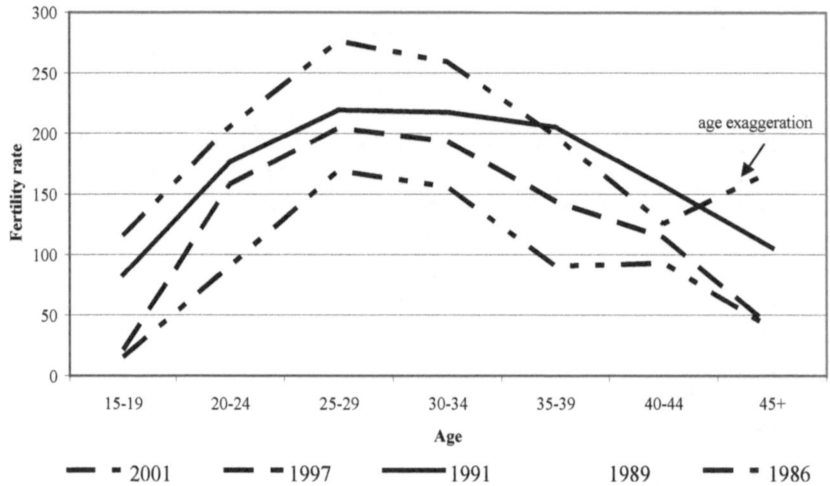

Figure 5.5
ASFR by period of immigration, immigrants from Ethiopia, 1996 and 2001

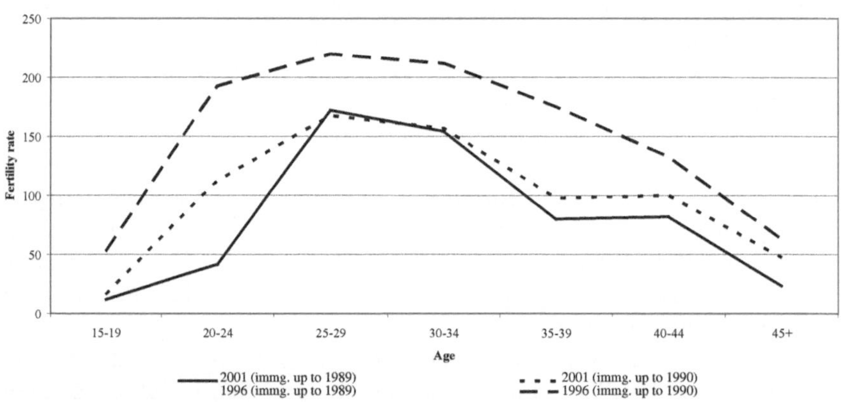

The average age at first birth is another indicator of the changing age-fertility function. All immigrants show an increasing average age at first birth as figure 5.7 shows. This demonstrates clearly that young immigrant women are increasingly delaying the commencement of childbearing. Interestingly, the veteran Ethiopian immigrants have overtaken veteran Jewish Israelis in the average age at first birth. Overall, the increase in age at first birth is more marked amongst immigrants from Ethiopia than amongst immigrants from the FSU. Amongst

Figure 5.6
15-19 ASFR by period of Immigration, Immigrants from Ethiopia, 1996-2001

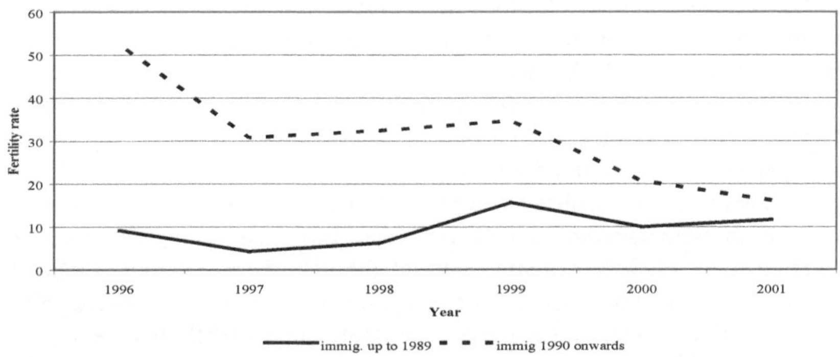

Figure 5.7
Average age at first birth, immigrants by country of birth, 1986-2001

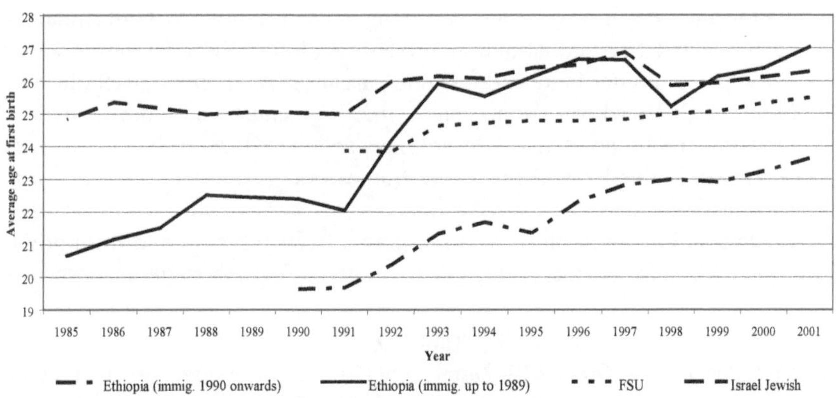

earlier immigrants from Ethiopia, each additional year in Israel adds 0.41 to the average age at first birth, while for later immigrants the figure is 0.37, and for immigrants from the FSU 0.15. In all cases time spent in Israel explains more than 80 percent of the variance in average age at first birth. A cohort analysis by year of immigration for FSU immigrants reveals similar trends. With the exception of the earliest immigrants (1990 immigration cohort), who arrived with relatively high average ages at first birth, all cohorts increased the average age at first birth. Interestingly, one sees an initial increase followed by a decrease, although not to the previous levels.

Changes in the Proximate Determinants of Fertility in Israel

While marriage is one of the most important proximate determinants of fertility, due to increasing births outside of marriage, its importance is decreasing. Figure 8 shows the changes in the mother's marital status of immigrants.

Overall, extra-martial childbearing is much less prevalent in Israel than in other developed countries, although the phenomenon is on the increase. Immigrants from the FSU show an increase in the percentage of unmarried mothers between 1990 and 2000 from 3.3 percent of all births in 1990 to nearly 10 percent in 2000, compared with only 3 percent of all births for veteran Jewish women. Although there is an overall trend amongst the veteran Jewish population of increasing births to unmarried mothers, the proportional increase amongst immigrants from the FSU is greater. Ethiopian immigrants who immigrated since 1990 show a similar trend although the rise is more moderate and fluctuates, increasing from 4 percent to 8 percent between 1990 and 2000. Amongst Ethiopian immigrants who immigrated up to 1989, there is no clear trend, with a decrease between 1990 and 1993, an increasing rate until 1998 when it reached a high of 8.7 percent, and a small decrease since then. In all cases the percentage of unmarried mothers is higher than in the overall Jewish population and there is no obvious narrowing of the differentials. Unfortunately, we do not have data on cohabitation at the time of birth, in other words we do not know if the mother is indeed a single parent or living in a household with the father of the newborn. Nonetheless, marriage cannot be ignored, even if only for the simple fact that we do not have accurate data on the age of entry into sexual union and it still forms the framework within which the majority of births take place.

As expected, veteran and new immigrants from Ethiopia and immigrants from the FSU have an increasing median age of first marriage, as shown in

Table 5.6
Average Age at First Birth, FSU Immigrants by Year of Immigration and Years since Migration, 1991-2001

	Years since migration										
Year of immigration	1	2	3	4	5	6	7	8	9	10	11
1990	25.1	25.1	25.33	25.44	25.8	25.58	25.94	24.73	24.8	25.11	25.1
1991	24.56	25.15	25.66	25.75	25.81	26.07	25.34	25.18	25.46	25.52	
1992	23.63	24.86	25.58	25.54	25.91	24.84	25.07	25.42	25.78		
1993	23.71	24.53	24.73	25.81	24.2	24.65	24.84	24.63			
1994	23.81	24.59	25.18	24.12	24.33	24.64	25.09				
1995	23.98	24.49	24.37	24.64	25.06	25.17					
1996	24.27	24.16	24.77	25.14	25.59						
1997	23.84	23.83	24.4	24.93							
1998	23.52	24.7	24.41								
1999	23.95	25.05									
2000	23.85										

Figure 5.8
Percentage of Births to Single Women, by Country of Birth, 1990-2000

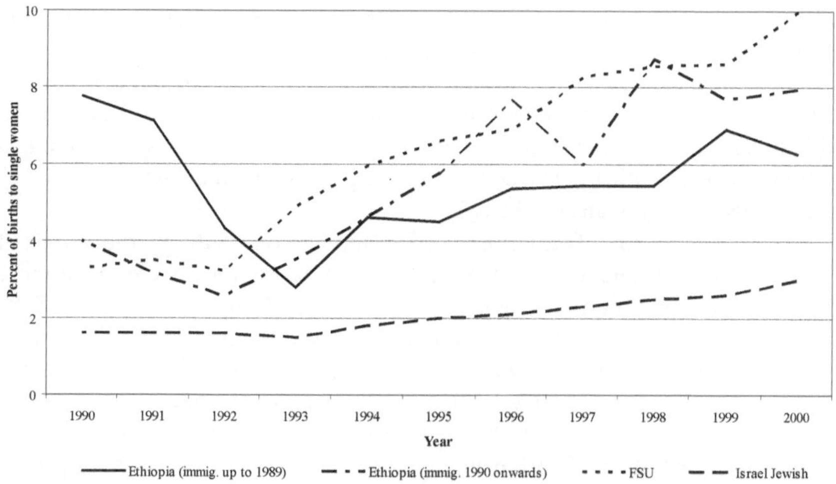

figure 5.9. Although the median age of marriage of Israeli Jewish women has also been increasing, the proportional increase of all the immigrants is greater. Additionally, the median age of marriage of veteran Ethiopian immigrants has overtaken that of veteran Israelis, indicating that veteran Ethiopian women are delaying marriage to the same extent that they are delaying childbearing. The increase in median age of first marriage is particularly impressive for new Ethiopian immigrants, which increased by six years between 1990 and 2000.

Abortion behavior is also showing signs of change, although the years available are more limited than with births (1994-2001). While abortion rates (abortions per thousand women of childbearing age) are interesting in their own right, the abortion ratio (percent of known pregnancies aborted) is more appropriate in this case, as it provides more information on the role of abortion as a proximate determinant. Amongst Israeli Jewish women, the percent of pregnancies aborted is declining slowly, from 11.3 percent in 1994 to 10.1 percent in 2001. The trend amongst all immigrant women is the opposite, with new Ethiopian immigrants clearly showing the greatest increase in the percentage of pregnancies aborted (from 10.5 percent in 1994 it nearly tripled to 29.2 percent in 2001).

In addition to the total abortion ratio, the age distribution of the abortion ratio also differs. Israeli Jewish women display a U-shaped curve, with the highest percentages of pregnancies aborted at the extremities of the fertility range, whereas immigrant women do not show this pattern. Ethiopian women have an I-shaped function. The percentage of pregnancies aborted amongst young women are extremely high and, especially amongst new immigrants, showing no signs of decreasing. The ratios are particularly high amongst veteran immigrants—in 1997 the percentage of pregnancies aborted amongst women under nineteen was over 90 percent (compared with around 30-40 percent for all Israeli Jewish women). FSU immigrants also have a unique age function. In this case it resembles a J-shaped function. There is a slight peak amongst younger women, but the percentages increase rapidly amongst older women. The function is slowly becoming similar to the Israeli Jewish function. However, this is through an increase in the percentage of pregnancies aborted amongst younger women rather than a decrease amongst older women, which fluctuates but shows no clear signs of change.

Another interesting feature of abortion applications is the marital status of the applicant. Throughout the 1990s, Ethiopian immigrants were much more likely to be never married women than either Israeli Jewish women or FSU immigrants, with new Ethiopian immigrants having the highest percentage (72 percent of all applicants were never married in 2001). On the other hand, FSU immigrants were less likely than Israeli Jewish to be never-married. This perhaps indicates the use of abortion by Ethiopian immigrants to delay the commencement of childbearing and by FSU immigrants to cease childbearing. By 2001, all groups (including Israeli Jewish women) had seen an increase in the percentage of never-married women amongst applicants.

Data on contraceptive use are particularly hard to come by. No nation-wide fertility surveys were conducted during the 1990s with the most recent nation-wide survey being conducted in 1987/1988. Unfortunately the data available do

Figure 5.9
Median Age at First Marriage, Immigrants by Country of Birth, 1990-2000

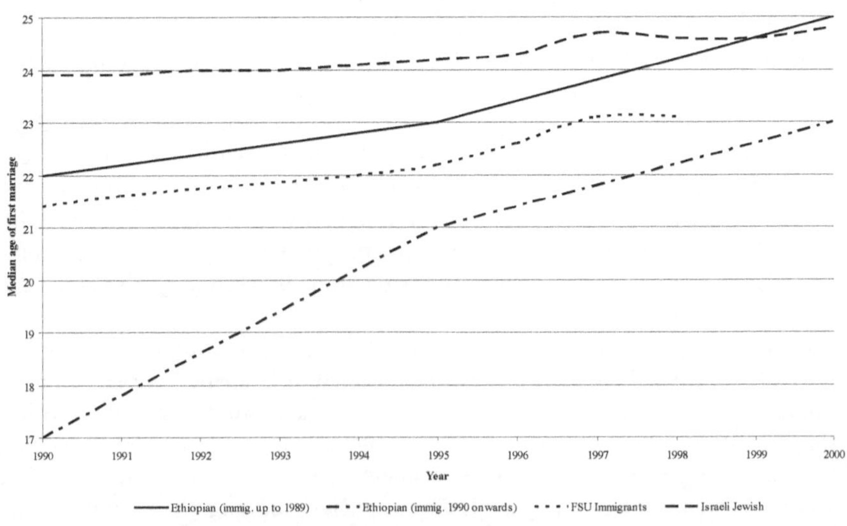

Figure 5.10
Abortion Ratios, Immigrants by Country of Birth, 1994-2001

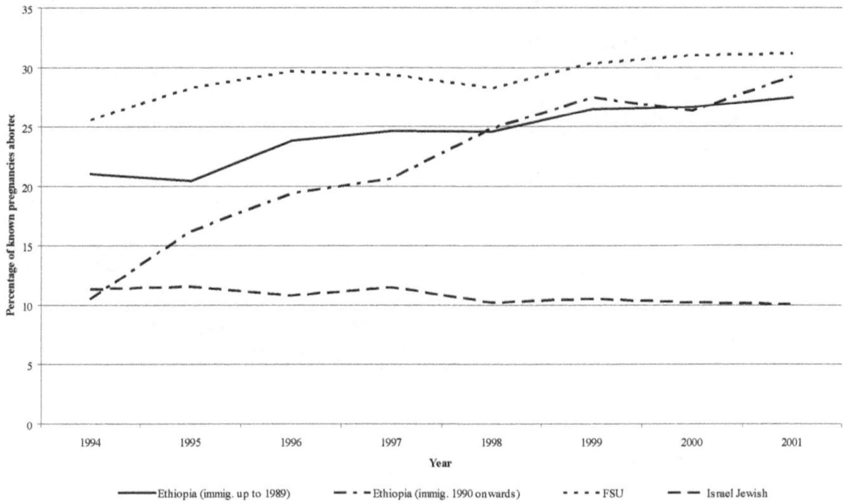

not include information on contraceptive use. However, we do have information on contraceptive use for women applying to pregnancy termination committees. Obviously women applying for pregnancy terminations are not representative of the whole population, and a higher representation of less reliable types of contraception is expected. Additionally, there are problems with the quality of responses to the questions on contraceptive use but, since information on contraceptive use is so sparse, it does at least allow us to compare respondents by their country of birth. Chi-square tests on use of contraceptives (whether contraceptives were used since the last period and which type of contraceptives) show no significant differences according to country of birth. In other words, there was no difference according to immigration group on the overall use of all kinds of contraceptives (both modem and traditional). Nonetheless, there are significant differences in the method mix amongst those reporting contraceptive use in 2001. Ethiopian applicants have high rates of Pill use (over 50 percent) and FSU applicants low usage rates (28.8 percent) compared with the Israel Jewish average (35.1 percent). Condom use for both FSU and Ethiopian applicants was lower than the Israel Jewish average (39.6 percent, 40.3 percent and 44.5 percent respectively). The I.D.D. was more popular amongst FSU immigrants (23.7 percent) than for Jewish women (10.8 percent) and its use was very low amongst Ethiopian women (less than 1 percent). Given that I.D.D. use is not user dependent, its failure rate tends to be low. Thus the fact that nearly a quarter of FSU applicants for an abortion reported I.D.D. use seems particularly high.

Figure 5.11
Abortion Ratios by Age, Immigrants by Country of Birth, 2001

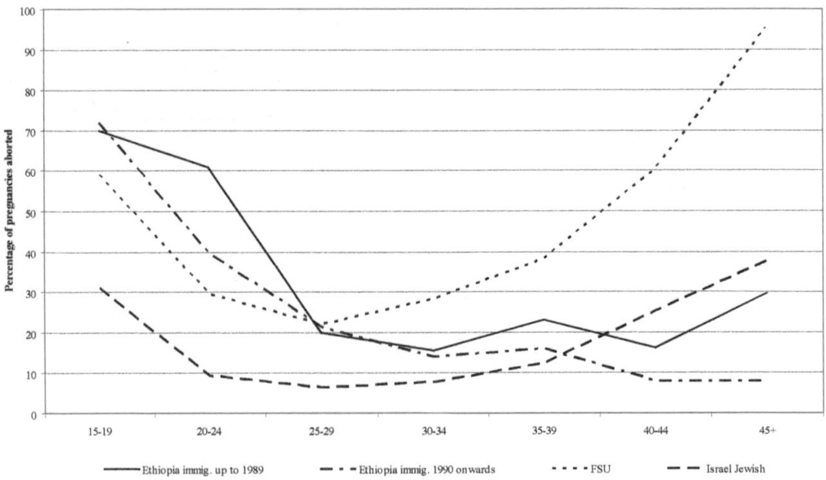

Discussion and Conclusions

Israel has an unusual fertility regime. On the one hand, it is a developed country with high levels of education and female labor force participation amongst secular Jewish women, but on the other hand fertility remains higher than countries of comparable status. The situation in Israel is unique since there are sub-populations with persistent high fertility cultures and there is also an emphasis on the demographic outcomes, in political and ethnic terms, of differences in fertility (Yishai 1978). Additionally, Israel is a reproductively paternalistic country with those in the establishment determining, to a large extent, what is correct reproductive behavior for women (Amir and Benjamin 1997). Within this framework, it is expected that Russian women cease using abortions as a means of birth control, now that they have the option of effective contraceptives and that Ethiopian women limit their family size to that prevalent in the absorbing society. Basker (1980) shows that the expected norm in Israel was (and is still maybe today) to have as many children as one could afford to have. In that context, Ethiopian women would be expected to reduce their fertility to a level that they could support in a modem economy.

As hypothesized, FSU immigrants are indeed increasing their fertility, although the increase is small and less than I would have predicted. However, there is no doubt that the age-fertility function has become much more similar to that of Israeli Jews. The decrease in the 15-19 age group is clearly seen. The changes in the age distribution of the births probably account for the lack of a clear trend in the TFR. I expect that in the future, as young women who

Figure 5.12
Percentage of Never-Married Women amongst Abortion Applicants, Immigrants by Country of Birth, 1991-2001

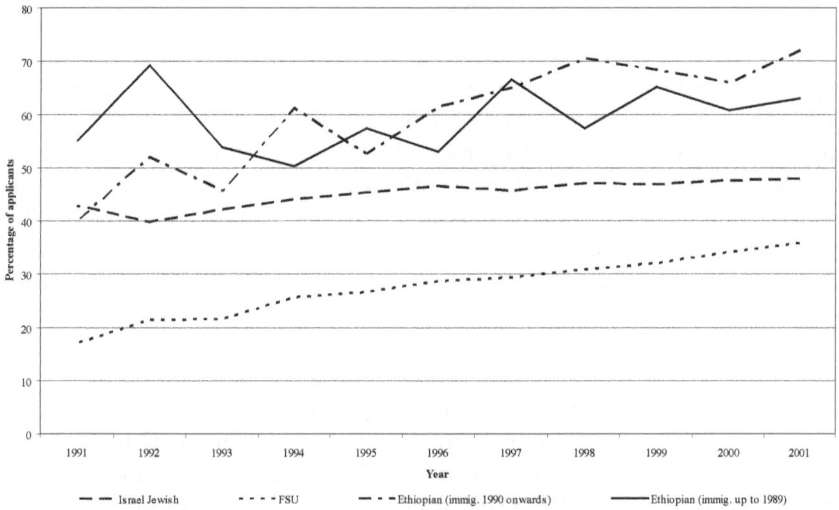

delayed childbearing enter the peak childbearing ages, there will be an increase in overall fertility.

The reasons for this increase in fertility are not immediately clear. The classic debate of culture as opposed to socio-economic conditions is apparent; but the two are not mutually exclusive, and the complex interacting reasons behind the increase in fertility are most likely a mixture of both cultural and socio-economic factors. In some ways the economic conditions in Israel allowed couples to have more children, assuming that the desire for more children existed previously and fertility was depressed due to the prevailing conditions in the FSU. For example, the shortage of housing in the FSU may have had a limiting effect on fertility rates, particularly in the big cities. However, many immigrants experienced a decrease in their relative standard of living and their status, which would probably lead to a desire to control fertility. It is unlikely that the child allowances (see appendix) in Israel had much effect on the fertility of FSU immigrants. The child allowances are graduated by parity of the child, with the percentage of the average net household income rising from less than 2 percent for the first child to 15 percent and above for the fourth and higher parity children. Since so few FSU families have four or more children, this is unlikely to provide an incentive. In 2001, only about 5 percent of FSU immigrants had four or more children, compared with 22.5 percent for Israeli Jewish mothers. Admittedly, there is an increase in higher parity births with time amongst FSU immigrants, but the increase is small. If anything, the child allowances would act as a support to the high fertility of the Ethiopian immigrants, both due to the larger families and also their relatively low income levels, which has not been the case.

The Israeli cultural milieu can contribute much to our understanding of the fertility changes of FSU immigrants. Higher fertility is both accepted and encouraged in Israel. Even amongst secular Jews, fertility rates are still above replacement level, with few one-child families. Much of the conflict in Israel is represented in demographic terms, with an emphasis on the need to increase the fertility of Jews in order to preserve the numerical majority. Additionally, Israel may be perceived as a more dangerous country, due to army service for young people and the threat of terrorist attacks. Thus parents may feel the need for an additional child to "insure" that their desired number reaches mature adulthood.

In contrast to the situation in the former USSR, abortion in Israel is a value laden process, with access controlled by committees effectively acting as gate keepers and determining, according to certain criteria, those who may abort their pregnancies (Basker 1980). Goldenberg and Saxe (1996) found that Russian immigrants to the U.S. remain much more pro-abortion than their American counterparts. Thus, there may be a conflict of values here with the Israeli establishment being anti-abortion but the Russian immigrants still holding on to pro-abortion views. Nonetheless, the data point to a marked decline in abortion rates amongst Russian women and in contrast to that predicted by Sabatello (1992). Based on a survey by Remennick et al. (1995) there has been a clear reduction in the use of all traditional methods of contraception, that is, withdrawal and rhythm method by FSU immigrants in Israel. Although there has been an increase in the use of condoms and oral pills, this has not been enough to account for the decrease in traditional methods. A much more positive attitude towards oral contraceptives has been noted amongst Russian immigrants. However, it is possible that sexual activity has decreased which may also partly account for the fact that overall contraceptive use has appeared to decrease (Remmenick 1995). This would also account for the extremely low known pregnancy rate (abortions and live births) amongst Russian immigrants, rather than illegal abortion being the main cause of the low rate.

The changes amongst Ethiopian immigrants are surprising, although the fact that the data are of poorer quality and the population smaller than immigrants from the FSU needs to be taken into account. A decrease in fertility is indeed being witnessed. This decrease is mainly accounted for by decreases in fertility at older ages, particularly forty and over. The proportional decrease in births amongst younger women is much less. As with FSU immigrants, the same issue of culture versus socio-economic conditions arises. However, in this case, the same environment is being used to explain a decrease in fertility. Ethiopian immigrants arrived from a rural, less developed country, where traditionally children have an important economic role to play. Obviously, within a developed urban economy, children are a net economic burden upon the parents until early adulthood and there is an emphasis on the future returns to investment in the education of children. Thus the economic incentive to reduce fertility exists. Additionally, infant and child mortality rates are low in Israel especially in comparison with Ethiopia (seven and 179 deaths of children under five per a thousand live births in Israel and Ethiopia, respectively (World Bank 2003)). Thus couples need to give birth to less children as "insurance" for death in early childhood. However, in addition to factors encouraging fertility decline, there are also incentives to preserve the high fertility rates. In the case of Ethiopian immigrants, where large families are common (in 2001, 45 percent of births to Ethiopian immigrants were parity four or greater), child allowances may provide a greater support to high fertility, than they do an incentive to FSU immigrants. Additionally, assuming that the prevailing cultural values in Israel are pro-natalistic, then we would expect further supports to the high fertility of Ethiopian immigrants. In fact, the opposite is true, with Ethiopian immigrants undergoing a rapid fertility decline. It is possible that, in the absence of the supports to high fertility, the fertility decline would be even faster.

It would appear that abortions are being increasingly relied upon as a form of pregnancy control, especially amongst younger Ethiopian women. The application rates for abortions are much higher than for veteran Jewish Israelis, and even higher than the FSU rates at all age groups but particularly amongst younger age groups. Young Ethiopian women may not possess the knowledge of, or access to, contraception especially considering their young age. Data shows that younger women (under nineteen) apply for abortions at significantly more advanced stages of pregnancy than older women. This is probably due to lack of awareness of the pregnancy or delay in applying for an abortion that results in more costly procedures with higher risks to the woman. This evidence points to deficient knowledge amongst younger women regarding sexual issues that seems to be exacerbated amongst young Ethiopian women. It must be remembered, however, that Ethiopian women arrived from a country with extremely low contraceptive prevalence, and even lower modem contraceptive usage (UNFPA 2001). Henshaw et al. (1999) point out that it is common during periods of rapid fertility decline for populations to increase their use of abortion and contraceptives to meet the desire for smaller families and to time births more exactly. Thus, for a substantial period of time, as fertility is declining, both the abortion rate and contraceptive prevalence may increase. This would indeed seem to be the case with immigrants from Ethiopia. Fertility is rapidly declining and this can be accounted for by both increasing abortion rates, but accompanied also by increasing use of contraceptives. Ethiopian immigrants are turning to abortion to regulate fertility, most likely in conjunction with contraceptive use. The declining fertility indicates an adaptation to the prevailing fertility regime in Israel with the Ethiopian immigrant population undergoing a transition from natural to controlled fertility. Many populations are thought to pass through a period of increased recourse to abortion during their demographic transition (Kulczychi 1999:7). This same trend was also witnessed in the decline to below-replacement fertility in Addis Ababa, in conditions where abortion is less accessible and more risky than in Israel (Ashagrea 2002) and in the transition of immigrants from Asia and Africa in the 1950s and 1960s (Friedlander et al. 1980). It is most likely that with increased contraceptive use, the abortion rate will eventually decline as witnessed in other populations that underwent a rapid fertility decline such as in South Korea. Taking the fertility and abortion rates of young Ethiopian women together, the known pregnancy rate is elevated, indicating a high level of sexual ignorance amongst young women.

Overall, both immigrant groups are undergoing significant changes in their fertility behavior. Russian immigrants are indeed behaving as would be expected in the hypothesis. Their fertility is increasing towards the Israeli norm, especially if one takes the Jewish secular fertility rate as the standard and not the average rate. On the other hand, the abortion rate is surprisingly low. This could indeed be a result of decreased sexual activity or the increased use of modern contraceptives. Migration is a traumatic event and the change in living conditions, the difficulties of adjustment, and even the drop in status and/or prestige, could all lead to a decrease in sexual activity. On the other hand, there is also the question of the extent of illegal abortions. Although this phenomenon is known to exist, by its very clandestine nature it is very difficult to estimate. Therefore it is impossible to tell whether the sharp decrease in legal abortions is due to a true decrease in abortion rates or the use of illegal abortions. The increased use of abortion by Ethiopians was predicted but the increase far exceeded expectations. However, this does concord with the experiences of other populations undergoing a rapid fertility decline. Finally, the fertility of Ethiopian immigrants is decreasing as expected. That being said, the age specific analysis shows that the majority of this decrease is accounted for by decreasing fertility amongst older age groups with the fertility of younger age groups high.

To conclude, the fertility of immigrants is changing towards the Israeli Jewish norm, although it is currently in a state of flux and it will still take some time until rates stabilize and converge with Israeli Jewish rates (if at all). Immigrants from the FSU seem to be fast approaching Israeli Jewish norms with increasing fertility rates at older ages and postponement of childbearing until older ages. This is being achieved by postponement of marriage and despite decreasing abortion rates. The fertility of Ethiopian immigrants is declining rapidly towards the Israeli Jewish norm. Although abortion rates are higher than expected, it is likely that the abortion rate will decline in the future as contraceptive use increases and the fertility rate stabilizes. It is important to emphasize that the fertility changes are not yet complete and are still ongoing. Due to the continuing changes in the fertility rates and in the proximate determinants, it is important to keep track of the changes in order to categorically determine whether the immigrants have indeed adopted the fertility patterns of the absorbing society.

Appendix: National Insurance Child Allowances

The table below shows the national insurance payments according to number of children in Israel. It should be noted that these payments have undergone a number of changes during the 1990s, although they have been fairly stable since 1992 until recently. Between 1989 and 1992 child allowances for the first two children were cancelled unless a family had at least three children. The allowances were reinstated in 1992, regardless of size. However, the graduated increase in the allowance for each child with increasing number of children remained. Only recently, with the economic downturn, have child allowances been cut, particularly those for larger families. Considering that the average monthly household income (from all sources) was nearly $2,000 in 2000, the child allowance represents a large percentage of household income, particularly for families in the lower income deciles (Central Bureau of Statistics 2001). For example, the child allowances represented more than 100 percent of the average household income of a six child or more family in the bottom three income deciles.

Table A.1
National Insurance Child Allowances, by Number of Children, 2000

Number of children	Child Allowance (US$) per month	Percent of average monthly net household income
1	36.5	1.8
2	73.0	3.6
3	145.3	7.3
4	292.0	14.8
5	473.1	23.9
6	654.2	33.1
Each additional child	181.1	9.2

Source: National Insurance Institute (2003), Central Bureau of Statistics [Israel], (2001)

Notes

1. The majority of Jews in Ethiopia lived in the Gonder and Tigray regions of Northwest Ethiopia (Hobart 1995).
2. The population group Jews and Others includes Jews, non-Arab Christians and those not classified by religion and the population group Arabs includes Moslems, Arab Christians, Druze, and Lebanese citizens who arrived in Israel in May 2000.
3. Both Basker (1980) and Portuguese (1998:125) have noted the difficulty in obtaining official statistics on the contraceptive use in Israel.
4. Unfortunately, the population data available do not allow a breakdown of the Ethiopian immigrants by year of immigration prior to 1996.

References

Abbasi-Shavazi, M.J., and P. MacDonald. 2000. "Fertility and multiculturalism: Immigrants fertility in Australia, 1977-1991." *International Migration Review* 2000 34: 215-242.

Agadjanian, V., and Z. C. Qian. 1997. "Ethnocultural identity and induced abortion in Kazakhstan." *Studies in Family Planning* 28(4):317-328.

Amir, D., and O. Benjamin. 1997. "Defining encounters: Who are the women entitled to join the Israeli collective?" *Women's Studies International Forum* 20: 639-650.

Amir, D., L. Remmenick and Y. Elimelech. 1997. "Educating Lena: Women immigrants and 'integration' policies in Israel - The politics of reproduction and family planning." In N. Lewin-Epstein, R. Yaacov and P. Ritterband (eds.), *Russian Jews on Three Continents*, 495-509. London: Frank Cass.

Ashagrea, Y. K. 2002. "The quiet revolution: An analysis of the change towards below-replacement fertility in Addis Ababa." Ph.D. thesis, Australia National University. http://thesis.anu.edu.au/uploads/approved/adt-ANU20011218.163822 /public/02whole.pdf (accessed 12/3/02).

Basker, E. 1980. "Belief systems, cultural milieu and reproductive behvaiour: Women seeking abortions in a hospital in Israel." Ph.D. thesis, Hebrew University of Jerusalem, Jerusalem.

Basker, E. 1986. "The 'natural' control of fertility." *Sociology of Health and Illness* 8: 3-25.

Bystydzienski, J. M. 1989. "Women and socialism: A comparative study of women in Poland and the USSR." *Signs* 14: 668-684.

Central Bureau of Statistics, 2001 "Statistical Abstract of Israel, 2000" Jerusalem: Central Bureau of Statistics.

Demographic and Health Surveys. 2002. "Survey indicators STAT compiler—Ethiopia 2000." www.measuredhs.com/data/indicators (accessed 1/7/2002).

Dinkel, R.H., and U.H. Lebok. 1997. "The fertility of migrants before and after crossing the border." *International Migration* 35: 253-270.

Feyera, T. Year unknown. "Ethiopia one stop center for young people." International Council on Management of Population Programmes - Adolescent Reproductive Health www.icomp.org.my/Arh/pmgr4/pm4_ethi02.htm (accessed 9/7/02).

Friedlander, D., and C. Goldscheider. 1978. "Immigration, social change and cohort fertility in Israel." *Population Studies* 32: 299-317.

Friedlander, D., Z. Eisenbach and C. Goldscheider. 1980. "Family-size limitation and birth spacing: The fertility transition of African and Asian immigrants in Israel." *Population and Development Review* 6: 581-593.

Goldenberg, V., and L. Saxe. 1996. "Social attitudes of Russian immigrants to the United States." *Journal of Social Psychology* 136: 451-434.

Henshaw, S. K., S. Singh and T. Hass. 1999. "Recent trends in abortion rates worldwide." *International Family Planning Perspectives* 25: 44-48.

Hobart, G. T. 1995. "The evolution of Ethiopian Jews: A history of the Beta Israel (Falasha) to 1920." www.sistahspace.com/jewish/evolu.html (accessed 10/8/02).

Imbrogno, S., and N. L. Imbogno. 1989. "Soviet women and the autonomous family." *International Journal of Sociology of the Family* 19: 1-20.

Jones, H. 1990. *Population Geography*, 2nd ed. London: Chapman Publishing.

Kebede, T. 2001. "Teens pay the deadly price of religious taboo." In Panos Institute, London, Features, July 2001. www.panos.org.uk/news/July2001/Ethiopiayouth.htm (accessed 8/7/02).

Kingkade, W. 1997. "Population Trends: Russia." United States Bureau of the Census. http://www.census.gov/ipc/prod/ib96-2.pdf (accessed 2/2/03).

Kohler, H., and I. Kohler. 2002. "Fertility decline in Russia in the early and mid-1990s: The role of economic uncertainty and labour market crises." *European Journal of Population* 18: 223-262.
Kostantinov, V. 1991. "Jewish population of the USSR on the eve of the great exodus." *Jews and Jewish Topics in the Soviet Union and Eastern Europe* 3 (16): 5-23.
Kulczychi, A. 1999. *The Abortion Debate in the World Arena*. New York: Routledge.
Mammo, A., and S. P. Morgan. 1986. "Childlessness in rural Ethiopia." *Population and Development Review* 12: 533-546.
Micevska, M. B. 2002. "Marriage, uncertainty and risk aversion in Russia." Paper presented at VII Spring Meeting of Young Economists. http://smye2002.univ-parisl.fr/program/paper/ c6 _mic. pdf (accessed 2/2/03).
National Insurance Institute. 2003. "Child insurance." www.bt1.gov.il (accessed 2/2/03).
Okun, B. 1997. "Family planning in the Jewish population of Israel: Correlates of withdrawal use." *Studies in Family Planning* 28: 215-227.
Paltiel, A. M., E. F. Sabatello and D. Tal. 1997. "Immigrants from the former USSR in Israel in the 1990s: Demographic characteristics and socio-economic absorption." In N. Lewin-Epstein, R. Yaacov and P. Ritterband (eds.), *Russian Jews on Three Continents*, 284-321. London: Frank Cass.
Popov, A. 1991. "Family planning and induced abortion in the USSR: Basic health and demographic characteristics." *Studies in Family Planning* 22: 368-377.
Popov, A. 1996. "Family planning and induced abortion in post-Soviet Russia of the early 1990s: Unmet needs in information supply." In J. DaVanzo (ed.), *Russia's Demographic "Crisis"*. Santa Monica, CA: RAND. www.rand.org/pubs/conf_proceedings/CF124/CF124.chap3.html (accessed 1/7/02).
Population Reference Bureau. 2001. "World population datasheet." www.prb.org (accessed 1/7/02).
Remmenick, L. 1993. "Patterns of birth control." in I. Kon and I. Riordan (eds.), *Sex and Russian Society*. Bloomington, IN: Indiana University Press.
Remmenick, L., D. Amir, Y. Elimelech and Y. Novikov. 1995. "Family planning practices and attitudes among former Soviet new immigrant women in Israel." *Social Science and Medicine* 41: 569-577.
Sabatello, E., and N. Yaffe. 1988. "Israel." in Paul Sachdev (ed.), *International Handbook on Abortion*. Westport, CT: Greenwood Press.
Sabatello, E. F. 1992. "Immigration from the former Soviet Union - How many additional abortions in the 1990s?" In *Health and Women in Israel*, 87-95. Jerusalem: Women's Lobby in Israel (in Hebrew).
Sabatello, E. F. 1995. "Continuity and change in reproductive and abortion patterns of Soviet immigrants in Israel." *Social Science and Medicine* 40: 117 -124.
Scherbov, S., and H. van Vianen. 2002. "Period fertility in Russia since 1930: An application of the Coale-Trussel fertility model." *Demographic Research* 6 (16). www.demographic-research.org (accessed 10/6/02).
Schoenmaeckers, R.C., E. Lodewijckx and S. Gadeyne. 1999. "Marriages and fertility among Turkish and Moroccan women in Belgium: Results from census data." *International Migration Review* 33: 901-928.
Tolts, M. 1997. "The interrelationship between emigration and the sociodemographic profile of Russian Jewry." In Noah Lewin-Epstein, Ro'i Yaacov and Paul Ritterband (eds.), *Russian Jews on Three Continents*, 147-176. London: Frank Cass.
United Nations. 1999. "Abortion policy: A global review." www.un.org/esa/population/publications/abortion (accessed 1/7/02).
Weinstein, B. 1985. "Ethiopian Jews in Israel: Socialization and re-education." *Journal of Negro Education* 54: 213-224.

World Bank. 2003. "World development indicators - Data query." http://www. worldbank. org/data/dataquery.html (accessed 1/4/03).

Yisia, Y. 1978. "Abortion in Israel: Social demand and political responses." *Policy Studies Journal* 7: 270-290.

Zakharov, S. V., and E. I. Ivanova. 1996. "Fertility decline and recent changes in Russia: On the threshold of the Second Demographic Transition." In J. DaVanzo (ed.), *Russia's Demographic "Crisis"*. Santa Monica, Calif.: RAND. www.rand.org/pubs/conf_proceedings/CF124/CF124.chap2.html (accessed 1/7/02).

Zbarskaya, I. 2001. "Child and family welfare in Russia: Trends and indicators." UNICEF background paper prepared for the Regional Monitoring Report No.8, *A Decade of Transition*. www.unicef-icdc.org/research/ESP/CountryReports2000_01/Russia00.pdf (accessed 2/2/03).

6

The Predecline Rise in Israeli Muslim Fertility

Jona Schellekens and Zvi Eisenbach

In the classical description of the "demographic transition," mortality decline precedes fertility decline, thus causing a period of increased population growth until fertility starts to decline as well. This classical portrayal of the demographic transition does not seem to be accurate for many countries. Often, a rise in fertility contributed to population growth in the early stages of the demographic transition, in addition to the contribution of mortality decline (Dyson and Murphy 1985). There are very few case studies of predecline rises in fertility. Usually, fertility studies focus on decline, although "a better appreciation of the changes that trigger such rises may enhance our understanding of the causes and timing of subsequent declines" (Dyson and Murphy 1985).

One of the largest predecline rises in fertility occurred among Israeli Muslims, from approximately 6.5 births among women born before 1900 to 8.5 births among women born in the 1920s and early 1930s. This rise culminated in a total fertility rate of well over nine births per woman during the 1960s.[1] In the early 1970s, the total fertility rate started to decline, reaching a level of 4.7 by the late 1980s. The major aim of this study is to try to explain this extraordinary rise. Improving social and economic conditions are usually associated with fertility decline. This study will try to show that this is not necessarily always the case.

Previous descriptions of the predecline rise were based on an incomplete series of period fertility measures (Bachi 1977). We used a continuous series of cohort fertility measures that suggest that the predecline rise started in the 1920s or 1930s. This would suggest that it was somehow related to the unprecedented economic growth that was recorded during the first fifteen years of the British Mandate. Jacob Metzer (1992), estimated that Arab income per capita in Palestine grew 4.4 percent annually between 1922 and 1935. The results of our analyses of a fertility survey and of the 1972 census are consistent with the hypothesis that a rise in income, as measured by male education, was responsible for the decline in breast-feeding to a considerable extent. This rise in income probably affected breast-feeding through the availability of breast milk substitutes and the parents' ability to acquire them.

Determinants of Rises in Fertility

Tim Dyson and Mike Murphy address four "proximate" determinants that seem especially important in the context of predecline increases: marriage patterns, breast-feeding, postpartum sexual abstinence, and disease-related sterility.[2] In Latin America, predecline increases seem to have resulted from a marriage surge at younger ages combined with increased marriage at later ages as a result of a decline in widowhood. In sub-Saharan Africa, declines in postpartum abstinence, breast-feeding, and the prevalence of venereal disease seem the most likely factors. In the rest of the developing world, predecline rises appear to have been comparatively limited. In most of these countries, early and universal marriage precluded a marriage surge at younger ages. However, the "widowhood effect" may apply in these countries. There also have been significant declines in breast-feeding in some parts of the Middle East and the Far East (Dyson and Murphy 1985: 427).[3] Thus, the "proximate" determinants responsible for predecline rises in fertility vary from region to region.

Much less is known about the "ultimate" determinants of predecline rises in fertility. To what extent did fertility rise as a result of improving social and economic conditions? Of course, when improving social and economic conditions cause fertility to rise, they must do so through the four "proximate" determinants mentioned above.[4] Perhaps the predecline rise that has received more scholarly attention than any other occurred in eighteenth-century England. This rise was due to a marriage surge at younger ages. There is evidence that connects the rise with the first Industrial Revolution (Schellekens 1997). However, the English experience may not be representative of similar rises in today's developing countries. The marriage surge at younger ages in Latin America may reflect improved economic conditions. Declines in widowhood are, of course, the result of mortality decline, which, in turn, is the result of improved economic conditions and/or the spread of medical technology. Disease-related sterility may also decline with the spread of medical technology. Finally, improved economic conditions probably influence breast-feeding through the availability of breast milk substitutes and the parents' ability to acquire them.

Data

In 1948, after Israeli independence, most of the Arab population of Palestine was scattered over several countries. A minority, mostly Muslims, remained in Israel. Pre-1948 data sets do not enable us to identify those who were to become

Israeli Muslims. However, as we will try to show below, Israeli Muslims do not seem to have differed very much from other Muslims in the former Mandate of Palestine. Hence, we will also use statistics from the Mandate to present our case. There was no predecline fertility rise among Israeli Christians. Therefore, this Arab subpopulation has been omitted from the analysis.

The first census in the British Mandate of Palestine was conducted in 1922. This census, however, does not enable us to estimate Muslim fertility. Vital registration started in the same year. The 1931 census of Palestine (Mills 1933), is the first to report marital status by age and religious group. Indirect estimates of fertility may be derived from the census and vital registration data (see appendix).

Reliable vital statistics for Israeli Muslims begin in 1954. We have made extensive use of the 1972 census because it is the first census to cover the whole predecline rise in fertility. The 1961 census should have been useful to measure fertility levels among early cohorts. Unfortunately, the exact number of children ever born is not available from this census in machine-readable form for women who gave birth to more than eight children. The 1983 census has not been used since a comparison of its retrospective fertility data with that of vital registration data suggests problems of selectivity and undercounting that seem to be more serious than those in the 1972 census. Census statistics are presented by birth cohort. It should be noted, however, that among older women age overstatement occurs to an unknown extent.

Finally, we used a detailed fertility survey carried out by the Department of Demography of the Hebrew University during 1974-1975. Approximately 3,000 Israeli Arab women were sampled, about 2,300 of who were Muslims. The sample included women who at the time of the survey were under age fifty-five and currently married in their first marriage. Bedouin women and women living in East Jerusalem were excluded. The women were asked about their birth

Table 1
Total Fertility Rate among Israeli Muslims

Year	Total Fertility Rate
1954	7.53
1955-59	8.17
1960-64	9.23
1965-69	9.22
1970-74	8.47
1975-79	7.25
1980-84	5.54
1985-89	4.70
1990-94	4.67

histories, use of family planning, socioeconomic characteristics, and other topics thought to be relevant to reproductive behavior (Eisenbach, 1978).

Fertility Trends

When did the predecline rise in fertility start? In 1954, when official Israeli figures become available, the total fertility rate (TFR) among Muslims in Israel was already above 7.5 per woman (table 6.1). Total fertility rate reached its highest levels in the 1960s. Total fertility rate measured about 9.2 during this period, with a maximum of 9.9 in 1965 (Central Bureau of Statistics 1996; Coale et al. 1975).

Cohort fertility never reached such a high level. The published age-specific fertility rates can be used to reconstruct cohort fertility trends (table 6.2). Women born in the 1930s had about 8.6 births. This figure is very close to that obtained from the 1972 census for women born in the 1920s (table 6.3). This cohort had more than 8.5 births. Thus it would seem that cohort fertility reached a peak of about 8.5 births among women who were born in the 1920s and 1930s.

To trace the beginnings of the rise, we computed completed fertility by birth cohort from the 1972 census (see table 6.3). These data suggest a prerise fertility level of between six and 6.5 births per woman. Table 6.3 suggests a sudden rise among women born after 1900 and, hence, that period fertility did not start to rise before the 1920s or before the British Mandate (figure 6.1). This is not inconsistent with the time of the beginning of the rise implied by Bachi's period fertility measures, if one allows for a certain degree of age overstatement in the cohort data. However, the steepness of the rise suggested by his estimates is not consistent with the cohort data (see appendix for a discussion of Bachi's estimates).

Of course, the fertility estimates for the earliest cohorts may be too low because the number of births in the 1972 census may have been underreported. Older women may have forgotten some children, in particular, those who died early. In any case, it would seem unlikely that the number of births exceeded seven before the rise.[5] Hence, we need to account for a rise in cohort fertility of 1.5 to two births.

Table 2
Total Fertility Rate for Selected Birth Cohorts

Year	Total Fertility Rate
1930	8.6
1935	8.6
1940	8.0
1945	7.2

Note: In order to compute the total fertility fate for the first two cohorts, we assumed that age-specific fertility rates below age 25 before 1955 were equal to those in 1955-59.

Table 3
Children Ever Born by Birth Cohort

Birth Cohort	Children Ever Born	Number of Cases
1875 – 84	6.18	45
1885 – 89	6.42	89
1890 – 94	6.48	100
1895 – 99	6.17	180
1900 – 1904	7.22	313
1905 – 9	7.37	454
1910 – 1914	7.89	492
1915 – 19	7.95	556
1920 – 24	8.56	771
1925 – 27	8.52	458

Source: –1972 census.

Israeli Muslims constitute only one of several groups that formerly made up the Muslim population of Mandate of Palestine. To what extent is the predecline rise a phenomenon shared by all the groups that made up the Muslim population of Palestine? A comparison with data published from the 1967 census in the West Bank and Gaza Strip suggests that the rise was shared by other groups as well. The number of children ever born in the 1913-1917 birth cohort in the West Bank and Gaza Strip was 7.9, while that in the 1918-1922 birth cohort was 8.3 (Central Bureau of Statistics 1968).[6] The latter is a lower bound because not all of the women in this cohort had finished their childbearing period and there may also be some recall errors. About 95 percent of the women in both

Figure 6.1
Total Fertility by Birth Cohort

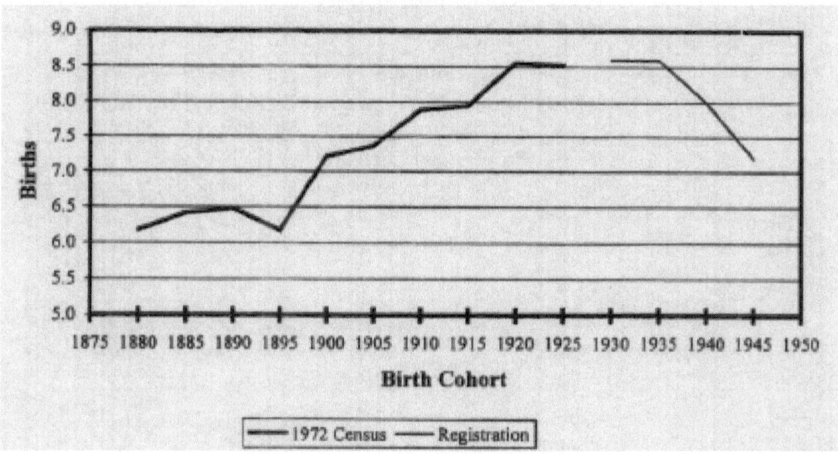

cohorts are Muslims. Despite all these reservations, the number of children ever born in these two birth cohorts resembles that in the 1915-1919 and 1920-1924 cohorts of Israeli Muslims rather closely (see table 6.3). This suggests that the predecline rise was a phenomenon common to most sections of the Muslim population of Palestine.[7]

Proximate Determinants of the Predecline Rise in Fertility

Previous research suggests two variables as the most likely proximate determinants responsible for a predecline rise: nuptiality and postpartum infecundability (Bongaarts and Potter 1983).

Nuptiality

Nuptiality may raise fertility in several ways. Age at first marriage may decline or proportions married at later ages may rise. Life expectancy at birth rose from an estimated 37.5 among Muslims in Palestine in 1926-1930 to over seventy years among the remaining Muslim population in Israel in 1960-1964 (Freidlander and Goldscheider 1979). A decline in mortality would imply a decline in widowhood and, hence, a rise in the proportions of currently married women at later ages, assuming that remarriage rates of widows did not change much over time (Eisenbach 1978).

Table 4 presents proportions currently married among Palestinian Muslims in 1931 and Israeli Muslims in 1961.[8] This table suggests that female age at first marriage among Israeli Muslims in 1961 is higher than that among Palestinian Muslims, while widowhood is lower.

We used J. Bongaarts's aggregate fertility model to evaluate the potential effect of changes in nuptiality on the total fertility rate. Bongaarts's index of marriage, C_m, is the weighted average of the age-specific proportions of females currently married, with the weights provided by age-specific marital fertility rates (Bongaarts and Potter 1983). Bongaarts's index of marriage, C_m, is .75 for

Table 6.4
Proportions Currently Married by Age and Marital Fertility Rates

	Proportions Currently Married		Marital Fertility Rates
Age Group	1931	1961	1961
15 – 19	33.7	16.5	531
20 – 24	76.6	72.8	490
25 – 29	90.0	88.9	467
30 – 34	91.8	93.0	394
35 – 39	89.3	91.3	332
40 – 44	80.2	85.2	151
45 – 49	71.0	81.6	84

1961 (Knodel and Wilson 1981).[9] If marital fertility rates in 1931 would have been equal to those in 1961, then C_m would have been .79. Apparently, a rise in age at first marriage more than compensates for the decline in widowhood. To explain the rise in fertility, the index of marriage would have had to rise. Clearly, nuptiality is unlikely to explain the predecline rise in fertility. This leaves postpartum infecundability as the most likely proximate determinant responsible for the rise.

Postpartum Infecundability

Table 6.5 presents, by decade, the average length of birth intervals that open with the birth of a child that survived infancy. Depending on the interval, the length of birth intervals declined from the 1940s to the 1960s by 3.4 to 5.6 months. The most likely explanation is a similar decline in the length of the postpartum period of infecundability. We estimated the length of the postpartum period of infecundability in the 1960s from the 1974 fertility survey using a simple method described by J. Knodel and C. Wilson (1981). We compared the interval between marriage and first birth with the subsequent interval between first and second births.

Marriage cohorts before 1965 reported very little use of contraceptive methods before the third birth interval (2 percent or less). Hence, the difference between the first two birth intervals should reflect the extent to which the second birth interval is extended by nonsusceptibility. We excluded all women who reported having lost their first child and those cases in which the first or second intervals were reported to have been less than seven or more than sixty months.[10]

Table 6.5
Average Length of Birth Intervals That Open with the Birth of a Child Who Survived Infancy by Period

	Interval			
Period	2	3	4	5
1940 – 49:				
Length	24.9	25.4	26.7	28.1
Number of cases	183	137	88	46
1950 – 59:				
Length	22.4	23.8	25.5	24.7
Number of cases	424	366	334	277
1960 – 69:				
Length	20..2	22.0	22.2	22.5
Number of cases	591	573	550	523

Note: –Only includes intervals up to 60 months. The period of the interval is determined by the timing of the birth that precedes the index birth.

The estimate for the length of the postpartum infecundable period for the 1930s birth cohort, which is based on 253 cases, is rather short: between two and 2.5 months. Of course, this is only a rough estimate. Nevertheless, this implies that very little breast-feeding occurred in the 1960s.

Unfortunately, no estimate could be obtained for women who were born before 1900. We did obtain an estimate of ten months for the 1930s marriage cohort, but the sample is too small—thirteen cases—and this estimate should therefore be treated with caution. A postpartum infecundable period of ten months is not high for a historical society characterized by a low frequency of wet-nursing (Bongaarts and Potter 1983). Hence, the postpartum infecundable period before the 1920s may have been even longer.

Using the rough estimates for the length of the postpartum infecundable period for the 1930s birth cohort, we computed Bongaarts's index of postpartum infecundability, C_i. The index is .95, which is much higher than any of the indices for other contemporary Arab populations, although it is surpassed by certain subpopulations, such as Syrian women who had some schooling (Hill 1981; Singh et al. 1985). On the other hand, our estimate for the 1930s marriage cohort, .70, is within the range of values for Arab populations in the 1970s. If Bongaarts's index of postpartum infecundability, C_i, would have been .70 instead of .95 among women born in the 1930s, then their fertility would have been only 6.3 births per woman. Thus, a change in breast-feeding patterns could account for much of the predecline rise in fertility.

Causes of the Decline in Breast-Feeding

Moni Nag (1983) proposed that the duration and intensity of breast-feeding depend on three main factors: 1) the perception of parents and the community of what benefits a child, 2) the availability of breast milk substitutes and the parents' ability to acquire them, and 3) the convenience of breast-feeding for the mother. Nag adds that the convenience of breast-feeding depends largely on the nature and location of the work mothers do. We were unable to measure any of these "proximate determinants" of the incidence and duration of breastfeeding. However, the first factor, parents' perception of what benefits a child, is not a persuasive possibility since we are probably dealing with a decline in breast-feeding.

Urbanization and a rise in income and in maternal education are often mentioned as factors that may affect the incidence and duration of breastfeeding through changes in the availability of breast milk substitutes and the convenience of breast-feeding (Huffman 1984). Urban residence and income are more likely to influence the availability of substitutes and the parents' ability to acquire them, while a rise in maternal education is more likely to influence the nature and location of work mothers do and, hence, the convenience of breast-feeding to the mother.

In a population that rarely uses contraceptive methods, changes in the length of the second birth interval are mostly determined by changes in breastfeeding

(Bongaarts and Potter 1983). We used data from the 1974-1975 fertility survey to fit a proportional hazard model to the length of the second birth interval. In the analysis, we controlled for the length of the first interval—a proxy for coital frequency. Socioeconomic variables in the analysis include a variable indicating whether the husband is literate (a rough proxy for income), a variable indicating whether the woman is literate, a variable indicating whether the family is urban (at the time of the survey), and several dummy variables indicating the birth cohort of the woman. The women in the survey were divided into five five-year cohorts starting in 1920. Thus, we are able to analyze changes in the length of the second interval from the 1940s through the 1960s approximately. We excluded those cases in which the first child died before its second birthday and cases in which first or second intervals were reported to have been less than seven or more than sixty months.[11]

The first model in table 6.6 presents the second interval as a function of education and urban residence. Maternal literacy has the strongest effect on

Table 6.6
Event History Analyses of the Second Birth Interval

	Model 1			Model 2		
	b	*p* Value	Risk Ratio	*b*	*p* Value	Risk Ratio
First interval	–.004	.18	1.00	–.002	.56	1.00
Urban residence	–.191	.01	.83	–.171	.02	.84
Father's literacy	.044	.63	1.05	–.011	.90	.99
Mother's literacy	.322	.00	1.38	.234	.00	1.26
Macro variable	...	...	...	2.591	.00	13.34

	Model 3			Model 4		
	b	*p* Value	Risk Ratio	*b*	*p* Value	Risk Ratio
First interval	...	...	...	–.002	.55	1.00
Urban residence	...	...	...	–.169	.02	.84
Father's literacy	...	...	...	.001	.99	1.00
Mother's literacy				.218	.01	1.24
Macro variable						
Birth cohort:						
1920–24*						
1925–29	.056	.74	1.06	.045	.79	1.05
1930–34	.177	.25	1.19	.170	.28	1.19
1935–39	.332	.02	1.39	.309	.04	1.36
1940–44	.530	.00	1.70	.450	.00	1.57
Number of women				843		

*Omitted category.

the length of the second interval, followed by that of urban residence. Maternal literacy has a positive effect on the hazard rate and, hence, a negative effect on the length of the second interval. Surprisingly, urban residence has a positive effect on the length of the second interval. The husband's literacy, our proxy for income, does not have a significant effect on the length of the second birth interval.

To what extent are maternal literacy and urban residence able to explain the decline in the length of the second birth interval? One way to check this is to compare a model with cohort dummy variables (model 3 in table 6.6) with a model that also includes the three socioeconomic variables mentioned above (model 4). A comparison of these models shows that the inclusion of the socioeconomic variables in the model causes the risk ratio for the last cohort to decline from 1.70 to 1.57, mostly owing to maternal literacy. Thus, it would seem that a rise in maternal literacy only partially accounts for the decline in breast-feeding.

Male literacy at the individual level may be a poor proxy for living standards in a fast-growing agricultural economy. Therefore, we experimented with macroindicators. Presumably, the rise in living standards raised the number of male children who received any education. Hence, at about the same time as living standards are thought to have influenced the reproductive history of women starting between age fifteen and twenty, they probably also influenced the education of boys between age five and ten. Accordingly, the second model in table 6.6 includes the percentage of literate men in the 1972 census in birth cohorts that are ten years younger then the cohort to which the woman belongs.

This macroindicator has a very significant negative effect on the length of the second interval. Table 6.7 presents risk ratios by birth cohort for the second model in table 6.6 as implied by the level of the macroindicator for each birth cohort. A comparison with those for model 4 suggests that the percentage of literate men, our proxy for income, is able to account for much of the change, although at a different pace.

Table 6.7
Risk Ratios by Women's Birth Cohort and Male Literacy by Men's Cohort

WOMEN'S COHORT	NUMBER OF WOMEN	RISK RATIO Model 2	RISK RATIO Model 4	MEN'S COHORT	MALE LITERACY
1920 – 24*	60	1.00	1.00	1930 – 34	73.1
1925 – 29	93	1.20	1.05	1935 – 39	80.0
1930 – 34	147	1.29	1.19	1940 – 44	83.0
1935 – 39	234	1.53	1.36	1945 – 49	89.4
1940 – 44	309	1.65	1.57	1950 – 54	92.4

Source:–The literacy data were taken from the 1972 census.

The survey only dates back to the birth cohort of the 1920s. To what extent is a rise in living standards as measured by male literacy able to account for the decline in breast-feeding among earlier cohorts? We found further support for the hypothesis that a rise in income accounts for part of the rise in fertility in the census. Figure 6.2 compares the trend in the percentage of literate men with that in cohort fertility among women who were about ten years older (see table 6.8 for data). This figure suggests that a rise in income, as measured by male literacy, may well have influenced the decline in breastfeeding. Of course, fertility cannot rise indefinitely. Thus, male literacy continued its rise after fertility had reached a ceiling.

These results are consistent with the hypothesis that a rise in income caused the decline in breast-feeding through the availability of breast milk substitutes and the parents' ability to acquire them. However, the rise in maternal education starting with the birth cohorts of the late 1920s may have contributed at a later stage, perhaps through the convenience of breast-feeding to the mother (see table 6.8).

Conclusion and Discussion

Often, predecline rises in fertility are of short duration and, hence, difficult to observe. Moreover, many predecline rises probably started before the period covered by World Fertility Survey and Demographic and Health Survey data, as is the case in most countries in Middle East. Hence, the importance of an Israeli Arab case study.

The census data seem to suggest that Israeli Muslim women who were born before 1900 had between six and seven births, on average. Cohort fertility reached a high of 8.5 births among women born in the 1920s and 1930s. Thus,

Figure 2
Children ever Born (CEB), and Male and Female Literacy

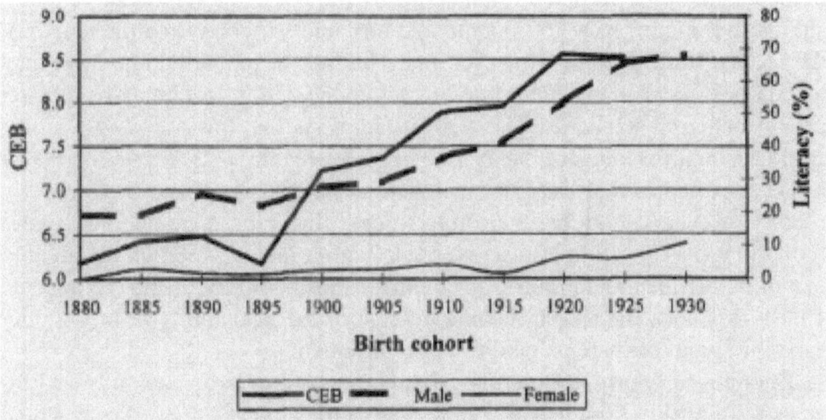

Table 6.8
Percentage of Literature Men and Women by Birth Cohort

BIRTH COHORT	MALES		FEMALES	
	Percentage	Number of Cases	Percentage	Number of Cases
1875 – 84	19.3	150	.0	171
1885 – 89	19.1	199	2.7	183
1890 – 94	25.7	214	1.7	171
1895 – 99	21.9	274	1.4	288
1900 – 1904	27.7	400	2.5	362
1905 – 9	29.1	333	2.8	423
1910 – 1914	36.5	373	4.2	452
1915 – 19	41.1	375	1.5	537
1920 – 24	53.2	624	6.3	665
1925 – 29	65.4	737	6.0	746
1930 – 34	67.9	1,043	10.6	1,010
1935 – 39	74.6	1,467	17.8	1,299
1940 – 44	76.6	1,746	30.8	1,564

Source: 1961 census

we need to account for a rise of 1.5 births at least. Nuptiality seems to have been declining despite a decline in widowhood. Hence, the proximate determinant that accounts for much of the rise in fertility is probably postpartum infecundability.

It is even more difficult to determine the ultimate causes for the rise. The literature suggests at least three variables associated with declines in breast-feeding: income, maternal education, and urbanization. Our results suggest that the rise in maternal education is able to account for a small part of the decline in the length of the second birth interval. We did not find a significant relationship between our proxy for income, the husband's literacy, and the length of the second birth interval. However, male literacy at the individual level may be a poor proxy for income. Male literacy at the cohort level may be a better proxy for living standards. The analysis suggests that this proxy for income could account for much of the decline in breast-feeding. Of course, there may be other variables that were not included in the analytic framework we have used. However, it may be interesting to note that John Akin and colleagues found that the only simple macrovariable with a rank correlation identical to that of breast-feeding in four Arab countries was income per head (Akin et al., 1986). Probably, the rise in income influenced the availability of breast milk substitutes and the parents' ability to acquire them.

Declines in breast-feeding may sometimes lead to large and sustained increases in fertility (Singh et al. 1985). One of the largest increases of this kind has been recorded among Palestinian and Israeli Muslims. This predecline rise in fertility was probably the result of special circumstances, namely, the close interaction of a developed Jewish economy with an underdeveloped Arab economy.[12] When Arab income rose, partly as result of a growing Jewish demand for agricultural produce, breast milk substitutes would have come increasingly within reach of the mostly rural Arab population. Women's education also benefited from the growth in income, contributing to the decline in breast-feeding at a later stage and, eventually, to the fertility decline, which started in the late 1970s.

Appendix

Bachi (1977: 196) published estimates of TFR for Palestinian Muslims for selected years during the Mandate (table A1).[13] Bachi's data would imply a much faster rise in fertility than suggested by the cohort data from the 1972 census (see table 6.3). Bachi corrected his fertility estimates for under registration of female births (Bachi, 1977: 385). However, his population estimates, which are based on the 1931 census, gradually deteriorate over time because they do not take into account immigration (Bromberger 1948; Gurevich, Gertz, and Bachi 1944: 110). Hence, his fertility estimates for the mid-1930s may be too high. In addition, there was considerable over registration of births after 1943 due to the wartime food control (Bromberger 1948). This probably explains Bachi's extremely high estimate of TFR for 1943-44.

Table 6. A1
Estimates of Total Fertility Rate among Palestinian Moslems

Period	Total Fertility Rate
1926 – 27	6.37
1928 – 30	6.56
1931 – 33	6.51
1937 – 39	7.51
1940 – 42	7.83
1943 – 44	9.42

Notes

* Thanks are due to Barbara Okun, Dov Friedlander, and an anonymous reviewer who made helpful comments on previous versions of this chapter.

1. The total fertility rate for a particular year is the number of births a woman aged fifteen is expected to have assuming that the age-specific fertility rates for that year do not change and that the woman does not die before she reaches age fifty. The total fertility rate is insensitive to changes in the age structure.
2. The proximate determinants of fertility are the biological and behavioral factors through which social, economic, and environmental variables affect fertility. Studies of the proximate determinants of fertility suggest that spontaneous miscarriage and,

probably also, increased frequency of intercourse are unlikely to explain much of the predecline rises in fertility. See Bongaarts and Potter (1983).

3. Perhaps the best-documented cases of predecline rises in fertility due to a decline in breast-feeding are actually North American. See, Romaniuk (1981); Blackwood (1981); Brainard and Overfield (1986).
4. The economic theory that, where the level of living improves, more babies are "purchased" until they come into more direct competition with consumer goods does not fit any of the cases of a predecline fertility rise because more babies are "purchased" through a decline in the use of contraceptive methods and not through any of the four "proximate" determinants thought to be responsible for most predecline rises in fertility. Contraceptive methods may have been used in the past, but if so, only on a marginal scale.
5. Women born in 1895-1899 reported an average of 6.17 live births. For much of their childbearing years, these women were exposed to a life expectancy at birth of about thirty-five years. This suggests an infant mortality rate in the range of 200-220. If one were to assume that they had forgotten every second infant death, then the true average number of live births would have been about seven. For estimates of life expectancy, see Friedlander and Goldscheider (1979).
6. Computed from Central Bureau of Statistics (1968), tables 7, 23, 34, and 50.
7. Compare Friedlander, Eisenbach, and Goldscheider (1979).
8. The proportions currently married in 1931 were computed from data in Mills (1933), p. 46; those in 1961 were computed from the census; and the marital fertility rates were taken from Eisenbach (1978: 99).
9. Compare Hill (1981).
10. Infant mortality declined over time. This decline would have caused a rise in fertility, others things being equal. However, this effect is small compared with the effect of a decline in breast-feeding. See Lesthaeghe (1983).
11. Compare Rodriguez et al. (1984)
12. The fertility level of Jewish immigrants from Yemen also rose after immigration, from 6.44 births among women born in 1915-1919 to 7.16 among those born in 1920-1922. Unfortunately, it is not known whether this was due to a decline in breastfeeding. See Schellekens (1977).
13. These estimates have been used by Hill (1983).

References

Akin, J. S., R. E. Bilsborrow, D. K. Guilkey and B. M. Popkin. 1986. "Breast-feeding patterns and determinants in the Near East: An analysis for four countries." *Population Studies* 40: 247-262.

Bachi, R. 1977. *The Population of Israel.* Jerusalem: Institute of Contemporary Jewry.

Blackwood, L. 1981. "Alaska native fertility trends, 1950-1978." *Demography* 18: 173-179.

Bongaarts, J. and R. G. Potter. 1983. *Fertility, Biology, and Behavior: An Analysis of the Proximate Determinants.* New York: Academic Press.

Brainard, J. M. and T. Overfield. 1986. "Transformation in the natural fertility regime of western Alaskan Eskimo. In W. P. Handwerker (ed.), *Culture and Reproduction: An Anthropological Critique of Demographic Transition Theory*, 112-124. Boulder, CO: Westview.

Bromberger, E. 1948. "The Growth of population in Palestine." *Population Studies* 2: 71-91.

Central Bureau of Statistics. 1968. *Demographic Characteristics of the Population in the Administered Areas: Data from Sample Enumeration.* Jerusalem: Central Bureau of Statistics.

Central Bureau of Statistics. 1996. *Statistical Abstract of Israel 1996*. Jerusalem: Central Bureau of Statistics.

Coale, A., A. G. Hill and T. J. Trussell. 1975. "A new method of estimating standard fertility measures from incomplete data." *Population Index* 41: 182-220.

Dyson, T., and M. Murphy. 1985. "The onset of fertility transition." *Population and Development Review* 11: 399-440.

Eisenbach, Z. 1978. "Trends and variations in Moslem fertility in Israel. Ph.D. dissertation, Hebrew University of Jerusalem (in Hebrew).

Friedlander, D., Z. Eisenbach and C. Goldscheider. 1979. "Modernization patterns and fertility change: The Arab populations of Israel and the Israel administered territories." *Population Studies* 33: 239-254.

Friedlander, D., and C. Goldscheider. 1979. *The Population of Israel*. New York: Columbia University Press.

Gurevich, D., A. Gertz and R. Bachi. 1944. *The Jewish Population of Palestine: Immigration, Demographic Structure and Natural Growth*. Jerusalem: Jewish Agency.

Hill, A. G. 1981. "Population growth in the Middle East since 1945 with special reference to the Arab countries of West Asia." In J. I. Clarke and H. Bowen-Jones (eds.), *Change and Development in the Middle East*, 130-153. London: Methuen.

Hill, A. G. 1983. "The Palestinian population of the Middle East." *Population and Development Review* 9: 293-316.

Huffman, S. 1984. "Determinants of breast-feeding in developing countries: Overview and policy implications." *Studies in Family Planning* 15: 170-183.

Knodel, J., and C. Wilson. 1981. "The secular increase in fecundity in German village populations: An analysis of reproductive histories of couples married 1750-1899." *Population Studies* 35: 53-84.

Lesthaeghe, R. 1983. "De borstvoedingshypothese als verklaring voor regionale verschillen in vruchtbaarheid en zuigelingensterfte: Nederland en België in het midden van de 19e eeuw" (The breast-feeding hypothesis as an explanation for regional variations in fertility and infant mortality: the Netherlands and Belgium in the middle of the 19th Century). *Bevolking en Gezin* 3: 61-84.

Metzer, J. 1992. "What kind of growth? A comparative look at the Arab economies in Mandatory Palestine and in the administered territories." *Economic Development and Cultural Change* 40: 843-65.

Mills, E. 1933. *Census of Palestine 1931*, vol. 2. Alexandria: Whitehead Morrison.

Nag, M. 1983. "The impact of sociocultural factors on breast-feeding and sexual behavior." In R. A. Bulatao and R. D. Lee (eds.), *Determinants of Fertility in Developing Countries*, vol. 1, *Supply and Demand for Children*, 163-198. New York: Academic Press.

Rodríguez, G., J. Hobcraft, J. McDonald, J. Menken and J. Trussell. 1984. "A comparative analysis of determinants of birth intervals." *WFS Comparative Studies* 30. Voorburg, Netherlands: International Statistical Institute.

Romaniuk, A. 1981. "Increase in natural fertility during the early stages of modernization: Canadian Indians case study." *Demography* 18: 157-172.

Schellekens, J. 2001. "Comparing demographic profiles of Jews and Moslems in Yemen." In S. DellaPergola and J. Even (eds.), *Papers in Jewish Demography, Selected Proceedings of the Demographic Sessions Held at the Twelfth World Congress of Jewish Studies, Jerusalem. July-August* 1997, 345-349. Jerusalem: Hebrew University of Jerusalem, Avraham Harman Institute of Contemporary Jewry.

Schellekens, J. 1997. "Nuptiality during the First Industrial Revolution in England: Explanations." *Journal of Interdisciplinary History* 27: 637-654.

Singh, S., J. B. Casterline and J. G. Cleland. 1985. "The proximate determinants of fertility: Sub-national variations." *Population Studies* 39: 113-135.

Part 2

Nuptially and Contraception

7

Age at Marriage, Sex-Ratios, and Ethnic Heterogamy

Haya Stier and Yossi Shavit

Introduction

Age at first marriage has risen dramatically in many industrialized societies (England and Farkas 1986; Oppenheimer 1988). This has been attributed to the expansion of labormarket opportunities for women that, in turn, created a demand by women for higher education. Prolonged schooling by women postponed their entry into marriage (Blossfeld and Huinink 1991; Blossfeld and Jaenichen 1992; Oppenheimer 1988). Researchers have studied the relationship between the delay of marriage and a host of other social and demographic processes. For example, Bumpass and Sweet (1972) studied the effect of age at marriage on marital stability; Marini (1978, 1984, 1985) studied its relationship to educational attainment, and Coale (1989) looked at its effect on fertility. The present study focuses on the relationship between age at marriage and patterns of mate selection. Specifically, we focus on the effect of age at marriage on ethnic homogany. Mate selection is, in part, a function of the differential availability of mates in different social categories that, in turn, is affected by the sex-ratio within them. Therefore, we also study the effect of the scx-ratio on ethnic intermarriage.

In the following section, we briefly summarize some of the main ideas in the literature on assortative mating, discussing the relationship between age at marriage and assortative mating. We then discuss the Israeli context and formulate our hypotheses. These hypotheses are then tested using census data. We conclude with a summary and discussion of our findings and their implications.

Homogamy in Marriage

A tendency for homogamous marriages is the rule in man (Epstein and Guttman 1984). This is not to say that all marriages are homogamous, but only that the odds for people to engage in homogamous marriages are usually greater than those for heterogamous ones. This is true whether homogamy/heterogamy is defined by ethnicity and race, or by the educational attainment and socio-economic origins of the spouses.

There are several plausible explanations for this empirical tendency. First, there are theories about people's preferences in mate and friend selection. Coombs (1961, cited in Epstein and Guttman 1984) proposes a value theory of mating, which states that people prefer friends and spouses with whom they share a common set of values. Similarly, DiMaggio and Mohr (1985) show that people tend to select mates who share similar cultural tastes with them (see also Kerckhoff 1964; Murstein 1976). Thus, the cultural distinctions of ethnic groups, religions, and socio-economic strata lead to a degree of endogamy along these dimensions.

The anthropologist Boas (1928) interpreted the overwhelming tendency towards ethnic endogamy in the groups he studied as an expression of ethnic-centrism—concern for the preservation of one's own cultural or racial group (Johnson 1980: 26). From a psychological point of view, Winch (1958) stresses the importance of preliminary needs as determinants of mate selection on the basis of traits (e.g., physical appearance, intelligence) or socio-economic background. Preferences in mate selection are also affected by economic considerations (Becker 1973, 1974; Oppenheimer 1988).

The Sex-ratio, Age and Marriage Patterns

Preference notwithstanding, mate selection is highly constrained by the availability of mates with preferred characteristics. Structural and demographic constraints may either enhance or inhibit intermarriage among groups.

A well-known demographic constraint on the availability of preferred spouses is the "marriage squeeze." In most societies, males marry women who are younger than they are by about two years. Thus, mate selection is constrained by the relative size of male and female birth cohorts (Schoen 1983; Schmeltz et al. 1991: 38; Guttentag and Secord 1983). A man belonging to a large cohort that is followed by smaller ones has a smaller chance of forming a homogamous marriage with a mate his junior by the "right" age-interval than a man belonging to a small cohort, and vice versa for women. Consequently, men of large cohorts that are followed by small ones would be forced to search for wives in ever-younger cohorts or engage in a heterogamous marriage (or both).

Although a marriage squeeze is expected to result in higher rates of out-marriage, men or women faced by a squeeze may either forgo marriage altogether, or select mates from different age-categories. Such is the case amongst blacks in the U.S. It has long been argued that black women face a serious problem of marriage squeeze, with relatively few marriageable men (Wilson 1987; Spanier and Glick 1980; Brien 1990). The marriage rate of blacks is indeed considerably lower than that of any other group in the U.S. Moreover, age and educational homogamy are low, as black women are more likely to marry men younger and less educated than themselves.

Why should age at marriage be related to patterns of mate selection? Ethnic groups and socio-economic strata tend to be geographically and socially concentrated. The ethnic and socio economic composition of most neighborhoods and schools is more homogeneous than the population at large. Researchers often assume that people who marry young often meet their future spouses in these relatively homogeneous social contexts. Therefore, young people are more likely to meet mates of like characteristics than those who are very different from themselves (e.g., Ramsoy 1966; Eckland 1968; Peach 1974; Blau and Schwartz 1984; Kerckhoff 1964). Furthermore, when they are young, people (but especially women) still face a relative abundance of potential mates of like characteristics. With age, the conditions in the marriage market deteriorate for women. The norm dictates that they should marry old men, but with age the pool of eligible older men is constantly shrinking as these men can marry ever-younger women. Consequently, older women suffer ever-greater squeezes which force them to compromise preferences and to cross ethnic and educational lines in pursuit of mates.

The Israeli Context

In Israel, age at marriage has risen by about two years since the 1950s (Central Bureau of Statistics 1991), and there are indications that this will accelerate for younger cohorts. Age-patterns of entry into marriage are similar among the different ethnic groups, with a median age of twenty-five for men and twenty-two for women (Friedlander and Goldscheider 1984: 10). Divorce-rates, although growing, are still at a relatively low level for homogamous as well as heterogamous marriages (Peres and Katz 1991). At the same time, there has been a rise in the rate of ethnic intermarriage from about 7 percent of all marriages in the early 1950s, to about 23 percent in the mid-1980s (Peres and Katz 1991). Is this the outcome of delaying the age at marriage, or a consequence of marriage squeezes which might have constrained marital choices by members of the different ethnic groups? We shall try to answer this question by comparing the ethnic homogamy of marriages which were formed early to thosc formed later in women's lives, looking at birthcohorts which experienced different degrees of marriage squeezes.

Jewish society in Israel is composed of two major ethnic groups: those of European or American origin and those of African or Asian origin. The two groups differ in their socioeconomic standing, and in their cultural and historical background. The Euro-American group was the first of the two to arrive in the land in large numbers and has dominated the political, economic, and cultural life until recently. The educational level of this group is high, and so is its members' socio-economic standing. Jews of Afro-Asian origin immigrated to Israel in the 1950s and 1960s. Their educational level is considerably lower than that of the Euro-American group and so is their occupational standing and level of income. Currently, the Israeli Jewish population is about equally divided between Afro-Asians and EuroAmericans.

Israel has absorbed massive immigration over the last fifty years, especially in the early 1950s. Immigration coupled with high fertility rates produced ever-growing birth-cohorts and, consequently, kept the sex-ratio at low levels (see below). Women who were born in the 1950s are in "oversupply." This is especially true for the Afro-Asian population, whose fertility rates were higher than those of Euro-Americans (Friedlander and Goldscheider 1984). Schmeltz and his associates (1991) argue that this has produced marriage squeezes for Asian-African females, many of whom were 'forced' to marry outside their ethnic group. Unfortunately, Schmeltz and associates do not present data supporting their plausible assertion. Nor do they show that the presumed squeezes affected rates of intermarriage among ethnic groups. One of the objectives of the present paper is to put this idea to an empirical test.

The discussion of the literature leads us to formulate three hypotheses:

1. Women of birth-cohorts with severe marriage squeezes are more likely to remain single.
2. Women of birth-cohorts with severe marriage squeezes are more likely to engage in heterogamous marriages. As noted, Afro-Asian women born during the 1950s faced a more severe marriage squeeze than females of Euro-American origin. We therefore expect the sex-ratio to have a stronger effect on the former than on the latter.
3. For women, later marriages are more likely than early marriages to be heterogamous, as the marriage market shifts from school to the workplace and as the squeeze becomes more severe.

Note that our first two hypotheses address the issue of sex-ratio effects on marriage patterns, while the third addresses the issue of age-at-marriage effects.

Cohorts and Squeezes

Data are drawn from the 20 percent public-use file of the 1983 Census. For the first part of the analysis, we employ data for Jewish men and women born between 1943 and 1958. We selected the 1943 cohort as our oldest cohort because among older cohorts a relatively high percentage of women had married prior to their immigration to Israel. This is especially true for Afro-Asians. Our choice of the youngest cohort was determined for us by the nature of the data-file. The public-use 20 percent files of the 1983 census do not classify people born between 1959 and 1966 by single years of birth. This is not a severe limitation from our perspective, because younger cohorts were still in the early stages of entry into marriage and many of their members were still single in 1983. Our older cohorts married primarily during the 1960s and the younger cohorts during the late 1970s and very early 1980s. Foreign-born individuals who married before immigrating to Israel were excluded from the analysis. The total number of cases in the file is 147,969. We employ these data to illustrate the demographic context for the marriage regime that we are about to study.

Figure 7.1 illustrates changes in cohort sizes for men and women of the two ethnic groups. As noted earlier, Afro-Asian birth-cohorts grew dramatically throughout the period. By contrast, Euro-American cohorts increased in size until the late 1940s and early 1950s and declined gradually thereafter. In figure 7.2 we present the sex-ratios for each ethnic group and for each cohort. The sex-ratio for a cohort born in year *t* is calculated as:

$$\frac{\text{(number of men of the ethnic group, who were born in } t\text{ - 2)}}{\text{(number of women of the ethnic group born in year } t\text{)}}$$

We note that the sex-ratio varies very differently across birth-cohorts for the two ethnic groups. For Euro-Americans the ratio was very unfavorable for the first three cohorts and then rose sharply, hovering around, but mostly above, unity. For Afro-Asians the ratio has been consistently below unity except for one cohort (the 1954 birth-cohort). For Afro-Asians it was least favorable for cohorts born in the very early 1950s and somewhat more favorable for those born in the late 1950s. In other words, Afro-Asian women have suffered a more consistently harsh marriage squeeze than EuroAmerican women.

Figure 7.1

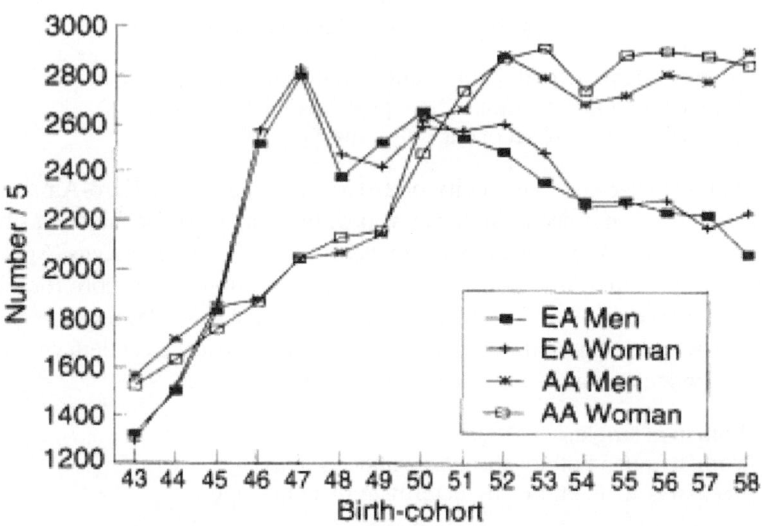

Age at Marriage, Marriage Squeeze and Homogamy

We now turn to testing our hypotheses. We do so using a sub-file drawn from the 1983 Census. It consists of a 10 percent random sample of women (i.e. 10 percent of the 20 percent census sample) born between 1945 and 1958 and who were either in their first marriage or had never married.[1] For each currently married woman, we retrieved and merged information on her husband's ethnicity and education. The file excludes divorced, widowed, and separated women, as well as those in a higher-order marriage because, for these women, information on first husbands is not available. The divorce-rate in Israel is low (Peres and Katz, 1991), thus the exclusion of divorced women amounts to 7 to 10 percent of the various cohorts. Since Peres and Katz report similar divorce-rates between ethnically homogamous and heterogamous marriages, we do not expect that the exclusion of divorced women will bias our results.

We use the information on age at marriage to estimate our models of the transition to marriage. Each woman's record was converted into multiple person-years representing her marital life-experience. Because the person-year is the unit of analysis, each woman can contribute a different number of person-years to the file. This is the number of years, from age seventeen until 1983, that she began as a single person. For example, a woman who married at the age of twenty-two, contributed six person-years to the file.

We employ four independent variables. The first is the age to which the person-year pertains. This variable is grouped into three categories: 17-20, 21-23, and over twenty-four, corresponding to early, intermediate, and late marriages. The second variable is the sex-ratio for each ethnic group and birth-cohort. For example, for Euro-American women born in 1945 the sex-ratio is 0.70 (see figure 7.2), and for Afro-Asian women born in 1947 the sex-ratio is 0.90. The third variable is woman's education, which is coded as follows:

1. all respondents who did not obtain a matriculation diploma;
2. those with a matriculation or any post secondary diploma;
3 those with any post-secondary diploma.[2]

The fourth variable is ethnicity, coded as Afro-Asians and Euro-Americans. Afro-Asians are defined as all those who were born, or whose father was born, in Asia or North Africa. All others are classified as Euro-Americans. Approximately 10 percent of the sample are second-generation Israeli-born for whom we cannot ascertain ethnic origins. We assume them to be descendants of Europeans who immigrated in the late-nineteenth and early-twentieth centuries. The dependent variable is a three-category variable:

1. Woman is single.
2. Woman is in an ethnically homogamous marriage.
3. Woman is in an ethnically heterogamous marriage.

Figure 7.2

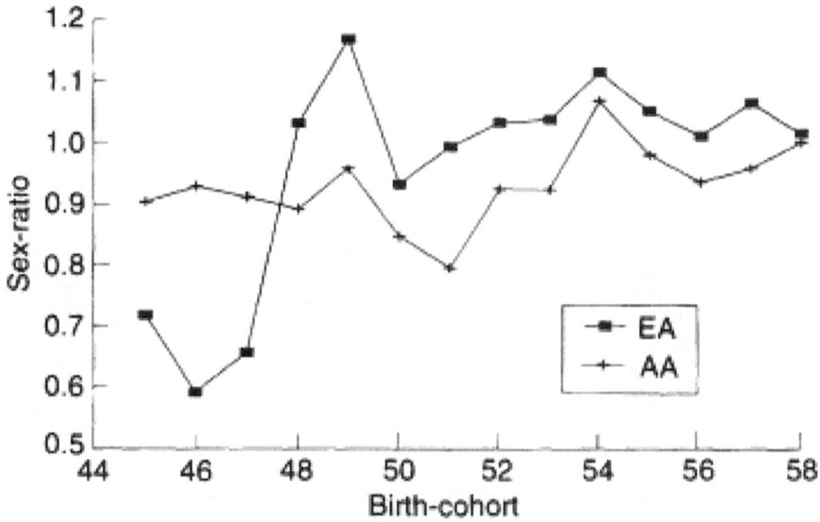

The distributions of the variables are presented in table 7.1. About half of the person-years in the sample pertain to the youngest age-category. This is to be expected because most women were still single in the earlier ages and contributed years to that category, but fewer women were still single by the age of twenty-one and fewer still by age twenty-four. (That there are more years in the oldest category than in the 21-23 category is due to the fact that the former spans many more years.) The age-distribution also shows that Afro-Asian females tend to marry somewhat earlier than women of Euro-American origin. The distribution of the education variables reflects the ethnic differences in educational attainment in Israel (e.g., Nahon 1987).

To test our first hypothesis concerning the effect of the sex-ratio on the odds of marriage, we estimate logistic regressions (Hanushek and Jackson 1977; Maddala 1983) for the log odds of getting married. In other words, the model contrasts getting married in a given person-year with staying single through that year. The results are presented in the left panels of tables 7.2a (for Euro-American women) and 7.2b (for Afro-Asian women). The left-hand model within each panel assumes that the log odds of marriage are only affected by age. The second model also includes women's education, and the third model includes the sex-ratio. For both Euro-Americans and Afro-Asians we find that the log odds of marriage increase with age (given that marriage had not occurred in previous ages). We also find that education (as measured by Matriculation and Post-Secondary Education) inhibits the log odds of marriage. This is a familiar finding from other settings which show that the pursuit of education by women

Table 7.1
Percentage Distribution of Variables in the Person-Years File by Ethnicity of Respondents

Variables	Ethnicity	
	Afro-Asian	Euro-American
Age		
17–20	54.8	50.4
21–23	18.2	19.5
24 +	27.0	30.1
Education		
Matriculation	27.0	61.1
Post-Secondary	4.9	24.2
Marital Status		
Single	48.4	55.8
Married	41.6	35.7
Homogamously		
Married	9.9	8.6
Heterogamously		
N of person-years	6158	6281

delays family formation (e.g., Oppenheimer 1988). In the third model we find that the sex-ratio enhances the log odds of getting married among Afro-Asians but does not significantly affect Euro-Americans' odds of marriage.

We now turn to test hypotheses 2 and 3 regarding the effects of the sex-ratio and age at marriage on homogamous versus heterogamous marriages. We do so within a multinomial logistic regression which contrasts the log odds of staying single and of marrying homogamously against the odds of marrying heterogamously. In the right panel of tables 7.2a and 7.2b we only present one of the two contrasts: homogamy versus heterogamy. As before, it is estimated under three models. The left-hand model in the panel of table 7.2a shows that Euro-American women who marry later are more likely than those who marry in the seventeen to twenty age-range to marry homogamously. This difference is reduced somewhat when we add education to the model and persists when we add the sex-ratio. For Afro-Asians the pattern is reversed: women who marry later are more inclined towards heterogamous marriages. Here too, the effects are slightly reduced when education is included in the model. Thus, interestingly, whereas among Euro-Americans education enhances homogamy, among Afro-Asians it enhances heterogamy.

The effect of the sex-ratio on homogamy among Afro-Asians is consistent with our third hypothesis (that an increase in the ratio of men to women will enhance homogamy). Among Euro-Americans however, the sex-ratio does not affect homogamy significantly.

To summarize, women who marry later, whether of Afro-Asian or Euro-American origin, are more likely than early-marriers to marry Euro-American

Table 7.2a
Logit regressions of marriage and of homogamous marriage: Euro-American women (standard errors in parentheses)

Independent variables	Married vs. single			Homogamous vs heterogamous marriages		
Intercept	−0.913[a]	−0.653[a]	−0.465[a]	1.193[a]	0.871[a]	1.276[a]
	(0.039)	(0.050)	(0.157)	(0.081)	(0.091)	(0.288)
Age 21–3[b]	1.252[a]	1.316[a]	1.315[a]	0.361[a]	0.295[a]	0.295[a]
	(0.061)	(0.062)	(0.062)	(0.114)	(0.115)	(0.116)
Age 24+	1.766[a]	1.871[a]	1.873[a]	0.332[a]	0.228	0.237
	(0.074)	(0.075)	(0.076)	(0.122)	(0.124)	(0.124)
Matriculation[c]		−0.283[a]	−0.286[a]		0.571[a]	0.581[a]
		(0.062)	(0.063)		(0.108)	(0.108)
Post-secondary education		−0.542[a]	−0.545[a]		0.538[a]	0.531[a]
		(0.073)	(0.073)		(0.167)	(0.167)
Sex-ratio			−0.202			0.434
			(0.160)			(0.292)

[a] Significant at the 0.05 level.
[b] Ages 17-20 are the omitted age-category.
[c] Women with less than a matricultaion constitute the omitted category of education.

Table 7.2b
Logit regressions of marriage and of homogamous marraige: Afo-Asian women (standard errors in parentheses)

Independent variables	Married vs. single			Homogamous vs heterogamous marriages		
Intercept	−0.354[a]	−0.247[a]	−1.331[a]	1.791[a]	2.059[a]	−0.069[a]
	(0.035)	(0.037)	(0.371)	(0.078)	(0.085)	(0.647)
Age 21–3[b]	0.875[a]	0.905[a]	0.914[a]	−0.578[a]	−0.520[a]	−0.508[a]
	(0.061)	(0.062)	(0.062)	(0.108)	(0.109)	(0.110)
Age 24+	1.280[a]	1.341[a]	1.342[a]	−0.583[a]	−0.461[a]	−0.462[a]
	(0.075)	(0.076)	(0.076)	(0.115)	(0.118)	(0.118)
Matriculation[c]		−0.393[a]	−0.408[a]		−0.965[a]	−0.995[a]
		(0.064)	(0.064)		(0.104)	(0.105)
Post-secondary education		−0.391[a]	−0.387[a]		−0.587[a]	−0.573[a]
		(0.135)	(0.134)		(0.203)	(0.204)
Sex-ratio			1.180[a]			2.319[a]
			(0.402)			(0.702)

[a] Significant at the 0.05 level.
[b] Ages 17-20 are the omitted age-category.
[c] Women with less than a matricultaion constitute the omitted category of education.

men. In addition, education enhances the marriage chances of Euro-American males. Finally, marriage squeezes affect the opportunities of Afro-Asian women to marry and to marry homogamously but do not affect either outcome among Euro-American women.

These findings suggest two questions: first, why do women tend to prefer Euro-American men as they get older and as they acquire an education? An obvious hypothesis is that the increased preference is not of Euro-American males *per se* but of educated mates. Educational inequalities between ethnic groups in Israel are such that educated Afro-Asian men are hard to come by. Less than 20 percent of Afro-Asian men attain post-secondary education as compared with over 30 percent of Afro-Asian women. Euro-Americans are more educated than Afro-Asians and there are virtually no gender differences in educational attainment among them. Over half of all Euro-Americans attend post-secondary schooling (e.g., Shavit 1989). If the increased preferences are for educated men rather than for men of Euro-American origin, we would expect these effects of age to be eliminated when we control for husband's education. We do so by estimating multinomial logit regressions which contrast marrying an educated Euro-American mate against each of the following possible outcomes: staying single; marrying an educated Afro-Asian man; marrying an uneducated Euro-American man; and marrying an uneducated Afro-Asian man. Husbands with a post-secondary degree (BA or higher) were defined as educated; all other husbands were defined as uneducated. In table 7.3 we present just one contrast: marrying an educated Euro-American man versus an educated Afro-Asian man. The model is estimated separately for Afro-Asian and Euro-American women. We find that the increased preference for Euro-American men with age diminishes. In other words, what seemed to be an increased preference for Euro-American men by older women, is now revealed to be a preference for educated men. And yet, among the educated women of both ethnic groups, there is still a tendency towards the Euro-Americans among the educated men (note the positive and significant effects of Post-Secondary Education in the left column

Table 7.3
Logit regression of marrying an educated Euro-American man versus marrying an educated Afro-Asian, by woman's ethnicity (standard errors in parentheses)

Independent variables	Woman's Ethnicity	
	Euro-American	Afro-Asian
Intercept	2.288[a]	0.350
	(0.806)	(2.553)
Age 21–3[b]	−0.259	0.776
	(0.416)	(0.524)
Age 24+	−0.641	0.610
	(0.414)	(0.516)
Matriculation[c]	−0.029	1.056[a]
	(0.365)	(0.502)
Post-secondary education	0.624[a]	−0.083
	(0.276)	(0.408)
Sex-ratio	−0.069	−1.877
	(0.840)	(2.763)

[a] Significant at the 0.05 level.
[b] Ages 17-20 are the omitted age-category.
[c] Women with less than a matricultaion constitute the omitted category of education.

and of Matriculation in the right column). We suspect that this simply reflects the much greater availability of Euro-Americans among educated men.

The second question is why Euro-American women are not affected by the sex-ratio? We suspect that this pattern simply reflects the ethnic difference in the magnitude of the marriage squeeze. We have shown that, whereas Afro-Asian women of all but one cohort faced a consistent shortage of men, the shortage of Euro-American men was severe only briefly, in the very early 1950s and was then compensated for throughout the 1950s. Thus, all Euro-American women had to do was wait a few years whereas for Afro-Asian women the shortage of like men was more acute.

Discussion

To summarize, we hypothesized that women who marry at a later age are more likely to enter ethnically heterogamous marriages. We also hypothesized that women belonging to birth-cohorts that face a low-sex-ratio are less likely to marry and, in addition, are more likely to marry heterogamously. Following Schmeltz and his associates (1991) we further hypothesized that the effects of the sex-ratio would be stronger for Afro-Asian than for Euro-American women.

We find that in and of itself, age at marriage does not enhance ethnic heterogamy. Women of both ethnic groups who marry later are more likely to marry men of Euro-American origin than those who marry early, but this seems to reflect educational rather than ethnic assortative mating. When education of mate is controlled for, we find no significant difference in ethnic heterogamy between early- and late-marriers.

We conclude that the trend towards a delay in the population's age at marriage is not likely to result in greater ethnic heterogamy. Older available women seek educated men. In past cohorts, educated men were overwhelmingly Euro-American, some of whom married educated Afro-Asian women. The recent increases in the educational attainment of Afro-Asian men may increase ethnic homogamy, as more women of this group will be able to find an educationally appropriate mate within their ethnic group.

We also find that Afro-Asian women born to cohorts which faced severe marriage squeezes were more likely to stay single than those born to better conditions in the marriage market. Furthermore, the marriage squeeze also enhanced their tendency towards heterogamy. By contrast, the demographic increase of the more recent birth-cohorts of the 1960s and 1970s was more moderate than those of the cohorts we have been studying. Consequently, the marriage squeeze faced by Afro-Asians, which we have shown to have contributed to ethnic intermarriage, has declined. We suspect that this decline, like the increased educational attainment of Afro-Asian men, may, *ceteris paribus,* inhibit ethnic heterogamy. In other words, we are suggesting that intermarriage between the ethnic groups was partly forced upon them by the uneven sex-ratio and by the educational inequality between Afro-Asian men and women.

Notes

1. As we explain below, the analysis consists of applying logit models to a file of person-years. The original 20 percent sample of women had over 100,000 person-years and the analysis (using SAS's Catmod Procedure) took a very long time. We resorted to a 10 percent sample to save time. We also constrained the age-range to those born in or after 1945 because this is the oldest cohort for which we now have a measure of the relevant sex-ratio (see figure 7.2).
2. Education is measured at the time of the census rather than at the ages during which women were exposed to the risk of marriage. This may bias our results because spouses' characteristics may affect women's education (Mare 1991). However, the vast majority of Israelis acquire their matriculation diploma by age eighteen, namely before the vast majority of marriages.

References

Becker, G. S. 1973. "A theory of marriage—Part I." *Journal of Political Economy* 81: 813-846.

Becker, G. S. 1974. "A theory of marriage—Part II." *Journal of Political Economy* 82: S11-S26.

Blau, P. M, and J. E. Schwartz. 1984. *Crosscutting Social Circles: Testing a Macrostructural Theory of Intergroup Relations.* Orlando, FL: Academic Press.

Blossfeld, H. P., and J. Huinink. 1991. "Human capital investments or norm of role transition?" *American Journal of Sociology* 97: 143-168.

Blossfeld, H. P., and U. Jaenichen. 1992. "Educational expansion and change in women's entry into marriage and motherhood in the Federal Republic of Germany." *Journal of Marriage and the Family* 54: 302-315.

Boas, F. 1928. *Anthropology and Modern Life.* New York: W. W. Norton.

Brien, M. J. 1990. "Economic determinants of family structure: Explaining black/white differences." Unpublished manuscript, University of Chicago.

Bumpass, L. L., and J. A. Sweet. 1972. "Differentials in marital stability: 1970." *American Sociological Review* 37: 754-766.

Central Bureau of Statistics. 1991. *Statistical Abstract of Israel.* Jerusalem: Central Bureau of Statistics.

Coale, A. 1989. "Marriage and childbearing in China since 1940." *Social Forces* 67: 833-850.

Coombs, W. P. 1961. "A value theory of mate selection." *Family Life Coordination* 10: 51-54.

DiMaggio, P., and J. Mohr. 1985. "Cultural capital, educational attainment, and marital selection." *American Journal of Sociology* 90: 1231-1261.

Eckland, B. C. 1968. "Theories of mate selection." *Eugenics Quarterly* 15: 71-84.

England, P., and J. Farkas. 1986. *Household, Employment, and Gender: A Social, Economic, and Demographic View.* New York: Aldine de Gruyter.

Epstein, E., and R. Guttman. 1984. "Mate selection in men: Evidence, theory, and outcome." *Social Biology* 31: 243-278.

Friedlander, D., and C. Goldscheider. 1984. "Israel's population: The challenge of pluralism." *Population Bulletin* 39 (2): 1-39.

Guttentag, M., and P. F. Secord. 1983. *Too Many Women: The Sex Ratio Question.* Beverly Hills, CA: Sage.

Hanushek, E. A., and J. E. Jackson. 1977. *Statistical Methods for Social Scientists.* Orlando, FL: Academic Press.

Johnson, R. A. 1980. *Religious Assortative Marriages in the United States.* New York: Academic Press.

Kerckhoff, A. C. 1964. "Patterns of homogamy and the field of eligibles." *Social Forces* 42: 289-297.

Maddala, G. S. 1983. *Limited-Dependent and Qualitative Variables in Econometrics.* New York: Cambridge University Press.

Mare, R. D. 1991. "Five decades of educational assortative mating." *American Sociological Review* 56: 15-32.

Marini, M. M. 1978. "The transition to adulthood: Sex differences in educational attainment and age at marriage." *American Sociological Review* 43: 483-507.

Marini, M. M. 1984. "The order of events in the transition to adulthood." *Sociology of Education* 57: 63-84.

Marini, M. M. 1985. "Determinants of the timing of adult role entry." *Social Science Research* 14: 309-50.

Murstein, B. I. 1976. *Who Will Marry Whom? Theories and Research in Marital Choice.* New York: Spring Publishing Company.

Nahon, Y. 1987. *Patterns of Educational Expansion and the Structure of Occupational Opportunities—The Ethnic Dimension.* Jerusalem: Jerusalem Institute for Israel Studies (in Hebrew).

Oppenheimer, V. K. 1988. "A theory of marriage timing." *American Journal of Sociology* 94: 563-591.

Peach, C. 1974. "Homogamy, propinquity, and segregation: A re-evaluation." *American Sociological Review* 39: 636-641.

Peres, Y., and R. Katz. 1991. "The family in Israel: Continuity and change." In Shamgar-L. Hendelman and R. Bar-Yosef (eds.), *Families in Israel*, 9-32. Jerusalem: Akademon (in Hebrew).

Ramsoy, N. 1966. "Assortative mating and the structure of cities." *American Sociological Review* 31: 773-786.

Schmeltz, U., S. DellaPergola and U. Avner. 1991. *Ethnic Differences Among Israeli Jews: A New Look.* Jerusalem: Institute of Contemporary Jewry.

Schoen, R. 1983. "Measuring the tightness of the marriage squeeze." *Demography* 20: 61-78.

Shavit, Y. 1989. "Tracking and the educational spiral: A comparison of Arab and Jewish educational expansion in Israel." *Comparative Education Review* 33: 216-231.

Spanier, G. B., and B. L. Glick. 1980. "Mate selection differences between whites and blacks in the U.S." *Social Forces* 58: 707-725.

Wilson, W. J. 1987. *The Truly Disadvantaged.* Chicago, IL: University of Chicago Press.

Winch, R. F. 1958. *Mate Selection: A Study of Complementary Needs.* New York: Harper and Brothers.

8

Insight into Ethnic Flux: Marriage Patterns Among Jews of Mixed Ancestry in Israel

Barbara S. Okun

Introduction

Increases in rates of ethnic and racial intermarriages, coupled with larger flows of immigrants from diverse countries of origin, have led to growing proportions of persons of mixed ancestry and backgrounds in many societies. Findings from the 2000 U.S. census indicate that 2.4 percent of all the respondents and 4.0 percent of the respondents under age eighteen identified themselves as belonging to more than one race (Jones and Smith 2001). Because ethnic and racial exogamy tends to be more common among second-generation than among first-generation immigrants, the growing size of the second generation in the United States will likely lead to larger proportions of multiracial and multiethnic individuals in the future (Gshur and Okun 2003; Portes 1994; Qian and Lichter 2001). Studies of intermarriage in the United Kingdom, France, Sweden, and Israel have suggested that future generations in these countries will also have significant proportions of multiracial and multiethnic persons (Coleman 1994; Cretser 1999; Okun 2001). Patterns of intermarriage are thus challenging concepts of race and ethnicity and are leading to complex views of ethnic and racial boundaries (Harris and Sim 2002; Hirschman 2003; Rockquemore and Brunsma 2002).

In this chapter, I tie together research on assimilation, ethnicity, and ethnic intermarriage by focusing for the first time on the marriage patterns of persons of mixed ethnic backgrounds, specifically the marriage patterns of Jews of mixed ancestry in Israel. There are several aspects of the Israeli case that make for interesting comparisons with other multiethnic societies. First, because of the fairly recent history of the first massive Jewish immigration to Israel, only a small minority of marriage-age Jews in Israel today can trace their roots in Israel past their grandparents' generation. Therefore, Israelis are at a much earlier stage in terms of generational effects than are European immigrant groups in the United States (Lieberson and Waters 1988). In contrast, Israelis are at a more advanced stage in terms of generational effects than are many of the recent immigrant groups to the United States, such as Koreans and Filipinos (Lopez and Espiritu 1990).

Second, in Israel, large socioeconomic gaps remain between major Jewish ancestry groups, and residential segregation is pronounced in certain regions of the country. This situation contrasts with the case of the Southern and Eastern European immigrants in the United States, who benefited from sustained economic expansion after 1940 and have been able to close socioeconomic gaps vis-à-vis earlier immigrants from Northern and Western Europe (Alba 1990). The gap in socioeconomic status between Jewish ancestry groups in Israel, however, is similar to that of some immigrant Hispanic and Asian groups in the United States today (Waters and Eschbach 1995).

Third, Israel may be unique in that its national ideology and governmental policy have been actively directed toward the realization of the "melting pot" ideology. In particular, Zionist ideology largely denies the importance of ethnicity that reflects the Jewish experience in the Diaspora. Rather, Zionism has idealized a new national Israeli Jewish culture, and official Israeli policy has envisioned the complete assimilation of Jews from diverse countries of origin within three generations (Goldscheider 1996).

A brief review of the history of immigration to Israel highlights the period between 1948, when the State of Israel was founded, and 1951, during which about 700,000 immigrants arrived and doubled the previous Jewish population.[1] Substantially lower, but still significant levels of immigration in the 1960s and 1970s, continued to contribute to the diversity of Israeli society. Differences in culture, language, and demographic characteristics were dramatic between Jews from Eastern and Central Europe, Muslim North Africa, and the Muslim Middle East (Friedlander and Goldscheider 1979). Following a lull during the 1980s, the early 1990s brought another substantial wave of immigration-from the former Soviet Union.

Despite the immigration of Jews from diverse origins, Israeli society has always been dominated by Ashkenazim (immigrants from Europe and their descendants). Some of these Jews were the first to immigrate to pre-independence Israel and were the founders of most political, economic, and cultural institutions. In general, Jewish immigrants from Muslim countries in North Africa and the Middle East were characterized by lower levels of socioeconomic status, as well as higher levels of fertility and mortality. For a variety of reasons, including the placement of newly arrived immigrants in different geographically and economically peripheral regions, as well as the differences in the timing of their arrival in Israel, Jews of North African and Middle Eastern ancestry have been disadvantaged socioeconomically (Cohen and Haberfeld 1998; Friedlander et al. 2002).

Over time, ethnic flux in Israel has led to the evolution of new ethnic groups (Goldscheider 1996; Matras 1973; Shavit and Stier 1997). For example, a broadening of the basis of ethnicity has resulted in the creation of a panethnic identity—Israelis of Middle Eastern or North African descent—known in Hebrew as Mizrahim (persons of Eastern origin). Consistent with a framework outlined by Lopez and Espiritu (1990), it is likely that the creation of the panethnic identity came about, despite cultural and socioeconomic diversity among Israelis of Middle Eastern and North African descent, because of broad differences between these groups and the Ashkenazi group in socioeconomic status, residential location, cultural and religious practices, and the generally darker skin phenotype of the Mizrahim. The split between Mizrahim and Ashkenazim has become dominant in Israeli Jewish society, especially because it is understood largely in terms of class inequality (Ben-Rafael 1982; Smooha 1993).

Ben- Rafael and Sharot (1991) discussed why the North African and Middle Eastern groups have a much greater ethnic consciousness than have the Ashkenazim. In coming to Israel, Ashkenazim made a conscious and desired break from the cultural and social features of the Jewish communities from which they originated. In contrast, Jews from North Africa and the Middle East conceived of immigration to Israel as a means of continuing their cultural practices and traditions.

Theoretical Considerations

Ethnicity and race are increasingly understood among social scientists as fluid social constructs, rather than as fixed or biologically determined characteristics. Identification with particular ethnic or racial groups is often viewed as stemming from economic or political interests in group or community membership or from advantages gained through social networks and other forms of social capital (Portes and Zhou 1993). Alternatively, identification can be seen in terms of "symbolic" ethnicity, which is increasingly "optional" for some multiethnic or multiracial groups. In cases of symbolic ethnicity, ethnic identity does not affect social behavior or life chances, but is understood as an individual choice that may be more or less salient at different stages of the life cycle (Gans 1979).

Alba (1990) suggested that among U.S. non-Hispanic whites, ethnicity is largely symbolic, and that ethnic intermarriage among U.S. non-Hispanic whites has contributed to the formation of a new European American ethnic group. This European American group, which is largely homogeneous across component groups with respect to a wide range of socioeconomic characteristics, is seen as partially replacing other more specific forms of ethnicity, such as German American or Polish American. Moreover, there has been evidence of growth in the proportion of non-Hispanic U.S. whites who have reported their ethnicity simply as "American" and speculation about the formation of a new American ethnic group (Lieberson and Waters 1988).

The evolution of symbolic ethnicity among non-Hispanic whites in the United States is largely consistent with classic assimilation theories, which suggest that persons of mixed ancestry are only weakly identified with their particular ethnic backgrounds (Gordon 1964). Among non-European Americans in the United States—such as some Hispanic or Asian groups—ethnicity is also seen as increasingly symbolic, particularly for those of mixed ancestries (Eschbach and Gómez 1998).

When ethnicity or race is symbolic, there may be individual- or family-level variation in ethnic or racial identity that is associated with socioeconomic status. The relationships between socioeconomic status and ethnic identity appear to depend on the aggregate socioeconomic status of relevant groups, as well as on the extent to which ethnic identity is seen as a cultural resource (Eschbach, Supple, and Snipp 1998; Qian 2003; Waters 1994). For example, among Hispanics in the United States, higher family status is associated with less-consistent positive responses to questions about Hispanic ethnicity (Eschbach and Gómez 1998; Qian 2003). In contrast, parents' greater educational attainment is associated with Asian racial identification among third-generation biracial Americans of Asian descent (Xie and Goyette 1997). The associations between educational attainment and ethnic identity are important for understanding patterns of intermarriage because education is an important direct factor in the selection of mates via well-known patterns of educational homogamy (Kalmijn 1991; Marc 1991), as well as a potentially important indirect factor via its associations with ethnicity and ethnic identity and, therefore, with ethnic endogamy (Qian, Blair, and Ruf 2001).

How is ethnicity among persons of mixed ancestry reflected in marriage behavior? It may be that over time, a new "Israeli" ethnicity is being created, and that there is a concomitant decline in the salience of a distinct "Mizrahi" ethnicity. If so, I hypothesize that there is a tendency for persons of mixed ancestry to marry among themselves, a tendency that I term "ethnic endogamy" among persons of mixed ancestry. There are at least two reasons why these changes may be expected. First, according to Zionist ideology, ethnic intermarriage is a means of creating a single, unified culture among Jews in Israel (Rosen 1982). Second, there has been little immigration to Israel from countries of North Africa and the Middle East since the mid-1960s, thereby cutting off, in Massey's (1995:642) words, "the supply of raw materials for the grist mill of ethnicity" and enabling generational effects to weaken ethnic identity.

In contrast, it may be that persons of ethnically mixed unions do not form a new "Israeli" identity, but rather identify, and are identified primarily, with one of the two major origin groups. If so, I hypothesize that persons of mixed ethnic ancestry exhibit *one-sided* marriage behavior in the sense that, among those who marry Mizrahim or Ashkenazim, marriage with one origin group is more common than marriage with the other. Consequently, the proportion of people who identify themselves with the "favored" group may actually increase more over time than if there were no ethnic intermarriage. This has been shown to be true in the case of Irish Americans (Hout and Goldstein 1994). The salience of Mizrahi identity could increase or decrease, depending on which is the favored group.

Another possibility is that persons of mixed ancestry marry with ethnic groups according to their educational attainment. Assimilation theories suggest that education tends to weaken ethnic attachments and to increase exposure to people of different ethnic origins, thereby leading to a loss of ethnic identity among upwardly mobile members of disadvantaged ethnic groups (Alba 1990; Qian et al. 2001). In the Israeli context, the assimilation hypothesis suggests that the greater contact of educated Mizrahim with Ashkenazim has led to the erosion of their Mizrahi ethnic consciousness, more frequent intermarriage, and the consequent concentration of Mizrahi ethnicity in the lower classes (Ben-Rafael 1982). If assimilation theory is applied to the case of persons of mixed ethnic ancestry, the more educated among them should be expected to have a less-well-defined Mizrahi ethnic consciousness and, therefore, to be less likely to marry Mizrahim, whereas those who are less educated should be expected to be more likely to marry Mizrahim.

In contrast to the assimilation hypothesis, the awareness hypothesis states that education may increase social sensitivity to ethnicity and ethnic distinctiveness, so that when ethnicity is optional, educated ethnics are more likely to have a stronger ethnic identity and are, thus, less likely to marry out of their ethnic groups (Qian 2003; Xie and Goyette 1997). In the case of Israel, the awareness hypothesis suggests that among Mizrahim and persons of mixed ancestry, the educated are more likely to have a strong Mizrahi ethnic identity and, hence, are more likely to marry Mizrahim.

Data and Variables

The source of data for this study was a file that contains linked records from the 1995 20 percent sample of the Israeli census and the 1983 100 percent sample of the Israeli census. As is explained later, the linked records were necessary to define the ethnicity of third-generation persons in 1995 (Friedlander et al. 2002). The data provide information on current marital status, number of times married, and year of first marriage as of 1995. I defined the sample of 15,997 married couples as husbands and wives who were living in the same household in 1995: 1) who married in Israel, 2) in which the wives married for the first and only time between 1986 and 1995, and 3) in which the wives were aged eighteen to forty in 1995. By restricting the study to marriages that occurred within a relatively short period prior to the census, I reduced potential biases that occur if marital dissolution of exogamous couples is more common than that of endogamous couples. According to Eisenbach (1992), such biases are not large, partially because overall rates of marital dissolution in Israel are still lower than those of other countries, such as the United States.[2]

Census data from 1995 contain information on the respondents' countries of birth, as well as the countries of birth of the respondents' parents. However, these data do not contain information on the grandparents' places of birth, and this omission poses a problem for defining ethnicity among third-generation Israelis (those with at least one native-born parent).[3] Therefore, I turned to the linked data file. In the 1995 census, persons were linked to the 1983 census records of their parents. In the 1983 records, parents responded to questions on *their* fathers' countries of birth (that is, the countries of birth of the grandfathers of the marriage-age persons in 1995). Because the data I analyzed provides objective information on the countries of birth of the respondents, their parents, and grandfathers, my research does not suffer from the distortion in reported ethnicity and race that is common in subjective questionnaires, such as that included in the U.S. census (Lieberson and Waters 1988).

I defined the ethnicity of persons in the married-couples sample as: 1) Middle Eastern or North African (Mizrahi); 2) European[4] (Ashkenazi); or 3) mixed, with one Mizrahi parent and one Ashkenazi parent. For first-generation Israelis (immigrants to Israel), I defined ethnicity as Mizrahi or Ashkenazi on the basis of information on the respondents' places of birth.[5] For persons in the married-couples sample who were born in Israel, I defined ethnicity as a function of both parents' ethnicity. In the case of persons who were second-generation Israelis (their parents were immigrants to Israel), I defined the parents' ethnicities as a function of their countries of birth. In the case of third-generation Israelis, the parents were themselves born in Israel, so that the parents' ethnicities had to be defined as a function of *their fathers'* places of birth (i.e., the places of birth of the grandfathers of those in the married-couples sample). My reliance on grandfathers' places of birth to define ethnicity among third-generation Israelis is potentially problematic, since it is possible that individuals' grandmothers may have had different places of birth. However, given the overwhelming prevalence of ethnically endogamous unions in the past, I do not believe that this problem is of practical significance (Okun 2001).

By this definition, persons of ethnically mixed ancestries were a minority in the sample. Among brides and grooms, 11 percent and 9 percent were of mixed ancestry, respectively. The proportions of brides and grooms who were of Mizrahi ethnicity were 58 percent and 60 percent, with the remaining 32 percent of the brides and grooms of Ashkenazi origin. The small proportions of ethnically mixed persons among recently married Israeli Jews reflects low levels of Ashkenazi-Mizrahi intermarriage in the more distant past. In the future, I expect to see large increases in these proportions as a consequence of significant increases in Ashkenazi-Mizrahi intermarriage over the past forty years (Okun 2001).

Explicit consideration of educational attainment is essential in an analysis of ethnic marriage patterns in Israel because of the strong association between ethnicity and educational attainment and because educational homogamy is a central feature of marriage patterns (Friedlander et al. 2002; Okun 2001). I categorized persons in the sample into five ascending groups of educational attainment, according to whether the highest degree or diploma they ever received was: 1) a primary or intermediate school diploma, 2) a high school diploma without matriculation certification, 3) a matriculation diploma, 4) a postsecondary school diploma (such as a teaching certificate), or 5) an academic degree (BA or higher). Attaining a matriculation diploma is a critical step in the Israeli educational system because this diploma is a prerequisite for most types of postsecondary education. The completion of high school does not guarantee attainment of the matriculation diploma because the latter requires passing a series of standardized national examinations. As can be seen in table 8.1, Ashkenazim are the most educated group and Mizrahim are the least educated, with persons of mixed ancestry in an intermediate position.[6]

To provide a descriptive assessment of marriage patterns, I present, in table 8.2, the distribution of persons in the married-couples sample by sex, ethnicity, educational attainment, and spouses' ethnicity. First, note that overall and within almost every sex-education group, the probability of marrying a spouse of Ashkenazi origin is the greatest among persons of Ashkenazi ancestry, the lowest among persons of Mizrahi ancestry, and intermediate among persons of mixed ancestry. Similarly, the probability of marrying a spouse of Mizrahi origin is the greatest among persons of Mizrahi ancestry and the lowest among persons of Ashkenazi ancestry. In contrast, the probability of marrying a spouse of mixed ancestry varies little by ethnic origin. Thus, there is a strong suggestion of ethnic endogamy among Ashkenazim and Mizrahim, but no prima facie evidence of endogamy among persons of mixed ancestry.

Second, the proportion of Mizrahim who marry other Mizrahim declines with educational attainment, while the proportion of Ashkenazim who marry other Ashkenazim tends to increase with educational attainment. Thus, it appears that the extent of ethnic endogamy may vary by educational attainment. The

Table 8.1
Distribution of Persons in the Married-Couples Sample, by the Highest Educational Level Attained, Ethnicity, and Sex (Percentage)

Ethnicity	Primary/ Intermediate School	High School Diploma	Matriculation Diploma	Post-Secondary Diploma	Academic Degree	Total	Total (N)
Brides							
Ashkenazi	3.0	15.5	24.0	16.7	40.7	100	5,095
Mixed ancestry	5.1	26.3	26.0	16.4	26.2	100	1,614
Mizrahi	8.8	39.3	26.7	14.2	11.0	100	9,288
Grooms							
Ashkenazi	6.6	19.7	19.3	18.3	36.1	100	5,090
Mixed ancestry	12.2	30.8	21.4	16.1	19.4	100	1,373
Mizrahi	20.4	41.3	13.7	15.3	9.2	100	9,534

Table 2

Distributions of Persons in the Married-Couples Sample, by Ethnicity, Educational Attainment, and Ethnicity, Educational Attainment, and Ethnicity of the Spouses

Educational Attainment	Persons of Ashkenazi Ancestry			Persons of Mixed Ancestry			Persons of Mizrahi Ancestry		
	Married to Ashkenazi	Married to Persons of Mixed Ancestry	Married to Mizrahi	Married to Ashkenazi	Married to Persons of Mixed Ancestry	Married to Mizrahi	Married to Ashkenazi	Married to Persons of Mixed Ancestry	Married to Mizrahi
Total									
Brides	58.9 (5,095)	10.3 (5,095)	30.8 (5,095)	35.8 (1,614)	10.8 (1,614)	53.3 (1,614)	16.3 (9,288)	7.2 (9,288)	76.5 (9,288)
Grooms	58.9 (5,090)	11.4 (5,090)	29.7 (5,090)	38.3 (1,373)	12.7 (1,373)	48.9 (1,373)	16.5 (9,534)	9.0 (9,534)	74.5 (9,534)
Primary or Intermediate School									
Brides	55.5 (155)	9.7 (155)	34.8 (155)	18.1 (83)	3.6 (83)	78.3 (83)	7.1 (815)	4.8 (815)	88.1 (815)
Grooms	55.0 (338)	6.8 (338)	38.2 (338)	19.6 (168)	9.5 (168)	70.8 (168)	8.6 (1946)	7.6 (1946)	83.8 (1946)
High School Diploma									
Brides	43.3 (792)	10.2 (792)	46.5 (792)	17.9 (424)	11.6 (424)	70.5 (424)	9.6 (3,654)	6.5 (3,654)	84.0 (3,654)
Grooms	46.9 (1,004)	10.1 (1,004)	43.0 (1,004)	22.2 (423)	15.1 (423)	62.6 (423)	11.9 (3,942)	8.6 (3,942)	79.5 (3,942)
Matriculation Diploma									
Brides	52.1 (1,222)	11.1 (1,222)	36.7 (1,222)	33.9 (419)	13.8 (419)	52.3 (419)	17.9 (2,478)	9.0 (2,478)	73.1 (2,478)
Grooms	59.0 (981)	13.1 (981)	27.8 (981)	44.2 (294)	11.9 (294)	43.9 (294)	20.9 (1,304)	9.3 (1,304)	69.9 (1,304)
Postsecondary Diploma									
Brides	60.6 (850)	10.0 (850)	29.4 (850)	38.5 (265)	7.9 (265)	53.6 (265)	20.1 (1,321)	6.7 (1,321)	73.1 (1,321)
Grooms	55.9 (931)	11.6 (931)	32.5 (931)	40.7 (221)	13.1 (221)	46.2 (221)	22.1 (1,463)	10.5 (1,463)	67.4 (1,463)
Academic Degree									
Brides	68.4 (2,076)	10.1 (2,076)	21.6 (2,076)	57.4 (423)	10.4 (423)	32.2 (423)	38.7 (1,020)	8.4 (1,020)	52.8 (1,020)
Grooms	67.8 (1,836)	11.8 (1,836)	20.4 (1,836)	67.0 (267)	11.6 (267)	21.3 (267)	38.3 (879)	11.4 (879)	50.3 (879)

Notes: Figures are percentages. The numbers in parentheses are the total number of marriages for each ethnic, education, and sex combination.

proportion of persons of mixed ancestry who marry others of mixed ancestry does not seem to vary systematically by education.

Third, there appears to be some one-sided behavior in the marriage patterns of persons of mixed ethnic ancestries. A larger proportion of these individuals marry spouses of Mizrahi ancestry than of Ashkenazi ancestry, but this pattern may be expected, given the larger proportion of Mizrahim than of Ashkenazim in the overall sample.

Fourth, it appears that one-sided behavior by persons of mixed ancestry is a function of education; as education increases, the proportion of persons of mixed ancestry who are married to Mizrahim declines relative to the proportion who are married to Ashkenazim.

Finally, marriage patterns are fairly similar for men and women. Men appear to be slightly more likely than women to marry spouses of mixed ancestry, overall and in most ethnicity-educational groups.

My interpretations of table 8.2 may not be reliable because of large ethnic differences in the sizes of groups and in sex-educational composition. I therefore used various log-linear models that control for the marginal distributions, by ethnicity and education, of married men and women. Log-linear models enabled me to distinguish marriage patterns that reflect the associations between spouses' traits from patterns that result from the marginal distributions of husbands' and wives' traits (Mare 1991).[7] In addition, multivariate log-linear models allowed me to describe the patterns of ethnic and educational assortative mating net of each other.

Log–Linear Models

The log-linear analyses describe mating patterns in a marriage table of 225 cells [$225 = (5 \times 3)^2$], that is, five categories of educational attainment and three categories of ethnicity for each of the sexes). Table 8.3 presents the fit statistics for eight models (the model equations are available from me on request). Baseline Model I involves random mating after marginal distributions of married persons by ethnicity and education are controlled. Model 1 also controls for the joint distribution of ethnicity and education among husbands, as well as among wives, but does not allow for cross-spouse interactions of any kind.

Model 2, a *quasi-symmetry* model of educational mating, adds to Model 1 ten sex-symmetric, off-diagonal parameters, each representing intermarriage patterns between pairs of different educational groups (Haberman 1979). This sex-symmetric approach assumes that fitted frequencies do not depend on whether the husband or wife is the more educated in each educationally heterogamous combination.[8] I selected this approach after I tested a variety of models, including models that allow for asymmetry, as well as crossing models (Mare 1991). The large reductions in the G^2 and BIC statistics[9] between Model 1, which does not allow for assortative mating of any kind, and Model 2, which allows for educational assortative mating, indicate that educational homogamy is an important element in Israeli marriage patterns. The values of the G^2 and BIC statistics remain large in Model 2, however, indicating that marriage patterns are not well described by a model that considers only educational assortative mating.

All further models build on Model 2. Therefore, patterns of ethnic assortative mating in Models 3-8 are described net of patterns of educational assortative mating, thus avoiding confounding between the two. Fits are substantially better in Models 3-8 than in Model 2. These improvements in fit indicate that ethnic assortative mating makes significant independent contributions to explaining marriage patterns, beyond the patterns described by educational assortative mating. Models 3-8 fit the data reasonably well according to the BIC statistics.

Model 3 adds to Model 2 three ethnic *variable diagonal* parameters to examine the varying extent of ethnic endogamy among the three different ethnic groups.[10] Model 4 differs from Model 3 in that it constrains the extent of ethnic endogamy among Ashkenazim to equal that among Mizrahim and allows only the extent of ethnic endogamy among persons of mixed ancestry to differ from the two. The parameterization in Model 4 thus saves one degree of freedom compared with Model 3.

In Models 3 and 4, no distinction is made between different types of ethnically exogamous unions. In contrast, Model 5 builds on Model 4 by adding an ethnic distance parameter, which allows the fitted frequency of ethnic intermarriages between Ashkenazim and Mizrahim to differ from the fitted frequency of ethnic intermarriages involving spouses of mixed ancestry. Model 5 allows for a cleaner test of the relative frequency of endogamous versus exogamous unions by persons of mixed ethnic ancestry.

Model 6 builds on Model 5 by allowing the fitted frequency of intermarriages between persons of mixed ancestry and Mizrahim to differ from the fitted frequency of intermarriages between persons of mixed ancestry and Ashkenazim. This model is useful for testing the one-sided hypothesis. Model 7 also builds on Model 5 and allows for gender asymmetry in one-sided behavior among persons of mixed ethnic ancestry.

To test the assimilation hypothesis, I constructed a more complex interaction model, which allows patterns of ethnic mating to vary by educational attainment. Model 8 allowed me to test, for example, whether the extent of ethnic endogamy varies by educational attainment, and whether one-sided behavior by persons of mixed ethnic ancestry varies by educational attainment. In this model, parameters of ethnic mating were estimated for couples in which both spouses had matriculation diplomas or higher degrees, while distinct ethnic mating parameters are estimated for all other couples. As table 8.3 shows, Model 8 offers the best fit, indicating that patterns of ethnic mating vary by the educational levels of spouses.

Table 8.3
Fit Statistics for Long-Linear Models

Model	G^2	*df*	BIC
Random Mating			
(1): base model	9,957	196	8,060
Educational Assortative Mating			
(2): (1) + quasi-symmetric educational intermarriage	3,027	186	1,226
Educational Assortative Mating and Ethnic Assortative Mating			
(3): (2) + ethnic variable diagonal using three degrees of freedom	756	183	–1,016
(4): (2) + ethnic variable diagonal using two degrees of freedom	763	184	–1,018
(5): (4) + ethnic distance parameter	763	183	–1,009
(6): (5) + parameter describing "one-sided" behavior	761	182	–1,001
(7): (5) + gender asymmetry among persons of mixed ancestry	756	182	–1,006
(8): (2) + ethnic mating varies by the educational level of couples	573	177	–1,140

Results

I turn to a test of my first hypothesis, which states that a new "Israeli" ethnic identity is manifest in the tendency of persons of mixed ancestry to marry among themselves, rather than among Ashkenazim and Mizrahim. I present here the relative fitted frequencies, net of marginal distributions, of ethnically endogamous unions among Ashkenazim, Mizrahim, and persons of mixed ancestry, based on Model 3.[11] The reference category is all exogamous marriages. I computed the relative fitted frequencies of endogamous unions separately for each ethnic group and found the following: while ethnically endogamous unions among Mizrahim and among Ashkenazim have much higher fitted frequencies (2.94 and 2.35, respectively) than all ethnically exogamous unions, ethnically endogamous unions among persons of mixed ancestry actually have lower fitted frequencies (0.72) than all ethnically exogamous unions.[12] These relative fitted frequencies differ from 1.00 at the .001 level of significance. Thus, I did not find support for the first hypothesis and suggest instead that persons of mixed ancestry do not tend to marry among themselves.

According to Model 3, the extent of ethnic endogamy among Ashkenazim appears to be similar to that of Mizrahim. In addition, a comparison of the BIC statistics for Models 3 and 4 in table 8.3 suggests that it is possible to save a degree of freedom without suffering a significant loss of fit by constraining the extent of ethnic endogamy among the two main ethnic groups to be equal. The exponentiated parameter estimate representing the relative fitted frequency of ethnically endogamous unions among Mizrahim and Ashkenazim is 2.64, while that among persons of mixed ancestry is 0.73. Again, reported fitted frequencies are relative to the fitted frequency of all ethnically exogamous unions and differ significantly from 1.00 at the .001 level. Thus, from Model 4, there is still no evidence that ethnically endogamous unions among persons of mixed ancestry are relatively more frequent than are all exogamous unions.

For a more direct comparison of ethnic endogamy versus ethnic exogamy among persons of mixed ancestry, I turn to the results of Model 5. The relative fitted frequency of ethnically endogamous unions versus ethnically exogamous unions, among couples involving at least one spouse of mixed ancestry, is 0.72 (not significantly different than 1 at the 10 percent level). Thus, among couples in which at least one spouse is of mixed ancestry, ethnically endogamous couples are no more common than are ethnically exogamous couples. Again the results are not supportive of the new Israeli-ethnicity hypothesis.

I now turn to Model 6 to test the one-sided hypothesis. Recall that this hypothesis states that among persons of mixed ethnic ancestry who marry either Mizrahim or Ashkenazim, marriage with one group is more common than marriage with the other group. The results from Model 6 are not consistent with the hypothesis. The fitted frequency of unions between persons of mixed ancestry and Mizrahim is 0.94 and is not significantly different from the fitted frequency of unions between persons of mixed ancestry and Ashkenazim (the reference category) at the 10 percent level. Likewise, table 8.3 indicates that there is no improvement in fit in Model 6 over Model 5, so that distinguishing between unions involving persons of mixed ancestry and Ashkenazim and unions involving persons of mixed ancestry and Mizrahim does not significantly improve the understanding of marriage patterns. Thus, the findings suggest that persons of mixed ethnic ancestry are not overwhelmingly identified as, and do not overwhelmingly identify with, either of the two major ethnic groups to the exclusion of the other.

I turn now to the results of Model 7, which allowed me to examine sex asymmetry in ethnic out-marriage among persons of mixed ancestry. There is some evidence that among persons of mixed ancestry who out-marry, men are more likely than women to marry an Ashkenazi, rather than a Mizrahi. In particular, the fitted frequency of unions between grooms of mixed ancestry and Ashkenazi brides relative to the fitted frequency of unions between grooms of mixed ancestry and Mizrahi brides is 26 percent greater than the analogous fitted frequency of unions between brides of mixed ancestry and Ashkenazi grooms relative to the fitted frequency of unions between brides of mixed ancestry and Mizrahi grooms. This ratio of relative frequencies is significantly different from 1.00 at the .01 level of significance.

Thus, it appears that men of mixed ancestry are closer in marriage behavior to Ashkenazim than are women of mixed ancestry. This finding may reflect broader gender issues, in that it suggests that men of mixed ancestry have greater opportunity to marry up than do women of mixed ancestry. This may be particularly true of educated men of mixed ancestry who are able to exchange their high educational status and presumably greater earnings potential for marriage with Ashkenazi women (Davis 1941; Fu 2001; Merton 1941). Although Model 7 does not provide direct evidence for this exchange theory, a closer look at table 8.2 supports this notion. Among persons of mixed ancestry who had academic degrees, 67.0 percent of the men were married to Ashkenazi women, and only 57.4 percent of the women were married to Ashkenazi men.

I now turn to a test of the assimilation hypothesis, basing my findings on Model 8. I focus on comparing several estimated parameters of ethnic mating among couples in which both spouses had matriculation diplomas or higher to estimated parameters of ethnic mating among couples involving one or more spouses who did not have at least matriculation diplomas.[13] The results are presented in table 8.4.

As I discussed earlier, the assimilation hypothesis suggests that more-educated persons of mixed ancestry are more likely to marry Ashkenazim than Mizrahim, while less-educated persons of mixed ancestry are more likely to marry Mizrahim than Ashkenazim. To test this hypothesis, I compared one-sided behavior among persons of mixed ancestry in more-educated couples with one-sided behavior among persons of mixed ancestry in less-educated couples. The fitted frequency of marriages between persons of mixed ancestry and Mizrahim relative to the fitted frequency of marriages between persons of mixed ancestry and Ashkenazim is 1.28 among less-educated couples (see the left-hand panel of table 8.4). The analogous relative fitted frequency is 0.57 among more-educated couples (see the right-hand panel of table 8.4). The difference in the relative fitted frequencies is statistically significant at the .001 level and indicates that among less-educated couples, persons of mixed ethnic ancestry are more likely to be married to Mizrahim than to Ashkenazim, while among more-educated couples, persons of mixed ethnic ancestry are more likely to be married to Ashkenazim than to Mizrahim.

The log-linear models I presented control for the marginal and joint marginal distributions of the sample, as well as for patterns of educational homogamy. Therefore, the finding that one-sided behavior among persons of mixed ancestry

Table 8.4
Exponentiated Estimates of Ethnic Mating Parameters, Model 8

	Less-Educated Couples			More-Educated Couples		
	Bride: Mizrahi	Bride: Ashkenazi	Bride: Mixed Ancestry	Bride: Mizrahi	Bride: Ashkenazi	Bride: Mixed Ancestry
Groom: Mizrahi	4.14**	1.41	1.28**	1.32	0.84	0.57**
Groom: Ashkenazi	1.41	4.14**	1.00 (Reference)	0.84	2.72**	1.00 (Reference)
Groom: Mixed ancestry	1.28**	1.00 (Reference)	0.79	0.57**	1.00 (Reference)	0.48**

Notes: More-educated couples are those in which both spouses hold at least a matriculation diploma. Less-educated couples are all other couples. All parameters for less-educated couples in the top panel of the table are ststistically different from the analogous parameter for for more-educated couples in the bottom panel at the 5% level.

** $p < .01$ in a test of statistical difference from 1.00. Unmarked figures are not statistically different from 1.00 at the 5% level.

differs as a function of educational attainment does not stem from the facts that Ashkenazim tend to be more educated in general and that persons tend to marry spouses with similar levels of education.

The assimilation hypothesis also suggests that, in the case of Israel, more-educated Mizrahim exhibit less ethnic endogamy than their less-educated counterparts. This indeed appears to be the case in that the relative fitted frequency of ethnically endogamous marriages among less-educated couples involving at least one Mizrahi spouse (4.14) is significantly greater at the .001 level than is the relative fitted frequency of ethnically endogamous marriages among more-educated couples involving at least one Mizrahi spouse (1.32). The difference in the extent of ethnic endogamy among Mizrahim in the two types of couples is striking and is substantively and statistically larger than the differences in the extent of ethnic endogamy by educational attainment among the other ethnic groups.[14] Overall, my empirical results are more consistent with the assimilation hypothesis than with the awareness hypothesis.

Summary and Discussion

My analyses lead to related findings regarding the marriage patterns of persons of mixed ancestry in Israel. There is no suggestion of ethnic endogamy among persons of mixed ancestry. That is, the as-yet small, but growing, group of marriage-age Israelis who are of mixed ethnic origins do not marry among themselves to any great extent. Rather, the findings suggest that ethnic mating among persons of mixed ancestry in Israel is largely a function of educational attainment. In particular, among persons of mixed ancestry, those who are more educated are more likely to marry persons of Ashkenazi origin, while those who are less educated are more likely to marry persons of Mizrahi origin.

That the structural integration of Mizrahim into the dominant society is imperfect as evidenced by the continuing existence of group differences in education, occupational status, income, and place of residence—despite a convergence in some types of social and demographic behavior over time (Friedlander et al. 2002). The continuing association between ethnicity and life chances is well known both in academic and popular circles. Indeed, the recent success of some Mizrahi politicians has often been a result of their appeal to disadvantaged Mizrahi ethnic groups, and much of Israeli politics has been ethnically based.

My findings suggest that if ethnicity is more than symbolic in nature—as is the case in Israel—then ethnic intermarriage may not have the effect of reducing the salience of ethnicity. This counterintuitive conclusion stems from two streams of research. The first, based on a well-established literature on Israel and other societies, shows that there is selective out-marriage of the more educated members of disadvantaged ethnic groups (Eisenbach 1992; Fu 2001; Goldscheider 1996; Qian 1997). The second, presented here, takes the literature one step further by examining the marriage behavior of the offspring of these interethnic marriages. I showed that the marriage behavior of persons of mixed ancestry concentrates more-educated persons of mixed ancestry in families with Ashkenazi spouses and less-educated persons in families with Mizrahi spouses. This pattern perpetuates the historically important association between Mizrahi ethnicity and low socioeconomic status, which is the basis of the popular understanding of current forms of Mizrahi ethnicity. Thus, I suggest that ethnic intermarriage itself should not necessarily be viewed as a vehicle for reducing group differences over time or for reducing the salience of ethnicity among disadvantaged groups.

To the extent that ethnic identification is reflected in marriage patterns, ethnic identity in Israel is conditioned on socioeconomic status, with more-educated persons of mixed ancestry indicating less identification with Mizrahim compared with their less-educated counterparts. My findings stand in contrast to the limited extant evidence on the effects of individual-level socioeconomic status on ethnic identity in cases in which ethnicity is symbolic or optional. In these instances, ethnic awareness among more-educated individuals may be stronger than assimilation effects that are associated with education (Eschbach 1995).

I now return to my negative finding—that I did *not* find evidence in marriage patterns of the formation of a new national Israeli ethnicity. My interpretation of this finding is that persons of mixed ancestry do not form a cohesive group and do not share a common identity. They may not do so partly because Jews of mixed Mizrahi-Ashkenazi origin are a group that knows no ethnic boundary among Jewish Israelis; there is no "other" group that defines them as distinct, since all other Jews fall into one of their component ancestries. In addition, I suggest that a necessary condition for the development of a new national ethnic identity in an immigrant country is the elimination of important structural differences between the various component groups. I suggest that gaps in socioeconomic status between Mizrahim and Ashkenazim have impeded the assimilation of Mizrahim along other dimensions, thus working to maintain the ethnic salience of Mizrahim and hindering the development of an assimilated Israeli ethnicity.

In contrast to the case of the Mizrahim in Israel, structural differences have been eliminated among U.S. non-Hispanic whites, and there are the makings of a new European American ethnicity (Alba 1990) and perhaps a new American ethnicity (Lieberson and Waters 1988). However, there are examples of recent immigrant groups in the United States whose future socioeconomic assimilation is still in doubt (Portes and Zhou 1993). In this sense, the relative socioeconomic status of these groups is similar to that of Mizrahim in Israel. Thus, the marriage behavior of some persons of mixed ancestry in the United States may parallel that of persons of mixed ancestry in Israel. Future research could investigate the marriage behavior of persons of mixed backgrounds in the United States and other countries to shed light on changes in the meaning of race and ethnicity in increasingly multiracial and multiethnic societies.

Notes

1. The extent of intermarriage between Jews and non-Jews who have married in Israel has been extremely limited. Because the marriage patterns of non-Jews (primarily Arabs) differ so markedly from those of Jews, the former are not discussed here.
2. Among couples who were married in Israel in the mid-1980s, approximately 10 percent had divorced within 10 years of marriage (Central Bureau of Statistics 2002). Period divorce rates in Israel have been consistently low. For example, in 1990, the crude divorce rate in Israel was 1.36 per 1,000, compared with 4.70, 2.94, and 2.50 in the United States, Canada, and Australia, respectively (United Nations 1994).
3. Approximately 30 percent of the couples in the sample included at least one spouse who was a third generation Israeli.
4. I categorized as Europeans all persons whose origins were in North or South America, as well as in Europe.
5. I did not include in the sample couples in which a spouse had immigrated to Israel in the period following 1983. Census data indicate that these recent immigrants form an essentially separate marriage market. Because the focus of this study was on the marriage behavior of persons of mixed ethnic backgrounds, I thought that the inclusion of post-1983 immigrants would complicate the analyses without further illuminating the topic of interest.
6. Because educational level is measured at the time of the census, rather than at the date of marriage, there is potential difficulty in identifying patterns of educational mating if there are substantial increases in educational attainment following marriage. However, increases in more than one or two educational categories between the marriage date and the census date are unlikely.
7. One well-recognized disadvantage of log-linear models is that they cannot account completely for the composition of a population because they do not control for the impact of individuals who remain unmarried during the period.
8. By "fitted frequencies," I mean fitted frequencies relative to the reference category of unions and net of the marginal and joint marginal distributions of the variables.
9. The BIC (Bayesian information criterion), developed by Raftery (1986), is a measure of goodness of fit that adjusts the G^2 statistic for sample size. More negative values of BIC indicate models that fit the data better.
10. I also estimated a model of ethnic mating with only one diagonal parameter fixing the extent of ethnic endogamy across ethnic groups, but found the fit of this model to be significantly inferior to that of Model 3. In addition, note that the variable diagonal model is also known as the *quasi-independence* model (Powers and Xie 2000).
11. Because of space considerations, statistical patterns of educational mating are not presented. The results in all models indicate that, as expected, the odds of marriage between persons with equal schooling are significantly higher than the odds of marriage between persons of unequal schooling, and the ratios of the odds increase as the difference in levels of schooling between spouses increases.
12. Relative fitted frequencies were computed by exponentiating estimated parameter values.
13. I also ran the model by categorizing couples by whether one or more spouses had matriculation diplomas or higher. In addition, I estimated various other types of models to test the assimilation hypothesis. Because of space considerations, these alternative models are not presented here. The substantive results in all estimated models were the same as those presented here. Details are available from me on request.

14. It is also the case that among Ashkenazim and persons of mixed ancestry, ethnic endogamy is significantly weaker among more-educated couples than among other couples. Thus, ethnicity appears to matter less among the more educated than among the less educated, as has been shown in other studies (see, e.g., Qian 1997).

References

Alba, R. D. 1990. *Ethnic Identity: The Transformation of White America.* New Haven, CT: Yale University Press.

Ben-Rafael, E. 1982. *The Emergence of Ethnicity: Cultural Groups and Social Conflict in Israel.* Westport, CT: Greenwood Press.

Ben-Rafael, E., and S. Sharot 1991. *Ethnicity, Religion, and Class in Israeli Society.* Cambridge, England: Cambridge University Press.

Central Bureau of Statistics. 2002. *Statistical Abstract of Israel, 2002.* Jerusalem: Israel Central Bureau of Statistics.

Cohen, Y., and Y. Haberfeld. 1998. "Second generation Jewish immigrants in Israel: Have the ethnic gaps in schooling and earnings declined?" *Ethnic and Racial Studies* 21: 507-528.

Coleman, D.A. 1994. "Trends in fertility and intermarriage among immigrant populations in Western-Europe as measures of integration." *Journal of Biosocial Science* 26: 107-136.

Cretser, G.A. 1999. "Cross-national marriage in Sweden: immigration and assimilation 1971-1993." *Journal of Comparative Family Studies* 30: 363-380.

Davis, K. 1941. "Intermarriage in caste societies." *American Anthropologist* 43: 388-395.

Eisenbach, Z. 1992. "Marriage and fertility in the process of integration: Intermarriage among origin groups in Israel." In Goldscheider (ed.), *Population and Social Change in Israel*, 131-147. Boulder, CO: Westview Press.

Eschbach, K. 1995. "The enduring and vanishing American Indian: American Indian population growth and intermarriage in 1990." *Ethnic and Racial Studies* 18: 89-108.

Eschbach, K. and C. Gómez. 1998. "Choosing Hispanic identity: Ethnic identity switching among respondents to high school and beyond." *Social Science Quarterly* 79: 74-90.

Eschbach, K., K. Supple and C.M. Snipp. 1998. "Changes in racial identification and the educational attainment of American Indians, 1970-1990." *Demography* 35: 35-43.

Friedlander, D., and C. Goldschcider. 1979. *The Population of Israel.* New York: Columbia University Press.

Friedlander, D., B. S. Okun, Z. Eisenbach and L. Lion Elmakias. 2002. "Immigration, social change and assimilation: Educational attainment among birth cohorts of Jewish ethnic groups in Israel, 1925-1929 to 1965-1969." *Population Studies* 56: 135-150.

Fu, Y. K. 2001. "Racial intermarriage pairings." *Demography* 38: 147-159.

Gans, H. 1979. "Symbolic ethnicity." *Ethnic and Racial Studies* 2: 1-20.

Goldscheider, C. 1996. *Israel's Changing Society: Population, Ethnicity, and Development.* Boulder, CO: Westview Press.

Gordon, M. M. 1964. *Assimilation in American Life: The Role of Race, Religion, and National Origins.* New York: Oxford University Press.

Gshur, B. and B. S. Okun. 2003. "Generational effects on marriage patterns: Jewish immigrants and their descendants in Israel." *Journal of Marriage and Family* 65: 287-301

Haberman, S.J. 1979. *Analysis of Qualitative Data,* Vol. 2. New York: Academic Press.

Harris, D. R. and J. J. Sim. 2002. "Who is multiracial? Assessing the complexity of lived race." *American Sociological Review* 67: 614-627.
Hirschman, C. 2003. "The rise and fall of the concept of race." Paper presented at the annual meeting of the Population Association of America, Minneapolis.
Hout, M., and J. Goldstein. 1994. "How 4.5 million Irish immigrants became 40 million Irish Americans: Demographic and subjective aspects of the ethnic composition of white Americans." *American Sociological Review* 59: 64-82.
Jones, N., and A. S. Smith. 2001. "The two or more races population: 2000." *Census 2000 Brief.* Washington, DC: U.S. Census Bureau. http://www.census.gov/prod/2001pubs/c2kbr01-6.pdf (accessed 1/8/06).
Kalmijn, M. 1991. "Shifting boundaries: Trends in religious and educational homogamy." *American Sociological Review* 56: 786-800.
Lieberson, S., and M. Waters. 1988. *From Many Strands: Ethnic and Racial Groups in Contemporary America.* New York: Russell Sage Foundation.
Lopez, D., and Y. Espiritu. 1990. "Panethnicity in the United States: A theoretical framework." *Ethnic and Racial Studies* 13: 198-224.
Marc, R. D. 1991. "Five decades of educational assortative mating." *American Sociological Review* 56: 15-32.
Massey, D. S. 1995. "The new immigration and ethnicity in the United States." *Population and Development Review* 21: 631-652.
Matras, J. 1973. "On changing matchmaking, marriage and fertility in Israel: Findings, problems and hypotheses." *American Sociological Review* 79: 364-388.
Merton, R. K. 1941. "Intermarriage and social structure." *Psychiatry* 4: 361-374.
Okun, B. S. 2001. "The effects of ethnicity and educational attainment on Jewish marriage patterns: Changes in Israel, 1957-1995." *Population Studies* 55: 49-64.
Partes, A. 1994. "Introduction: immigration and its aftermath." *International Migration Review* 28: 632-639.
Portes, A., and M. Zhou. 1993. "The new second generation: Segmented assimilation and its variants." *Annals of the American Academy of Political and Social Sciences* 530: 74-96.
Powers, D. A., and Y. Xie. 2000. *Statistical Models for Categorical Data Analysis.* San Diego, CA: Academic Press.
Qian, Z. 1997. "Breaking the racial barriers: Variations in interracial marriage between 1980 and 1990." *Demography* 34: 263-276.
Qian, Z. 2003. "Racial options: Racial identification of children of intermarried couples." Paper presented at the annual meeting of the Population Association of America, Minneapolis, MN.
Qian, Z., S. L. Blair and S. D. Ruf. 2001. "Asian American interracial and interethnic marriages: differences by education and nativity." *International Migration Review* 35: 557-586.
Qian, Z., and D. T. Lichter. 2001. "Measuring marital assimilation: Intermarriage among natives and immigrants." *Social Science Research* 30: 289-312.
Raftery, A. E. 1986. "Choosing models for cross-classifications." *American Sociological Review* 51: 145-146.
Rockquemore, K. A., and D. L. Brunsma. 2002. *Beyond Black: Biracial Identity in America.* Thousand Oaks, CA: Sage.
Rosen, S. 1982. "Intermarriage and the 'blending of exiles' in Israel." *Research in Race and Ethnic Relations* 3: 79-102.
Shavit, Y., and H. Stier. 1997. "Ethnicity and education in patterns of marriage in Israel: changes over time." *Megamot* 2: 207-225 (in Hebrew).

Smooha, S. 1993. "Class, ethnic and national cleavages and democracy in Israel." In E. Sprinzak and L. Diamond (eds.), *Israeli Democracy Under Stress,* 309-342. Boulder, CO: Lynne Rienner.

United Nations. 1994. *Demographic Yearbook,* 46th issue. New York: United Nations.

Waters, M. C. 1994. "Ethnic and racial identities of second-generation black immigrants in New York City." *International Migration Review* 28: 795-820.

Waters, M. C., and K. Eschbach. 1995. "Immigration and ethnic and racial inequality in the United States." *Annual Review of Sociology* 21: 419-446.

Xie, Y., and K. Goyette. 1997. "The racial identification of biracial children with one Asian parent: Evidence from the 1990 Census." *Social Forces* 76: 547-570.

9

Religiosity and Contraceptive Method Choice: The Jewish Population of Israel

Barbara S. Okun

Introduction and Background

The Jewish population of Israel comprises religiosity subgroups that are numerically important and that vary widely in fertility behavior. The primary purpose of this paper is to explore the relationship between religiosity and contraceptive method choice among married Jewish users of contraception in Israel.

Theoretical Considerations

There are a variety of possible effects of religion, religious denomination, and religiosity on fertility and contraceptive practices (see Goldscheider (1971) for a more complete discussion). The "characteristics" hypothesis states that differences in behavior among religious or ethnic groups are a function of the different social and economic characteristics of the groups. The "characteristics" hypothesis implies that no systematic behavioral differences remain once there are controls for socio-economic factors known to be important in determining fertility behavior.

The "particularized theology" proposition, also known as the "doctrine" hypothesis (DeJong 1965), posits that specific religious doctrines or teachings concerning fertility and contraceptive use influence behavior. An implication of the "particularized theology" hypothesis is that the effects of the doctrines are larger among the more religious sectors of the population, since these sectors are more likely to be influenced by the religious teachings. For example, DeJong (1965) suggested that Fundamentalist Protestants in rural Appalachian communities are influenced by their literal interpretation of the Biblical teaching to "be fruitful and multiply."

A different proposition, known as the "cultural" hypothesis, is that membership in a racial, ethnic, religious or religiosity group implies being part of a *social* community that may have pro-natalist or anti birth-control norms which increase fertility (Forste and Tienda 1996). The "cultural" hypothesis is distinct from the "particularized theology" hypothesis in the context of religious or religiosity differentials, in that group norms that affect fertility and contraceptive behavior are not necessarily operating through or driven by theological factors. Rather, the "cultural" hypothesis emphasizes that the effects of membership in certain ethnic, racial, religious, or religiosity groups operate through factors such as family and gender roles and the power of peer and community influence (Goldscheider and Mosher 1991). According to the "cultural" hypothesis, religious beliefs are part of a social system that shapes normative fertility and fertility control behaviors.

The "minority group status" hypothesis essentially states that there are interaction effects between membership in a minority group (racial, ethnic, or religious) and factors associated with the "particularized theology" and "cultural" hypotheses. That is, the effects of being affiliated with a specific religious group may differ depending upon whether that religious group comprises a minority or majority subpopulation within the greater society. The direction of the effect of minority group status on fertility is thought to depend on the desire and opportunity for upward social and economic mobility on the part of the minority group in question (Goldscheider 1971).

In addition to these hypotheses, we propose that religiosity may influence contraceptive prevalence and method choice by affecting the suitability of specific contraceptive methods to fertility control needs. For example, it is well-known that considerations of better health for mothers and children often motivate a desire for birth spacing, in a wide variety of contemporary and historical populations (Santow 1995). Contraceptive use for birth spacing (delaying the next birth), as opposed to limiting (preventing all future births), often requires the use of different birth control methods. It is clear, for example, that sterilization cannot be used for birth spacing. Similarly, use of the IUD for spacing is rather impractical, given its relatively large fixed costs in Israel: a doctor's visit for the purpose of insertion, the cost of which, approximately $125, is paid out-of-pocket by the woman, followed by another doctor's visit for the purpose of removal. Since religious women have different family-building strategies from secular women in that they may put different emphases on the relative importance of spacing and limiting, we posit that religiosity influences contraceptive method choice indirectly through its effects on the suitability of particular methods for contraceptive needs. We call this the "spacing versus limiting" hypothesis.

It is important to note that in general, the different hypotheses discussed above are not mutually exclusive. Only an extreme version of the "characteristics" hypothesis excludes the possibility of any of the others. Any or all of the hypotheses may contribute to an explanation of differentials in contraceptive practices by religiosity. Moreover, it may not be possible in every context to reach an unambiguous conclusion concerning the presence or absence of effects of each of the hypotheses. These considerations must be kept in mind in our analyses and interpretations below.

In one of the few recent studies of religion, religiosity, and contraceptive use, Goldscheider and Mosher (1991) essentially reject the "characteristics" and "particularized theology" hypotheses and conclude in support of the "cultural" hypothesis in the context of Christians in the United States. They conclude that there exist substantial net effects of religion and religiosity on sexual behavior and contraceptive practices that are not theologically derived. For example, Goldscheider and Mosher do not, in general, find a positive relationship among Catholic contraceptors between religiosity and rhythm use, despite the fact that the Catholic Church has condoned only the use of the rhythm method to prevent conception. Rather, they find evidence that greater religiosity among Catholics and Protestants is associated with greater use of male methods such as condoms and male sterilization, and less use of the birth control pill. Goldscheider and Mosher emphasize that the effects of religion and religiosity operate through gender relations and differ in various racial and ethnic groups.

The Setting

Differences in religiosity are associated with severe discordance among major segments of the Jewish population of Israel. Political, economic, and social conflicts are becoming increasingly dominant among the secular, religious, and ultra-orthodox segments of the population. Many conflicts revolve around differences in demographic patterns and labor market activities among the various groups.

Variation in fertility across Jewish subpopulations defined by religiosity is striking. Coupled with low, homogeneous levels of mortality across all sectors of the Jewish population, these fertility differentials lead to dramatic differences in natural growth rates across religiosity subgroups.

Friedlander and Feldmann (see chapter 2) write that the total fertility of secular women, particularly those of Eastern European descent, was at approximately replacement-level in the mid-1980s, while that of religious women was much higher. There is also a great deal of diversity within the religious sector. Of the roughly 20 percent of the Jewish population who are considered religious, the majority are well-integrated into Israeli society in terms of residential patterns, participation in military service, and patterns of labor force participation, and have high levels of total fertility of around 4.5. While there is no information on religiosity collected in censuses or large, nationally representative samples, it is believed that approximately one-third of the religious are ultra-orthodox.

The ultra-orthodox communities, which are in many senses separate from the mainstream of Israeli society, have extremely high total fertility, estimated at around 7.0 in the mid-1980s (Friedlander and Feldmann, see chapter 2). Members of these communities live in largely segregated neighborhoods and attend schools that are part of a separate educational system whose curricula contain few or no secular subjects. Moreover, ultra-orthodox males generally receive exemptions from otherwise mandatory three-year military service participation because they report organized religious study in yeshivas as their full-time vocation. In addition, prime-aged males have very low official rates of labor force participation as they continue studying in yeshivas for a substantial part of their active lives.

Differences in contraceptive use are of importance in explaining differentials in fertility by religiosity. A limited number of studies have been directed at exploring the relationship between contraceptive practices and religiosity within the Jewish population of Israel in the late 1960s and mid-1970s. While Hartman (1984) finds no evidence of a relationship between ever-use of contraception and religiosity in his sample of urban Israelis in the mid-1970s, Neuman and Ziderman (1986) conclude that current contraceptive prevalence declines with increasing religiosity in a 1968 sample of salaried workers. Schmelz (1989) also reports a negative relationship between religiosity and contraceptive use since last pregnancy among respondents to a maternity ward interview study in Jerusalem in the mid-1970s. Harlap (1980), using data collected in maternity wards in Jerusalem hospitals between November 1974 and December 1975, discusses differential contraceptive practices of postpartum mothers by religiosity. There has been no research that has focused on differentials by religiosity in *contraceptive method choice among contraceptors* using more recent, representative data sources. This is the primary purpose of our paper.

An abundant history, both ancient and modem, of rabbinical writings on the subjects of birth control and contraceptive methods provides us with a standard against which we can judge whether the use of various contraceptive methods is consistent with rabbinical teachings. The "particularized theology" proposition implies that the acceptability of the methods in the religious teachings will affect contraceptive choices, especially among the religious. Thus, the case of Judaism provides us with an excellent opportunity to test the "particularized theology" hypothesis.

An alternative proposition, in line with the "cultural" hypothesis, is that the specific teachings of the rabbinical writers on contraceptive use may have a less important effect on individual behavior than do community norms concerning fertility and fertility control. Although these indirect effects of religiosity on individual behavior via social norms are more difficult to test in a statistical sense, we are able to come to some preliminary understanding about these effects below.

In order to test for the "characteristics" hypothesis, we control for social and economic background factors, which may affect contraceptive method choice.

If net effects of religiosity remain even after we control for other background characteristics, then the "characteristics" hypothesis does not fully explain the relationship between religiosity and contraceptive method choice. In addition, we discuss the effects of the "spacing versus limiting" hypothesis. We do not deal with the "minority group status" hypothesis here since such considerations can best be made through comparative studies of religious groups in different contexts (see Anson and Meir, chapter 3) for a discussion of this issue in relation to differentials in Jewish fertility in Israel).

Jewish Teachings on Selected Reproductive Issues

The Acceptability of Various Contraceptive Methods According to Rabbinical Teachings

Our exposition on Judaism's teachings on contraceptive method choice is based on Feldman's (1995) text, which draws on a large literature of centuries of rabbinical writings. It is important to note at the start that there is no single source in Judaism concerning correct and proper behavior; rather there are multiple interpretations and scholarly interchanges concerning the Biblical teachings and oral traditions. Thus, there is often no consensus about any single issue, including contraceptive behavior. This said, we present here Feldman's main points, which characterize the essence of the rabbinical teachings.

Rabbinical writings note two fundamentally different purposes of marital sexual relations: 1) the commandment (*mitzvah*) of procreation (Be fruitful and multiply—*p'ru ur'vu*); and 2) the commandment of providing sexual pleasure for the wife (*onah*). Both commandments are directed only at the husbands, who are responsible for their fulfillment. While these two purposes of marital sexual relations are not generally at odds with each other, fulfillment of the second commandment of providing marital sexual pleasure is essential even when procreation is not feasible, as is the case, for example, when the wife is known to be sterile or pregnant. Further, specific acts of marital intercourse may be performed in fulfillment of sexual pleasure for the wife, even when pregnancy is a possible, though undesirable, consequence.

Pregnancy is seen as undesirable in a variety of circumstances, such as those involving a nursing mother whose young child would be prematurely weaned as a consequence of her becoming pregnant, or in other situations where pregnancy would threaten the fundamental health and welfare of existing children, or when pregnancy poses a threat to the health of the potential mother. In these cases, certain types of birth control may be used within marriage in order to fulfill the commandment of sexual pleasure, without the risk of pregnancy. Clearly, fertility control may be necessary for contraceptive spacing as well as limiting; the need for child spacing is generally motivated by consideration for the health of children and mothers. As Santow (1995) discusses, these motivations for child spacing are known to be widely held, in both historical and contemporary populations.

When the need for birth control is justified by any of the reasons discussed above, contraception should be used to prevent pregnancy and allow fulfillment of the commandment of providing sexual pleasure. Use of various forms of birth control is deemed acceptable, to the extent that the contraceptive methods do not involve improper emission of semen (*hash-hatat zera*), which is considered a terrible sin in rabbinical writings. The definition of what constitutes improper emission of semen is a matter of interpretation, and may be viewed in a variety of ways. According to a broad definition, improper emission is said to occur when sperm is "brought forth in vain." Since sperm is thought to be involved in the two functions of marital sex (procreation and marital sexual pleasure), some rabbinical writers conclude that improper emission has occurred only when *both* purposes of the semen have been frustrated. Thus, remarkably, the acceptability of a specific method of contraception depends upon the extent to which it is thought not to interfere with the sexual pleasure of the wife (Feldman 1995: 130)! Fulfillment of normal sexual relations and sexual pleasure is thought to require unimpeded physical contact between the man's sperm and the vaginal canal as is described by " ... he shall cleave unto his wife and they shall become as one flesh" (Genesis 2:24).

Feldman describes the acceptability of various contraceptive methods in terms of avoidance of improper emission of semen. At the bottom of the list in terms of acceptability is *coitus interruptus* (withdrawal) that is thought to interfere with normal sexual relations. Similarly, condoms are thought to interfere with the normal sex act, in the sense that there is no direct contact between the man's sperm and the vaginal canal. The diaphragm and cervical cap are much more acceptable, since they do not impede such contact. Even spermicides are better than condoms because coitus is thought to occur ". . . in the normal manner . . . , that is, unimpeded contact, with its normal gratifications" (Feldman 1995: 231). Rhythm certainly is free of any mechanical impediment to the sex act, but, like abstinence, rhythm frustrates the attainment of a woman's sexual pleasure, which is a serious shortcoming. The IUD poses a difficult problem because the mechanism by which the method operates is considered controversial by the rabbinical authorities. Therefore it is not entirely clear whether the IUD should be judged as a method of birth control or as a form of abortion. Post-coital contraception practiced by the woman, following "normal" sexual relations, is allowable by many rabbinical writers, since improper emission has not occurred. Thus, contraceptive douching, for example, would be allowable. Female sterilization (tubal ligation) is also permitted by Jewish law, since women, unlike men, are not required to procreate. However, female sterilization has the disadvantage of being permanent, which the rabbinical writers consider undesirable since the circumstances surrounding a desire to prevent childbearing may be only temporary. Male sterilization (vasectomy) is strictly forbidden as technical castration (Feldman 1995: 241). Finally, oral contraceptives (the birth control pill) are considered to be at the apex of the hierarchy of contraceptive methods because they absolutely do not interfere with coitus, and therefore allow unimpeded fulfillment of the wife's desire for sexual pleasure.

Other Religious Teachings on Reproductive Behavior, and their Applications

Another important point about rabbinical teachings on sexual affairs concerns regular attendance by women at a ritual bath (*mikveh*), where she is thought to be purified following the complete cessation of the menstrual period. During her menstrual period, and until she attends the ritual bath, the woman is considered "unclean" and must not engage in sexual relations. To change her status to one of purity, the woman must attend the bath, usually on the seventh day following the last day of the period. It is expected that couples will have intercourse immediately after the wife's immersion (Heilman 1992: 320).

Assuming that the menstrual period lasts approximately five days, and that the wife participates in the bath seven days after the end of the period, the first act of sexual intercourse following participation in the bath would likely occur just prior to the wife's ovulation, which is usually around the middle of the menstrual cycle. Acts of sexual intercourse just prior to ovulation have higher probabilities of resulting in pregnancy than acts timed differently. Thus, traditional mikveh attendance and subsequent sexual relations would increase the likelihood of pregnancy in each month. In an anthropological study of ultra-orthodox women in Jerusalem, Simon (1978) reports, however, that religious women exercise some discretion as to the exact timing of the bath attendance after the complete cessation of the menses. In particular, women who wish to avoid pregnancy in a particular month postpone attending the bath until after the fertile days have passed. A 1975-1976 study of fertility and contraceptive practices of maternity ward patients in Jerusalem found that, among the highly religious, postponement of the wife's attendance at the bath was the most widely reported method of contraception used in the last interpregnancy interval (Schmelz 1989). The ritual bath is a convenient method of contraception unnoticed by friends, neighbors, and possibly even husbands. In this way the contraceptive function is carried out, while there is still a semblance of appropriate behavior. This behavior is known to occur, despite the fact that, as mentioned above, periodic abstinence is a less rabbinically sanctioned method than others, such as oral contraceptives.

Also, breastfeeding for the purpose of fertility control was found to be comparatively frequent among the highly religious (Schmelz 1989). Extensive breastfeeding is promoted in rabbinical writings as beneficial to the health and development of the child (Feldman 1995). We see here again an interesting twist that women take on rabbinical teachings; they may breastfeed in accordance to the religious teachings, but for purposes in addition to, or in lieu of, those that were originally intended.

Popular Understanding and Behavior

Given the multitude of different interpretations of biblical law and oral tradition written by the rabbinical scholars, and the many subtleties of the arguments and counter-arguments presented by them, it is likely that popular understandings of rabbinical teachings may not coincide exactly with actual teachings, or may be applied selectively when convenient (Goldscheider 1971). For example, although use of birth control is acceptable under certain circumstances, and even recommended in situations such as those mentioned above, in ultra-orthodox communities there may be a general understanding that use of contraceptives is forbidden in all cases, simply because the practice is not generally permitted. Moreover, there may be a reluctance on the part of couples to make it seem as if they are controlling fertility, since this practice is not understood to be generally acceptable.

In addition, individual behavior among religious subpopulations may not be consistent with either rabbinical teachings, or with popular understandings of rabbinical teachings. We suggest, rather, that individual behavior may affect, as well as be affected by, rabbinical teachings and popular understandings of them. Conflicts that may arise between individual motivations and rabbinical teachings, or popular understandings thereof, may result in adjustments in behavior and norms that are a compromise between these elements. The role of local rabbis, who interpret the law in the context of the members of their community and advise the members accordingly, may be important in understanding the ongoing dynamic between individual behavior and socio-religious norms.

Data, Variables and Methods

The principle source of data used in this paper is a survey entitled "The 1987-1988 Study of Fertility and Family Formation," carried out by the Hebrew University School of Public Health. A description of the survey and various analyses that focus on Israeli fertility can be found in Peritz and Baras (1992). Contraceptive prevalence rates computed from the survey data are reported in Okun (1997). The survey provides the most recent, publicly-available data on contraceptive use among a representative sample of married Jewish women in Israel. Conducted in Hebrew, the survey included 1,751 Jewish, urban, currently-married women aged 22-39 and contains information on current contraceptive method used at the time of the survey. Since approximately 90 percent of the Jewish population in Israel reside in urban areas, the exclusion of rural women from the survey is largely immaterial. Indeed, given the great differences between Israel's rural and urban populations, (for example, special kibbutz populations are included as rural), an analysis of the urban population separately is desirable.

Women were shown a list of contraceptive methods, and were asked to select one of the following as their current method: withdrawal (coitus interruptus, outside); safe days (rhythm); condom (rubber); spermicides (jelly, suppositories, foams, paste); diaphragm or cervical cap; IUD (loop); oral contraceptives (pills); sterilization (male or female); other; none. This information allows us to report on levels of contraceptive prevalence and the distribution of use by method.

In addition to the information on contraceptive use, much detailed information was collected concerning other behavioral, attitudinal, demographic, and socioeconomic factors. In our analyses of contraceptive method choice, our focus, beyond socioeconomic factors and sex role attitudes and behaviors shown to be important in previous research (Okun 1997), will be on the effects of religiosity.

The survey contains detailed information concerning the religiosity of the female respondent and that of her husband. The information includes self-reported religiosity of the respondent and the respondent's report on the religiosity of her husband in four categories of increasing religiosity (secular, traditional, religious, and ultra-orthodox). Also, the survey contains respondents' reports on her and her husband's behavioral adherence to several specific commandments of Judaism. Women were asked whether they adhere to commandments (*mitzvot*) by: 1) not traveling on the Sabbath; 2) separating meat and dairy dishes in the home (an indicator of a kosher home); 3) fasting on the Holy Day of Yom Kippur; 4) refraining from eating leavened foods during the Passover holiday; and 5) attending the ritual bath regularly. Women were also asked how often their husbands pray at the synagogue (daily, weekly, at holidays only, at high holidays only, not at all, don't know), and whether it is customary to recite prayers (kiddush) in their home on Friday nights.

Table 9.1 provides distributional information regarding respondents' self-reported religiosity, respondents' reports of husband's religiosity, and fulfillment of some of the behavioral commandments, for the 1,732 respondents with valid data on religiosity variables. As is indicated in Panel A, approximately 50 percent of women defined themselves as secular, an additional 36 percent as traditional, 10 percent as religious, and 4 percent as ultra-orthodox. Respondents' reports on their husbands' religiosity reveal a similar distribution. Panel A indicates that there is a large positive association between the religiosity of spouses. Panel B indicates general consistency between self-reported religiosity and reported adherence to selected commandments, in that the proportion of women who fulfill commandments increases with the self-reported religiosity.

However, some of the questions on specific commandments were less informative than others, simply because a large majority of all women, even those who considered themselves secular, adhered to them. For example, fasting on Yom Kippur was performed by over 80 percent of the respondents, including nearly two-thirds of the self-reported secular respondents. Performance of this ritual is so firmly entrenched among virtually all Jewish Israelis, that it cannot be used effectively to identify the degree of religiosity.

Also, the data indicate that the fulfillment of certain commandments is a more refined indicator of religiosity than is the fulfillment of others. For example, nearly 95 percent of women who do not travel on Sabbath also separate meat from dairy dishes (not shown in the table). The converse, however, does not hold; only about 50 percent of women who separate meat from dairy dishes refrain from traveling on the Sabbath. Thus, we conclude that not traveling on the Sabbath indicates greater religiosity than does separating meat and dairy dishes. Similarly, the vast majority of women who attend the ritual bath regularly also separate meat and dairy dishes, while the converse is true only 50 percent of the time.

Clearly, religiosity takes on a continuum of values, and is not uni-dimensional in character. Theoretical considerations discussed above along with results from a variety of data analyses suggested that we present here two alternative

Table 9.1
Indicators of Religiosity: Descriptive Statisitcs

Panel A: Percent distribution of paired responses of interviewees' self-reported religiosity and interviewees' reports on husbands' religiosity

	Respondents' reports on husbands' religiosity				
	Secular	Traditional	Religious	Ultra-orthodox	Row total (in percents)
Respondents' self-reported religiosity					
Secular	47.3	2.4	0.1	0.0	49.8
Traditional	6.2	28.0	1.6	0.0	35.9
Religious	0.5	0.5	8.9	0.2	10.1
Ultra-orthodox	0.0	0.1	0.0	4.2	4.2
Column total (in percents)	54.1	31.0	10.6	4.3	100.0

Note: N = 1732.

Panel B: Association between respondents' self-reported religiosity and fulfillment of selected religious commandments. Figures are row percentages

	Respondents' reports on fulfillment of religious commandments			
	Regularly attend ritual bath (mikveh)	Do not travel on the Sabbath	Separate meat and dairy dishes	Fast on the Holy Day of Atonement
Respondents' self-reported religiosity				
Secular (N = 863)	3	2	14	64
Traditional (N = 621)	22	23	63	97
Religious (N = 175)	82	96	100	99
Ultra-orthodox (N = 73)	99	96	100	100
All respondents (N = 1732)	22	23	44	81

measures of religiosity in our models of contraceptive method choice. These two measures are self-reported religiosity of the respondent, and whether the respondent reports that she regularly attends the ritual bath. The measure of adherence to the rabbinical teachings regarding ritual bath attendance has particular relevance to contraceptive issues, particularly use of the rhythm method, as described above. Other measures of religiosity which were used in analyses not presented here depend on: 1) reported fulfillment of commandments such as refraining from traveling on the Sabbath; 2) fulfillment of different combinations of commandments, and 3) amalgamations of self-reported religiosity and commandment fulfillment. These other measures of religiosity led to generally similar results, although parameter coefficients on the religiosity covariates were sometimes smaller in size and had lower statistical significance.

Our first step is to estimate contraceptive prevalence by religiosity, and then to utilize Bongaarts' model of the proximate determinants of fertility in order to check consistency of reported contraceptive use with information about fertility and its other proximate determinants (Bongaarts 1978). Then we consider how women from different religiosity subgroups differ from each other with regard to socioeconomic and other explanatory variables. Finally, we rely on logistic regression methods for our multivariate analyses of method choice among current contraceptive users, by religiosity.

Results

Descriptive Statistics

Tables 9.2a and 9.2b present contraceptive prevalence, and the distribution of users by method, for married, urban, Israeli Jews, and for subsamples defined by various measures of religiosity. Table 9.2a indicates that, as can be expected, contraceptive prevalence declines with increasing religiosity, whether religiosity is self-reported or defined by ritual bath attendance. Since the number of ultra-orthodox women in the sample was small, we were not always able to analyze this subgroup separately. We therefore generally present results for the combined sample of religious and ultra-orthodox women. Heterogeneity in this subsample must be kept in mind during the analyses presented below.

While there is no specific information collected in the survey concerning breastfeeding that is intentionally prolonged or intensified for the purpose of birth spacing, we have little evidence to support the widespread existence of this behavior. Breastfeeding is fairly short among Israeli Jews, even among the ultra-orthodox, who tend to breastfeed longer than other Jewish mothers. Median duration of full (partial) breastfeeding of the penultimate child is approximately four (eight) weeks for secular women, six (eight) weeks for traditional women, eight (twelve) weeks for religious women, and eight (fifteen) weeks for ultra-orthodox women. Fewer than 10 percent of the ultra-orthodox women reported even partially breastfeeding their penultimate child for more than nine months, and more than half of the ultra-orthodox women reported initiating some bottle-feeding within two months.

The information presented in table 9.2, supplemented with information from the survey concerning breastfeeding behavior and use of abortion, and estimates concerning proportions married in five-year intervals by religiosity allow for the application of Bongaarts' (1978) framework of proximate determinants. In

Table 9.2
Contraceptive Prevalence and Use by Method, Jewish Population of Israel (1987-88), by Various Indicators of Religiosity

Religiosity subgroup	All methods	With-drawal	Condom	IUD	Vaginal barrier methods or spermicides	Rhythm	Sterili-zation[b]	Pill	All other methods[c]
A. Percentage distribution of married couples[a]									
All women (N = 1703)	68	11	4	30	4	4	0.9	13	1.1
Secular[d] (N = 849)	74	12	5	35	4	3	0.6	14	0.8
Traditional[d] (N = 614)	69	12	4	28	3	5	1.5	13	1.5
Religious[d] (N = 172)	62	8	2	27	8	4	1.2	10	1.7
Religious and ultra-orthodox[d,e] (N = 240)	48	5	2	21	6	4	0.8	8	1.3
Does not attend mikveh regularly (N = 1330)	73	12	5	34	4	4	0.8	13	1.1
Attends mikveh regularly (N = 373)	54	7	2	19	5	5	1.6	13	1.3
B. Percentage distribution of married contraceptive users									
All users (N = 1165)	100	16	6	45	6	6	1.4	19	1.6
Secular[d] (N = 625)	100	16	6	47	5	5	0.8	19	1.1
Traditional[d] (N = 424)	100	17	6	41	4	8	2.1	19	2.1
Religious[d] (N = 106)	100	12	4	43	12	7	2.0	17	3.0
Religious and ultra-orthodox[d,e] (N = 116)	100	11	3	43	13	9	1.7	16	2.6
Does not attend mikveh regularly (N = 965)	100	16	6	46	5	6	1.0	18	1.5
Attends mikveh regularly (N = 200)	100	13	5	36	9	9	3.0	25	2.5

[a] The figures are based on current contraceptive practices of 1703 married women aged 22–39 in the 1987–88 survey. This number includes women who are currently pregnant, and therefore not practicing contraception. These women were included in the analysis to make the results comparable to other studies of contraceptive prevalence, which do not exclude pregnant women. The 1703 women excludes those with missing information on current method or religiosity, but includes others who are excluded from analyses in the rest of the paper because they had missing values for at least one of the explanatory variables, other than religiosity.

[b] Includes male and female sterilization.

[c] Includes deliberate postponement of mikveh.

[d] Respondent's self-reported religiosity.

[e] The sample of ultra-orthodox women was too small to be analyzed separately, so they are grouped here with religious women. Among ultra-orthodox women, 15% reported using a contraceptive method at the time of the survey.

results not presented here, we find that the reported contraceptive prevalence of approximately 60 percent among women who define themselves as religious is consistent with estimates from Friedlander and Feldmann (see chapter 2), based on entirely different sources, of total fertility among this subgroup of approximately 4.5. The small number of women who define themselves as ultra-orthodox report contraceptive prevalence of 15 percent which, according to Bongaarts' model, is too low to be consistent with Friedlander and Feldmann's estimate of total fertility of around 7.0. Thus, there is probably under-reporting of contraceptive use among this subgroup of women. This finding is not surprising, given the religious and social norms in favor of high fertility among this very selected subgroup. However, since the ultra-orthodox women are a small part of the sample, and since the focus of our research is on method choice among contraceptive users, rather than on contraceptive prevalence itself, we feel that this under-reporting does not seriously bias our results.

Table 9.2b presents the distribution of current contraceptive use by method among current users of contraception. Overall, we see that Israeli Jews do not use sterilization to any significant extent; only about 1 percent of married Israeli Jews relied on either male or female sterilization in 1987-1988. Instead, Israeli reliance on the IUD is substantial; approximately 45 percent of current Jewish contraceptors use the IUD. Use of withdrawal in 1987-1988 among current Jewish users (about 16 percent) is rather high for a developed country. In contrast, use of another male method, the condom, is relatively limited among Israeli Jews. Reliance on rhythm and vaginal barrier methods or spermicides is also not widespread, but as we shall see, their use is more common among certain subsamples. Pill use is about average for a developed country. For a more detailed discussion of general trends in contraceptive use among married Israeli Jews, see Okun (1997).

Statistics presented in table 9.2b suggest that the use of withdrawal, and perhaps condoms, is less common among contraceptive users who define themselves as religious or ultra-orthodox, or who regularly attend the ritual baths, than among other users. Also, reported reliance on the IUD is less common among contraceptive users who regularly attend the ritual bath than among other users. In contrast, use of vaginal barrier methods or spermicides, and use of the rhythm method, appear more common among self-described religious and ultra-orthodox contraceptive users, and among those who regularly attend the ritual baths, than among other contraceptive users. Finally, reported pill use is higher among contracepting ritual bath attenders than among other contraceptive users.

The results in table 9.2b suggest that religious users of contraception tend to rely more heavily on certain methods of birth control and less on other methods, compared with other users of contraception. However, these findings do not control for socioeconomic and other explanatory variables that may affect contraceptive method choice. To the extent that contraceptive users in different religiosity subgroups differ from one another with respect to socioeconomic and other factors, the bivariate relationships suggested in table 9.2 may be spurious. In table 9.3, we examine the characteristics of contraceptive users in different religiosity subgroups. The table shows that users of contraceptives in different religiosity subgroups are roughly similar to each other in terms of their average age and proportion with less than twelve years of completed schooling, but are quite different from each other in terms of other factors. Relative to other birth controllers, religious users of contraception have, on average, a larger number of children as of the survey date, are more likely to be planning an additional child within the next three years, and are more likely to live in a household with family income in the bottom fortieth percentile of the distribution. In terms of gender system variables, religious users of contraception are more likely to view men as the authority in fertility-control decision-making—that is, they are less likely to disagree fully with the statement that wives may use birth control only with their husbands' consent. Also, religious users of contraception tend to exhibit a slightly greater degree of gender specialization in household/childcare responsibilities—that is, in their households, it is more often the case that as many household/childcare responsibilities are performed solely or primarily by one spouse as are shared equally by the spouses.

Table 9.3
Characterisitcs of Married Contraceptive Users, by Degree of Religiosity. Figures are Means (Standard Deviations in Parentheses)

	All women (N = 1043)	Secular and traditional women (N = 941)	Religious and ultra-orthodox women (N = 102)	Do not regularly attend ritual ritual bath (N = 863)	Regularly attend bath (N = 180)
Demographic factors					
Age	32.4 (4.7)	32.4 (4.7)	32.4 (5.2)	32.6 (4.7)	31.2 (5.0)
Parity	2.7 (1.1)	2.6 (1.1)	3.5 (1.4)	2.6 (1.0)	3.2 (1.5)
Low motivation for family planning					
Plan to have a(nother) child within the next 3 years (1 if Yes, 0 if No)	0.29 (0.45)	0.28 (0.45)	0.39 (0.49)	0.28 (0.45)	0.33 (0.47)
Socio-economic status					
Low household income (1 if Yes, 0 if No)	0.42 (0.49)	0.39 (0.49)	0.61 (0.49)	0.37 (0.48)	0.65 (0.48)
Respondent has less than 12 years education (1 if Yes, 0 if No)	0.35 (0.48)	0.34 (0.48)	0.38 (0.49)	0.34 (0.47)	0.38 (0.49)
Gender system					
Specialization in household/ childcare responsibilities (1 if Yes, 0 if No)	0.86 (0.35)	0.85 (0.36)	0.88 (0.32)	0.85 (0.36)	0.88 (0.33)
Respondent views men as authority in fertility-control decision-making (1 if Yes, 0 if No)	0.40 (0.49)	0.37 (0.48)	0.65 (0.48)	0.36 (0.48)	0.57 (0.50)

Notes: N = 1043.

Logistic Regression Analyses—Effects of Religiosity on Contraceptive Method Choice

Tables 9.4a and 9.4b present parameter estimates from logistic regression models of current contraceptive method choice. Use of each major method of contraception discussed above is analyzed in separate models. In each model, independent variables are used to predict the odds of use of a particular method versus use of any other method.

We note that only women who report that they are currently using a method of contraception are included in the analyses; non-users are not of interest to us here, because our focus is on *method choice.* Thus, we are, in some sense, assuming a two-stage decision-making model whereby women (or couples) initially decide whether they will currently use a contraceptive method, and then subsequently choose a method from the available selection. Of course, this simple model may be inaccurate if, for example, the availability or accessibility of certain methods affects the decision of whether to contracept.

In the upper panel of the table, models include only the religiosity factors as explanatory variables. In the lower panel, all of the other explanatory variables are included as well. Therefore, comparisons between the coefficients on the religiosity factors in the upper and lower panels show the extent to which socioeconomic and other differences among religiosity subgroups may lead to spurious relationships between religiosity and contraceptive method choice.

Table 9.4a

Logistic regression models of current contraceptive methos choice. Figures are parameter estimates (p-values in parentheses)

	Effect on log Odds of					
	Withdrawal vs. All other methods		Condom vs. All other methods		IUD vs. All other methods	
	(1)	(2)	(3)	(4)	(5)	(6)
Models with religiosity factors only:						
Religious or ultra-orthodox	−0.56* (0.10)	NIM	−0.53 (0.31)	NIM	−0.07 (0.73)	NIM
Attends ritual bath regularly	NIM	−0.45* (0.25)	NIM	−0.28 (0.45)	NIM	−0.40** (0.02)
Models with all explanatory factors included:						
Religiosity						
Religious or ultra-orthodox	−0.72** (0.05)	NIM	−0.24 (0.66)	NIM	0.01 (0.97)	NIM
Attends ritual bath regularly	NIM	−0.59** (0.03)	NIM	0.03 (0.94)	NIM	−0.30 (0.11)
Demographic factors						
Age 22–24	0.12 (0.77)	0.15 (0.72)	−0.14 (0.84)	−0.15 (0.83)	−0.81** (0.03)	−0.77** (0.05)
Age 30–34	0.40 (0.13)	0.38 (0.15)	0.50 (0.20)	0.51 (0.19)	0.08 (0.67)	0.04 (0.81)
Age 35–39	0.55** (0.05)	0.51* (0.07)	0.29 (0.48)	0.30 (0.47)	0.27 (0.18)	0.23 (0.25)
CEB 0–1	−0.03 (0.94)	−0.02 (0.97)	0.15 (0.77)	0.17 (0.74)	−0.87*** (0.00)	−0.90*** (0.00)
CEB 3 plus	−0.54** (0.02)	−0.53** (0.02)	−0.36 (0.25)	−0.39 (0.22)	0.29* (0.07)	0.34** (0.04)
Low motivation for family planning						
Plan to have a(nother) child within the next 3 years	0.22 (0.32)	0.19 (0.39)	−0.43 (0.22)	−0.45 (0.20)	−0.31* (0.06)	−0.30* (0.07)
Socio-economic status						
Low household income	0.33* (0.08)	0.37** (0.05)	−0.38 (0.21)	−0.40 (0.20)	−0.22 (0.12)	−0.18 (0.20)
Respondent has less than 12 years education	0.87*** (0.00)	0.87*** (0.00)	−0.61* (0.08)	−0.60* (0.08)	−0.07 (0.62)	−0.09 (0.55)
Gender system						
Specialization in household/ childcare responsibilities	0.41 (0.07)	0.40 (0.16)	−0.49 (0.12)	−0.49 (0.12)	0.13 (0.50)	0.13 (0.50)
Respondent views men as authority in fertility-control decision-making	0.44*** (0.01)	0.44*** (0.01)	−0.09 (0.74)	−0.11 (0.69)	−0.33*** (0.01)	−0.30** (0.02)

Notes: N = 1043. NIM = Not in model.

*** $p <= 0.01$; ** $p <= 0.05$; * $p <= 0.10$ for two-sided tests.

Table 9.4b
Logistic Regression Models of Current Contreceptive Method Choice. Figures are Parameter estimates (p-values in Parentheses)

Explanatory variables	Effect on log Odds of					
	Rhythm vs. All other methods		Vaginal barriers or spermicides vs. All other methods		Phill vs. All other methods	
	(7)	(8)	(9)	(10)	(11)	(12)
Models with religioisity factors only:						
Religious or ultra-orthodox	0.28 (0.48)	NIM	0.95** (0.01)	NIM	−0.05 (0.27)	NIM
Attends ritual bath regularly	NIM	0.57** (0.05)	NIM	0.45 (0.16)	NIM	0.44** (0.02)
Models with all explanatory factors included:						
Religiosity						
Religious or ultra-orthodox	0.02 (0.96)	NIM	0.94*** (0.01)	NIM	-0.03 (0.92)	NIM
Attends ritual bath regularly	NIM	0.50 (0.12)	NIM	0.48 (0.16)	NIM	0.30 (0.17)
Demographic factors						
Age 22–24	1.18** (0.05)	1.11* (0.07)	0.25 (0.66)	0.23 (0.68)	0.28 (0.35)	0.25 (0.42)
Age 30–34	0.61 (0.15)	0.68 (0.11)	−0.15 (0.72)	−0.17 (0.68)	−0.68*** (0.00)	−0.65*** (0.00)
Age 35–39	0.65 (0.15)	0.73 (0.11)	0.48 (0.26)	0.50 (0.24)	−1.78*** (0.00)	−1.73*** (0.00)
CEB 0–1	−0.89 (0.15)	−0.82 (0.18)	0.09 (0.85)	0.02 (0.96)	0.80*** (0.00)	0.83*** (0.00)
CEB 3 plus	0.40 (0.23)	0.30 (0.36)	−0.27 (0.45)	−0.20 (0.56)	−0.01 (0.96)	−0.07 (0.74)
Low motivation for family planning						
Plan to have a(nother) child within the next 3 years	0.65** (0.04)	0.62** (0.05)	0.61* (0.06)	0.70** (0.03)	0.00 (0.99)	−0.01 (0.96)
Socio-economic status						
Low household income	0.02 (0.94)	−0.06 (0.83)	−0.20 (0.51)	−0.20 (0.52)	0.25 (0.17)	0.20 (0.26)
Respondent has less than 12 years education	−0.43 (0.15)	−0.39 (0.20)	−0.13 (0.68)	−0.15 (0.64)	−0.21 (0.31)	−0.18 (0.37)
Gender system						
Specialization in household/ childcare responsibilities	0.05 (0.90)	0.05 (0.88)	−0.38 (0.27)	−0.36 (0.29)	−0.10 (0.68)	−0.10 (0.67)
Respondent views men as authority in fertility-control decision-making	0.22 (0.40)	0.17 (0.53)	0.24 (0.40)	0.29 (0.30)	−0.08 (0.66)	−0.12 (0.51)

Notes: N = 1043. NIM = Not in model.
*** p <= 0.01; ** p <= 0.05; * p <= 0.10 for two-sided tests.

In each panel, we report the results of two separate models for each major method. In the first model for each method, a woman is defined as having a high degree of religiosity if her self-description is religious or ultra-orthodox. We note that while table 9.1 reports that 14.3 percent of the overall sample of women described themselves as religious or ultra-orthodox, only 10.2 percent of *current contraceptive users* describe themselves in this way. This finding clearly follows from the fact that religious women are less likely to report currently using contraceptives than other women. Further, women who described themselves as "traditional" did not appear to behave differently from the "secular" women with regards to contraceptive method choice, in almost every model examined. Thus, we chose not to present the models that include a dummy variable set equal to one if the respondent described herself as "traditional." In the first models presented for each major method in each panel, the reference category of women is, therefore, all those who do not describe themselves as either religious or ultra-orthodox.

In the second model, religiosity is defined by whether the woman reports regular attendance at monthly ritual baths. We note that reported ritual bath attendance is apparently a less selective criterion than is self-reporting as religious or ultra-orthodox. Approximately 17 percent of current contraceptive users regularly attend the ritual baths, while only about 10 percent of current users describe themselves as religious or ultra-orthodox. In addition to a large majority of the self-reported religious or ultra-orthodox women who attend the ritual baths, approximately 22 percent of current users who describe themselves as traditional also attend regularly. Fewer than 3 percent of self-described secular users report that they attend the ritual baths regularly. Since self-described traditional women are more numerous than religious or ultra-orthodox women among all contraceptive users, just over 45 percent of ritual bath attendees who use contraceptives do not describe themselves as religious or ultra-orthodox. Thus, for some women who regularly attend ritual baths, their behavior may be better understood as a cultural practice than as a strict identifier of religiosity.

Table 9.4a reports parameter estimates from logistic regression models of withdrawal use, condom use, and IUD use, while table 9.4b reports estimates from models of use of rhythm, vaginal barrier methods or spermicides, and the pill. In each model, the dependent variable takes on the value one if the woman reports that she is currently using the specific method under analysis, and it takes on the value zero if she reports using a different method.

In all of the models, we include a number of other explanatory variables known to be of importance in contraceptive method choice. Current age is split into categories: 22-24, 30-34 and 35-39 (25-29 is the reference category). Current parity is categorized as zero or one live birth, or three or more live births, with two live births as the reference category. If respondents report that they plan to have a(nother) child within the next three years, then we code them as having low motivation for family planning. Indicators of low socioeconomic status are whether the female respondent lacks at least twelve years of education (dummy variable set to one if so), and whether the respondent lives in a household with family income in the bottom fortieth percentile of the distribution (dummy variable set to one if so). We also include the two gender system dummy variables described above in the discussion of table 9.3. These two variables were shown to be important in models of withdrawal use, as reported in Okun (1997). The construction of these variables was motivated by Santow's (1993) suggestion that certain aspects of the gender system may be related to withdrawal use in low fertility countries where other means of fertility control are available.

Models that included other explanatory variables, in addition to those described above, were estimated; however, in almost every case, the estimated coefficients for these variables were not statistically significant or sizable. In addition, their inclusion did not significantly affect the estimated coefficients on the religiosity variables. These other explanatory variables, not included in the final models presented in tables 9.4a and 9.4b, were: 1) whether the respondent was employed in the week prior to the survey; 2) whether the respondent had served in the military; 3) whether the respondent's husband had less than twelve years of formal education; and 4) country of origin of the respondent or the respondent's father (ethnicity). In addition, we did not find any significant interaction effects between ethnicity and measures of religiosity, in contrast to previous research, based on data in the 1960s, which did suggest that such effects may be present (Matras and Auerbach 1962).

Our main interest centers on the effects of the two measures of religiosity on the dependent variables. We note that in both the upper and lower panels, model: 1) suggests that the use of withdrawal rather than another method is significantly less likely among religious or ultra-orthodox users of contraception than among other users of birth control. The same result holds in both panels of model: 2) where religiosity is parameterized by attendance at the ritual bath; that is, the husbands of women who regularly attend the baths are significantly less likely than other men to practice withdrawal. In the lower panel, the parameter estimates in models (1) and (2) translate into 51 percent lower odds and 45 percent lower odds of withdrawal use.

It is interesting that in the upper and lower panels, models (3) and (4) show no effects of religiosity on the odds of condom use in our sample, despite as strict religious objections to its use as to withdrawal. We note that our multivariate models of condom use are poor in that there is only one statistically significant explanatory variable in each (women's education). Apparently, condom use is determined by factors unavailable to us in this analysis.

In the upper panel, model (6) suggests that ritual bath attendance significantly reduces the odds of IUD use relative to use of other methods, based on two-tailed tests. Although the effect is weaker in the lower panel, we can still reject the hypothesis that ritual bath attendance increases the odds of IUD use, in a one-tailed test. In neither the upper or lower panel, does model (5) indicate that self-described religiosity affects the odds of IUD use.

In neither the upper or lower panels does model (7) indicate that self-described religiosity affects the odds of rhythm use. Further investigation reveals, however, that a different multivariate model that includes three separate dummy variables for self-reports of being "traditional," "religious," and "ultra-orthodox" results in highly significant and sizable positive coefficients on the "traditional" and "ultra-orthodox" dummy variables, and only a weakly positive coefficient on the "religious" dummy variable. Thus, it appears that ultra-orthodox users of contraception are more likely to rely on rhythm than other users, while religious, but not extremely religious women, who are much more modernized and integrated into Israeli society, do not. It seems likely that rhythm may be practiced by the ultra-orthodox in the context of postponement of the ritual bath attendance, although we do not have direct evidence from the survey to indicate that this is the case. In addition to ultra-orthodox women who use rhythm, a relatively large proportion of "traditional" women who attend the ritual baths also use rhythm, though probably not for the same reasons as the ultra-orthodox women. The "traditional" women may feel more comfortable with a method such as rhythm which they may consider more "natural," and therefore more desirable than more medical or "artificial" methods such as the pill or IUD (Basker 1986). In the upper panel, model (8) shows that women who regularly attend the ritual bath are more likely to rely on rhythm than other birth controllers, but this effect does not retain its statistical significance in the multivariate analysis in the lower panel.

Models (9) and (10) in table 9.4b report results of our analyses of use of vaginal barrier methods (the diaphragm or cervical cap) or spermicides. Here we note a very strong and significant, positive effect of self-described religiosity in both the upper and lower panels. The coefficient on self-report as religious or ultra-orthodox translates into 156 percent greater odds of use of these methods in the multivariate model. Also, while the coefficients on ritual bath attendance are not statistically significant from zero at conventional levels in a two-sided test, we can reject the null hypothesis that the coefficient in the multivariate model is less than or equal to zero in a one-sided test, at the 10 percent level of significance.

Finally, models (11) and (12) report results from the analyses of pill use. Neither multivariate model shows any strong effect of religiosity on pill use, despite the rabbinical writings in favor of their use. We note, however, that in the upper panel, model (12) indicates that contraceptive users who attend the ritual baths are more likely to use the pill than other birth controllers. Also, in a one-sided test, we can reject the null hypothesis that the coefficient on ritual bath attendance in the lower panel is less than or equal to zero, at the 10 percent level of significance. In all, though, we have only weak support for the proposition that religiosity is positively associated with pill use among current contraceptors. These results will be discussed in the next section.

We briefly note here other important effects on contraceptive method choice that appear in the various models. A further discussion of the correlates of contraceptive method choice among the Jewish population of Israel can be found in Okun (1997). Age is an important determinant, in almost every model. Women aged 22-24 are less likely to use the IUD and more likely to use rhythm than women aged 25-29 (the reference category). Women aged thirty and older are more likely to use withdrawal and less likely to use the pill than women aged 25-29. Women with no or one live birth are less likely than women with two births to be using the IUD, which is understandable in light of medical recommendations against IUD use among nulliparous women. Women with three or more children arc the most likely to be using the IUD, possibly because they desire long-term contraception for the purpose of stopping or significantly delaying further childbearing. Women who report planning another child within the next three years are less likely than other women to be using the IUD. These women are more likely to use vaginal barrier methods, spermicides, or rhythm. Women with less than twelve years of education are much more likely to rely on men to practice withdrawal than are other women. Finally, women whose marriages are characterized by greater specialization in household/childcare tasks, and who view men as the authority in fertility-control decision-making, are more likely to be rely on men to practice withdrawal. Interestingly, these women are no more likely than other women to rely on men to use condoms.

Discussion

The multivariate results presented above indicate that religious and ultra-orthodox women, as well as women who regularly attend the ritual bath, are significantly less likely than other women to rely on men to practice withdrawal, and are much more likely to use vaginal barrier methods or spermicides, as well as rhythm. There seems to be no significant effect of religiosity on condom or pill use. We return now to a consideration of the hypotheses that relate religiosity to contraceptive method choice, in light of these empirical results.

Clearly, the "characteristics" hypothesis does not fully explain the association between greater religiosity and contraceptive method choice, since strong effects of religiosity remain, after controlling for various socio-economic characteristics in the sample. Comparisons between the upper and lower panels of the different models indicate that in only three of the twelve cases does the statistical significance of the parameter estimates differ in the bivariate and multivariate models. Even in these cases, the directions of the effects are consistent in both types of models. Therefore, we conclude that controlling for various explanatory variables does not affect our qualitative conclusions, and that the "characteristics" hypothesis explains little of the association between religiosity and contraceptive method choice among Jewish Israelis.

When we consider the "particularized theology" hypothesis, we note that some of our results are consistent with this hypothesis, while others are not. Our interpretation, discussed below, is that the effects of the "particularized theology" hypothesis are sometimes reinforced and sometimes counterbalanced by effects of the "cultural" and "spacing versus limiting" hypotheses. With large desired family sizes, religious birth controllers are more often motivated by a desire for fairly short-term birth spacing than for limiting the total number of births. In contrast, secular Jews, who have smaller desired family sizes, may more often be motivated by the desire to postpone the onset of childbearing for a significant period of time, and later to stop childbearing altogether. Therefore, religious Jews, more so than secular Jews, may prefer methods of contraception that are easily used sporadically and for relatively short periods of time. More generally, the specific fertility control needs of couples must be kept in mind in analyses of contraceptive method choice.

We will now interpret the results of our statistical analyses, in light of these considerations. The strong negative effects of religiosity on use of withdrawal are consistent with religious teachings, and thus provide support for the "particularized theology" hypothesis. It is interesting to note that while Goldscheider and Mosher (1991) report greater use of male methods (condom and male sterilization) among religious Catholics and Protestants in the U.S., we find here significantly less use of the male method of withdrawal among religious subgroups of Israeli Jews.

Our results do not indicate consistent effects of religiosity on IUD use. There were no significant effects of self-described religiosity on the odds of IUD use, and there was a significant negative effect of ritual bath attendance only in the bivariate model. As mentioned above, there is little rabbinical writing that details opinion on the IUD, since its precise mechanisms of action are open to debate. It is important to keep in mind, however, that there are relatively large fixed costs involved in IUD use. Therefore, women who are interested only in short-term or sporadic use of contraception would not likely be interested in the IUD. Thus, it is possible that the dummy variable for ritual bath attendance may be capturing some unmeasured desire for short-term or sporadic contraceptive use. While we do include in our analyses a dummy variable coded one if the respondent reports that she plans to have a(nother) child within three years, this variable cannot capture fertility plans for the more short-term future.

An alternative interpretation of the negative effect of ritual bath attendance on IUD use revolves around a common side effect associated with IUD use—bleeding and spotting between periods. Since ritual bath attendance is permitted only when the woman is not bleeding, troublesome irregular spotting between periods can be a reason that ritual bath attenders prefer not to use the IUD (Dr. Elchanan Bar-On, obtetrician and gynecologist, Jerusalem, Israel, Personal Communication, 1999).

Rhythm presents an interesting case. Our results indicate greater use of rhythm by more religious women. While rhythm is not an ideal method by rabbinical standards, since it frustrates the mitzvah of marital sexual pleasure, it is nonetheless a highly convenient method, particularly for those women who regularly attend the monthly ritual baths. Rhythm is amenable to use for birth spacing. Its use can be short-term and sporadic. It requires no trips to the doctor or pharmacy. For ultra-orthodox women, trained at the time of marriage to be alert to the timing of the end of menstruation, which is generally followed shortly thereafter by attendance at the bath and a resumption of sexual relations, no simpler method presents itself than postponement of ritual bath attendance by a few days in order to avoid the period of ovulation. This explanation may be behind the very large association between ultra-orthodoxy and rhythm use.

As discussed above, rabbinical writers condone use of vaginal barrier methods and spermicides, since they are thought not to interfere with normal sexual relations, as does withdrawal. Our results indicate that use of the vaginal barrier methods and spermicides is, indeed, more common among religious contraceptors than among other users. However, the "spacing versus limiting" hypothesis offers a plausible alternative to the interpretation that the women's behavior is strictly theologically derived. For example, for religious women, vaginal barrier methods and spermicides may be particularly convenient, since, like the rhythm method, they are well-suited to fertility control behavior motivated by a desire for short-term spacing of births. Vaginal barrier methods and spermicides can easily be used sporadically, and for short spans of time, and thus require no long-term commitment to contraceptive use on the part of the respondent. No insertion or medical follow-up is necessary, and discontinuation of use is followed immediately by a return to full fecundability. In the case of the diaphragm or cap, use is not directly noticeable by the husband; thus, for women who need short-term contraception that can be used without husband's knowledge or consent, these methods are practical, and considered acceptable by rabbinical authorities.

In terms of pill use, we note that, in contrast to expectations based on rabbinical writings, there seems to be at most a weak positive effect of religiosity on pill use among contracepting women. Our interpretation of this finding is that religious women who are interested in sporadic and short-term birth control may find the pill inconvenient. The pill must be used regularly and consistently, is not fully effective immediately upon initiation of use, and generally comes with a medical recommendation for a waiting period of a few months following cessation of use (in order to restore the normal cycle of menses) before a woman attempts to get pregnant. Thus, it appears that specific fertility control needs may counterbalance religious teachings in determining pill use among religious women.

In conclusion, we find that neither the "characteristics" nor the "particularized theology" hypotheses provide complete and consistent explanations of the observed behavior of Israeli Jews. With respect to the "characteristics" hypothesis, we note that important differences in contraceptive method choice by religiosity remain even after controlling for socioeconomic variables. With respect to the "particularized theology" hypothesis, results concerning withdrawal use and reliance on vaginal barrier methods and spermicides are as predicted by the hypothesis, but findings concerning condom, rhythm, and pill use are not consistent with the hypothesis. Our conclusion is that the contraceptive choices of religious women are determined largely by considerations unrelated to religious doctrine. A combination of factors, including the suitability of specific methods to fertility control needs, peer influences, and other cultural effects, appear to modify the acceptance and application of a particular religious theology.

Acknowledgments

This research was supported by Grant 0321212 from the Israel Academy of Sciences and Humanities. The author acknowledges the helpful comments of Zvi Eisenbach, Dov Friedlander, Calvin Goldscheider and Guy Stecklov on previous versions of this paper. Particular thanks are due to Jona Schellekens for suggesting this general line of research.

References

Basker, Eileen. 1986. "The 'natural' control of fertility." *Sociology of Illness and Health* 8: 3-25.

Bongaarts, John. 1978. "A framework for analyzing the proximate determinants of fertility." *Population and Development Review* 4: 105-132.

DeJong, Gordon E. 1965. "Religious fundamentalism, socio-economic status, and fertility attitudes in the Southern Appalachians." *Demography* 2: 540-548.
Feldman, David M. 1995. *Birth Control in Jewish Law.* New York: New York University Press.
Forste, Renata, and Marta Tienda. 1996. "What's behind racial and ethnic fertility differentials?" *Population and Development Review* 22 (Supplement): 109-133.
Goldscheider, Calvin. 1971. *Population, Modernization, and Social Structure.* Boston, MA: Little, Brown and Company.
Goldscheider, Calvin, and William D. Mosher. 1991. "Patterns of contraceptive use in the United States: The importance of religious factors." *Studies in Family Planning* 22: 102-115.
Harlap, Susan. 1980. "Contraceptive use by Jerusalem mothers with special reference to orthodoxy, ethnic group and husband's and wife's education." In U. O. Schmelz, P. Glikson and S. DellaPergola (eds.), *Papers in Jewish Demography* 1977. Jerusalem: Institute of Contemporary Jewry, Hebrew University of Jerusalem.
Hartman, Moshe. 1984. "Pronatalistic tendencies and religiosity in Israel." *Sociology and Social Research* 68: 247-258.
Heilman, Samuel. 1992. *Defenders of the Faith: Inside Ultra-Orthodox Jewry.* New York: Schocken Books.
Matras, Judah, and Chana Auerbach. 1962. "On rationalization of family formation in Israel." *The Milbank Memorial Fund Quarterly* 40: 453-480.
Neuman, Shoshana, and Adrian Ziderman. 1986. "How does fertility relate to religiosity: Survey evidence from Israel." *Sociology and Social Research* 70: 178-180.
Okun, Barbara S. 1997. "Family planning in the Jewish population of Israel: Correlates of withdrawal use." *Studies in Family Planning* 28: 215-227.
Peritz, Eric, and Mario Baras (eds.). 1992. *Studies in the Fertility of Israel.* Jerusalem: Institute of Contemporary Jewry, Hebrew University of Jerusalem.
Santow, Gigi. 1993. "*Coitus interruptus* in the twentieth century." *Population and Development Review* 19: 767-792.
Santow, Gigi. 1995. "*Coitus interruptus* and the control of natural fertility." *Population Studies* 49: 19-43.
Schmelz, Uziel O.1989. "Religiosity and fertility among Jews of Jerusalem." In Uziel O. Schmelz and Sergio DellaPergola (eds.), *Papers in Jewish Demography* 1985, 157-185. Jerusalem: Institute of Contemporary Jewry, Hebrew University of Jerusalem.
Simon, Rita James, 1978. *Continuity and Change: A Study of Two Ethnic Communities in Israel.* Cambridge: Cambridge University Press.

10

Socioeconomic and Cultural Determinants of Abortion Among Jewish Women in Israel

Esther I. Wilder

Introduction

Abortion is a sensitive topic that has evoked strong reactions from women's rights advocates, political leaders, and religious authorities in Israel. The political establishment has generally regarded the practice of induced abortion with disfavor, and while abortion is legal in Israel, an authorized abortion is difficult to obtain in a city such as Jerusalem where the religious authorities exercise considerable influence and there is notable anti-abortion activity (Golan 1987). For example, the Jerusalem-based organization Efrat, the International Organization for Saving Jewish Babies, actively lobbies against abortion. The abortion issue is further complicated by the reluctance of the Israeli government to take a strong stance in favor of family planning. Previous studies of reproductive behavior in Israel have indicated an inverse association between abortion rates and contraceptive use (Sabatello 1990; Slonim-Nevo 1988). To the extent that abortion rates are high among certain groups, further efforts to promote family planning are warranted.

Israeli society provides an ideal setting for exploring the relationship between immigration, ethnicity, and patterns of induced abortion. The population of Israel has been formed largely through successive waves of immigration from several continents. The country, therefore, constitutes a demographic laboratory, as it includes ethnic and religious subpopulations at varying stages of socioeconomic development ranging from traditional to modem. In this setting it is possible to analyze the interacting effects of religion, ethnicity, socioeconomic development, and international migration on patterns of fertility control and population growth (Nigem and Nagi 1988). The combination of geocultural origin and length of residence in Israel has been central to the analysis of fertility differentiation and transition within the country's Jewish population.

Over the years, Israel's ethnic groups have experienced dramatic declines (and accompanying convergences) in both fertility desires and family size. While considerable research has been devoted to the fertility behavior and contraceptive practices of ethnic and religious subpopulations in Israel, few studies have examined the determinants of variation in the practice of abortion. Most early work was limited to univariate description or standardized estimates that did not control for the full range of variables affecting the likelihood of having an induced abortion. This study fills a void in the literature by: 1) documenting the role of socioeconomic and cultural variables in shaping patterns of abortion among Jewish women in Israel at different stages of the development process, and 2) identifying trends in the practice of induced abortion over time. In addressing these key concerns, this analysis indicates where resources should be channeled to further reduce abortion rates in Israel.

Induced Abortion in Israel

For a timeline of legislation and important developments regarding the practice of induced abortion in Israel, see table 10.1. Until the 1970s abortion in Israel was regulated by the Mandatory Palestine legislation based on a British anti-abortion law of 1861. Regulations concerning abortion were extremely strict, as they stemmed from the British Offences Against the Person Act of 1861. Under this law, both performing and receiving an abortion were offences punishable by imprisonment (for fourteen and five years, respectively) (Bachi 1970; Sabatello and Yaffe 1988; Yishai 1978). In 1936 the Criminal Code Ordinance of Mandatory Palestine legislation, based on the British anti-abortion law of 1861, made it illegal to request or perform an abortion (Slater et al. 1978; Yishai 1993). The conditions under which an abortion might be allowed—safeguarding the woman's life or health—were not specified in the law; they were the result of court decisions (Yishai 1993).

Through the years, a variety of changes have occurred in the law regulating induced abortion in Israel. In 1952, the Haifa District Court declared abortions permissible if performed for medical reasons (Bachi 1970; Sabatello and Yaffe 1988; Slater et al. 1978; Yishai 1978). The Attorney General recommended that no prosecutions should be made on charges involving induced abortions except in special circumstances (such as abortions terminating in the death of the woman) because such prosecution "did not constitute an act of public interest" (Sabatello and Yaffe 1988). In 1963 these instructions were repealed. Three years later the abortion law was liberalized so that it was no longer illegal for women to seek an abortion and the maximum term of imprisonment for the person performing the abortion was reduced to five years (Yishai 1978).

Because abortions were permitted for "medical reasons" after 1952, many hospitals established pregnancy termination committees to consider requests

Table 10.1
Abortion in Israel, 1861-1980

Year	Political Development/Legislation
1861	UK Parliament Offences Against the Person Act of 1861: Abortion is illegal.
1936	Abortion is regulated by the Criminal Code Ordinance of 1936 Mandatory Palestine legislation based on the British anti-abortion law of 1861. It is illegal to request or perform an abortion.
1948	The British act is incorporated into the Israeli system.
1952	The Haifa District Court declares abortions permissible if performed for 'bona fide medical reasons' and without concealment. After this judgment, the Attorney General recommends that no prosecutions should be made on charges involving induced abortions except in special circumstances, such as abortions terminating in the death of the woman.
1963	Instructions from the Attorney General are repealed.
1966	The abortion law is liberalized so that it is no longer a crime for a woman to seek an abortion. The maximum term of imprisonment for the person performing the abortion is reduced to five years.
1971	A private member bill submitted by a member of a small liberal party demands legalization of abortion.
1973	The 1971 bill is struck down.
1975	Two private member bills on abortion are placed on the Knesset agenda. The first bill cites 'the basic human right of deciding whether or not to bring a child into the world.' Accordingly, any woman would have the right to ask her physician to terminate her pregnancy within the first trimester. The second bill stipulates that abortions would be permissible under specified circumstances if authorized by a board of experts and carried out in a recognized medical institution.
1977	The second of the two 1975 bills is passed. Committees composed of two qualified medical practitioners and a social worker are established in authorized hospitals and clinics and can grant a woman an abortion under one or more of the following conditions: 1. The woman is under legal age (17 years) or over forty. 2. The pregnancy resulted from an illicit (rape, incest) or non-marital relationship, irrespective of the woman's marital status. 3. The foetus is suspected to have physical or mental malformations. 4. Continuing the pregnancy may endanger the woman's life or health (either physical or mental). 5. Family or social circumstances (economic conditions of the woman, the presence of numerous or very young children, etc.) dictate an abortion. Duration of pregnancy is not a factor in the decision to allow an abortion, nor is parental permission required for minors.
1978	The 1977 law is enacted.
1979	It is decided that at least one member of every abortion committee must be a woman. The government presents a bill to repeal Article 5 of the Abortion Law. A tie vote in Parliament (Knesset) defeats this proposal. However, one month later (on 11 December 1979) the clause is repealed.
1980	The Abortion Law is amended as a result of the December 1979 ruling. Article 5 (the social clause) of the 1977 law is abolished.

Sources: Bachi 1970; Friedlander 1973; Sabatello 1992; Sabatello and Yaffe 1988; Schiff 1981; Slater et al. 1978; Yishai 1993.

for abortions, and by the early 1970s the majority of hospitals had established such committees, consisting of gynecologists, psychiatrists, and social workers (Slater et al. 1978). Although the committees were fairly liberal in granting abortions, a number of problems remained: relatively few requests were brought forth, since the existence of the committees was not publicized or well-known; abortion decisions were often quick and arbitrary; and if the woman was married, the husband's consent was required (Yishai 1978). As a result, many women resorted to private and illegal abortions.

Although illegal abortions were widespread during Israel's formative years, the parties involved were seldom prosecuted (Sabatello 1992, 1995). The glaring disparity between Israel's law and actual practice was considered undesirable by policy makers and led to demands from various quarters to enact a new abortion law entirely (Bachi 1970, 1977; Schiff 1981). In 1971, a member of a small, liberal party submitted a private member bill demanding the legalization of abortion. The bill was struck down two years later (Yishai 1993). At that time, a Committee on the Study of Abortion, appointed by the Health Minister, recommended that under certain specified conditions and with the approval of a professional board, abortions should be allowed if performed by qualified physicians in authorized medical institutions (Yishai 1993).

In January 1975 two private member bills on abortion were brought before the Knesset. The first bill cited "the basic human right of deciding whether or not to bring a child into the world" (Yishai 1993). Accordingly, any woman would have the right to a first trimester abortion. The second bill favored allowing abortions under certain conditions if authorized by a board of experts and performed in a recognized medical institution. In 1977, the second of the two bills was approved. Although abortion was banned in principle, physicians were authorized to perform the operation at General Sick Fund clinics for a wide range of medical, personal, and socioeconomic reasons (Sabatello and Yaffe 1988). The bill, enacted in February 1978, stated that committees composed of two qualified medical practitioners and a social worker could be established in any authorized hospital or clinic and could grant a woman an abortion after obtaining her informed consent under one or more of the following conditions:

1. The woman is under the legal marriage age (seventeen years) or over forty.
2. The pregnancy resulted from an illicit (rape, incest) or non-marital relationship, irrespective of the woman's marital status.
3. The fetus is suspected to have physical or mental malformations.
4. Continuing the pregnancy may endanger the woman's life or health (physical, mental, or both).
5. Family or social circumstances (economic hardship, the presence of numerous or very young children, etc.) dictate an abortion.

Informed consent was defined as "written consent to the abortion after the physical and mental risks involved [had] been explained to the woman" ("Abortion in Israel" 1978). Minors were not required to obtain parental permission. A qualified medical practitioner could not perform an abortion unless he notified the Director General of the Ministry of Health within five days that the operation was necessary to save the life of the woman or that the abortion occurred in the course of other medical treatment ("Abortion in Israel" 1978). Any person who performed an abortion beyond the law was liable to five years' imprisonment.

The legalization of abortion did not, however, mark the end of the abortion issue on the political agenda. In November 1979, at the behest of a small but powerful Orthodox religious party, the government presented a bill to repeal Article 5, which allowed abortions for "social" reasons. Although a tie vote in the Parliament defeated this proposal, the clause was repealed one month later and in February 1980 the new policy disallowed abortions for social reasons. This occurred despite the fact that public opinion polls showed that a sizable majority of Israelis favored a woman's right to terminate a pregnancy on social grounds (Yishai 1993). The law enacted in 1978, with the 1980 amendment, remains in effect today.

The 1977 Law of Pregnancy Interruption requires those hospitals that have authorized committees for pregnancy termination to report their monthly activities to the Ministry of Health (Central Bureau of Statistics 1993). Until 1987, these reports consisted of the number of pregnancy interruptions, the clinic where the abortion occurred, the ownership of the clinic, and the legal article on which the approval of the abortion was based. Beginning in 1988 the reports also included the number of applications and the number of approvals (Central Bureau of Statistics 1993). These data reveal very high rates of approval (over 90 percent) and in 1997 approximately 95 percent of applications were approved (Central Bureau of Statistics 1998). At the same time, there has been a moderate decline in abortion rates over time. Figure 10.1 presents rates of pregnancy terminations in hospitals from 1979 to 1997.

While over 300,000 Soviet Jews arrived in Israel during the early 1990s, these data do not reveal any increase in abortion rates associated with this influx. This is surprising given the widespread use of abortion among Soviet women. During the late 1980s the total abortion rate (TAR) in the U.S.S.R was close to 3.0 (Sabatello 1992).

It is possible that higher rates of abortion among foreign-born women have been counterbalanced by declines in abortion rates among native-born Israeli women. It is also the case that data from the Central Bureau of Statistics do not fully reveal trends in abortion rates since these figures include only legal abortions. Along with those women who do not have a legitimate (legal) reason for seeking an abortion, there are probably many others who opt for illegal abortions rather than going through the formal application process. While estimates of the number of illegal abortions are controversial and vary widely, Sabatello

Figure 10.1
Rates of Pregnancy Termination in Hospitals in Israel, 1979-1997.

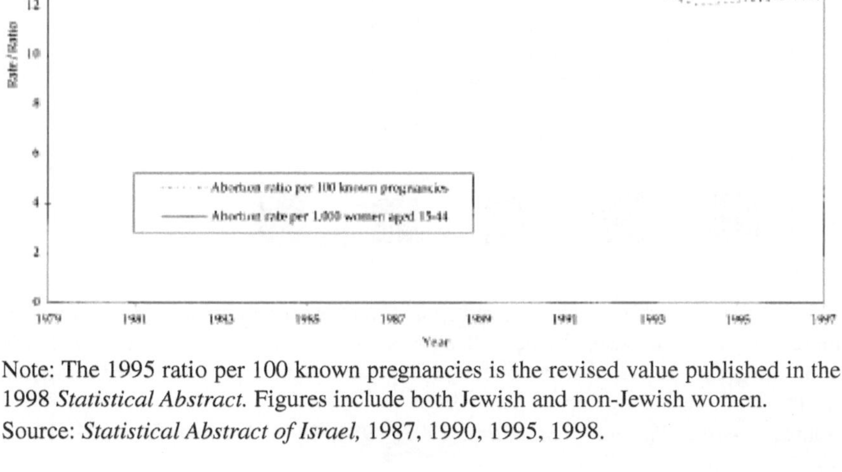

Note: The 1995 ratio per 100 known pregnancies is the revised value published in the 1998 *Statistical Abstract.* Figures include both Jewish and non-Jewish women.
Source: *Statistical Abstract of Israel,* 1987, 1990, 1995, 1998.

(1990) estimated that illegal abortions constituted between 25 and 30 percent of the total number of abortions in Israel from 1980 and 1983. Moreover, Slater and associates (1978) report that the overwhelming majority of women who are denied legal abortions in Israel do obtain illegal abortions.

As abortion rates have declined, there has also been a shift in the conditions under which the abortions are approved. (See figure 10.2.) For example, from 1981 to 1984, 34 percent of approved pregnancy terminations were in response to "danger to a woman's life"; from 1995 to 1997, only 24 percent. At the same time, there has been a sizeable growth in the proportion of abortions that are authorized for "out of wedlock pregnancies." From 1981 to 1984, out of wedlock pregnancies comprised 40 percent of actual terminations, whereas they constituted 50 percent during the 1995-1997 period.

In 1997, the ultra-Orthodox Shas party introduced (but failed to pass) a bill that defined an embryo as a human being from the day of conception. If the law were approved, it would have allowed abortion practitioners to be tried for first-degree murder (Osborne 1997). In contrast, the current abortion law does not limit abortion to the early months of pregnancy (Sabatello 1992). Sick funds typically cover the costs of the procedure for minors and for women who have

Figure 10.2
Hospital Abortions in Israel by Reason for Pregnancy Termination, 1981-1997.

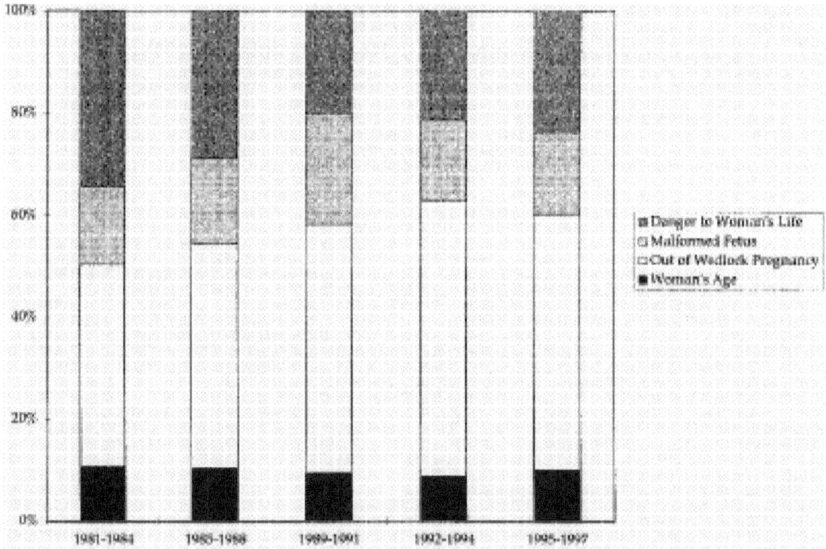

Note: Data for abortion by articles of law are available for 1979 and 1980, but during these years abortions were also permitted for family or social circumstances. The 1979-1980 categories are therefore not directly comparable to those presented above. Figures include both Jewish and non-Jewish women.
Source: *Central Bureau of Statistics,* 1983, 1984, 1986, 1987, 1990, 1991, 1995, 1998.

medical grounds for abortion. Abortions due to rape are funded by government welfare agencies, although full payment has been provided only since October 1991 (Sabatello 1995). Otherwise, the woman pays the equivalent of U.S. $250-400, depending on the hospital, for the procedure and associated care (Sabatello 1992, 1995). Abortion is widely available in Israel, and 95 percent of Israeli women have access to moderately priced abortion (Population Crisis Committee 1991).

Determinants of Abortion and Research Hypotheses

The likelihood of having an induced abortion is shaped by macro-level structural factors (family planning policies and contraceptive availability) as well as the individual socio-demographic characteristics of the women and their partners. In Israel, abortion was used extensively in the 1950s and 1960s as a standard method of limiting births. This has been attributed in part to insufficient knowledge of other birth control methods. While general social acceptance of abortion as a means of regulating fertility is likely to have grown over the years, reliance on induced abortion has probably declined due to the widespread adoption of efficient contraceptive practices.

Meanwhile, the extent to which Israel's subpopulations resort to induced abortion varies by ethnicity. Early studies of family planning in Israel indicated that Jewish childbearing women of European origin were more likely to have practiced abortion than women from the less developed countries of the Middle East, Asia, and Africa (Bachi 1970; Bachi and Matras 1962; Matras and Auerbach 1962; Yaffe 1976). While suggestive, these studies have been primarily descriptive. Further research is required to reveal the independent effects of ethnicity in a multivariate framework.

One of the fundamental problems in the study of abortion among ethno-religious groups in Israel is the lack of consensus about the best way to define and characterize ethnicity within the country's Jewish population. There are disagreements among sociologists concerning the relative importance of religious-cultural and economic factors in the identity and formation of ethnic groups. This debate about the strength of ethnic boundaries is also complicated by disagreement over the relative importance of boundaries based on the many communities of origin (e.g., Moroccans, Yemenites, etc.), broad regions of origin (Eastern Europe or Asia), and even larger continental groups (e.g., Europe-America or Asia-Africa) (Goldscheider 1995). An understanding of ethnic variation in rates of abortion in Israel requires an examination of the diverse political and socio-cultural environments of the state's ethno-immigrant communities, both in Israel and abroad.

Israeli women trace their origins to a diverse group of countries that—both historically and today—vary tremendously in social norms regarding the practice of induced abortion. The majority of African and Asian immigrants arrived from countries where abortion remained illegal or restricted to the termination of pregnancies on medical grounds. Even today abortion is permitted only to save a woman's life in several African and Arab Middle Eastern countries (e.g., Libya, Syria) and it is allowed only under strict indications such as safeguarding the mother's physical (e.g., Kuwait, Morocco) and/or mental (e.g., Algeria, Iraq) well-being in many other countries in the region (Rahman et al. 1998). In many of these cultures, abortion has not gained acceptance as a legitimate mode of fertility regulation.

In contrast, many of the countries of Eastern Europe have had liberal abortion laws for many decades. Following the example of the USSR, the socialist countries of Eastern Europe, with the exception of Albania and the German Democratic Republic, liberalized their abortion laws throughout the 1950s and 1960s (Tietze 1983). More recent data reveal that Soviet immigrants to Israel initially exhibit abortion rates considerably higher than those observed nationwide. Within a relatively short time, however, they make the transition to more efficient methods of birth control and reduce their abortion rates accordingly (Sabatello 1995).

In Western Europe until the mid-1970s, abortion was legally available only when the pregnancy threatened the woman's life (van der Tak 1974). The nations of Western Europe, with the exception of the Nordic countries and Great Britain, had restrictive abortion laws until January 1974, but shortly thereafter Austria, France, the German Federal Republic, and Italy eased their abortion laws (Tietze 1983). Although abortion was socially unacceptable—even viewed with hostility—Western European women are thought to have relied upon abortion to prevent births (as a supplement to abstinence, withdrawal, and traditional forms of birth control) prior to the liberalization of abortion laws in the region. Over time, the social disapproval of abortion has subsided. Due to the importance of immigrant ancestry, abortion rates in Israel are likely to vary according to ethnicity. Specifically, ethno-immigrant groups with liberal views toward abortion are likely to make greater use of the procedure to eliminate unwanted pregnancies.

Jewish religious doctrines also circumscribe appropriate roles for men and women, stipulating the conditions under which induced abortion is justifiable. Although Jewish law condones the use of abortion when the fetus poses a serious physical or psychological threat to the well-being of the mother, the use of abortion as a method of birth control is proscribed (Biale 1995; Feldman 1975, 1984; Margolies 1970; Silber 1980). Although many Jews are probably unaware of these specific guidelines, the religious population maintains strong social norms against abortion. Previous research has documented an inverse association between religiosity and the acceptance of abortion (Notzer et al. 1984), and highly religious Jewish women may be less likely to admit having had an abortion because of the social ban on the practice (Schmelz 1989). Overall, there is likely to be an inverse association between religiosity and the practice of induced abortion.

Women's education is another component of female status and autonomy with important implications for the practice of induced abortion. The inverse association between women's education and fertility is generally attributed to the higher opportunity costs of childbearing as well as an expanded knowledge of effective contraceptive methods. Meanwhile, the effects of education on the likelihood of obtaining an abortion are less straightforward. Judith Blake (1971) found education to be a very strong correlate of attitudes toward abortion; both men and women with high levels of education exhibited more liberal views. It is unclear, however, whether these favorable attitudes toward abortion result in higher abortion rates among the educated. It has been suggested that better educated women experience greater opportunity costs in carrying a pregnancy to term (Gober 1994) and that the desire for fewer children among the educated may result in a lowered tolerance for unplanned births, thereby increasing the likelihood of abortion (Powell-Griner and Trent 1987). Moreover, better-educated women tend to have more information about abortion services as well as greater financial resources with which to obtain these services.

The positive association between education and abortion is likely to be mediated by the use of contraception, however. In a situation of limited access to contraception, women with higher socioeconomic status are often the first to control their fertility with abortion (Humphries 1980). As efficient methods of birth control become increasingly available, educated women are likely to be the first to rely on such techniques and, consequently, the least likely to experience unwanted pregnancies. Thus, while educated women are likely to have more liberal attitudes toward abortion as well as greater information about the procedure, they are also more likely to use efficient contraception, thereby avoiding unwanted pregnancies. In Israel, therefore, we expect the effect of education to have varied over time due to changes in the availability of modem contraceptives. Specifically, the effect of education in reducing rates of abortion is likely to be more pronounced in 1987-1988 than in 1974-1975.

Like education, women's employment is expected to influence fertility desires and to provide a channel for the acquisition of knowledge about the various methods of fertility control, including abortion. Specifically, working women may gain knowledge about abortion services through friends and associates at the workplace. They may also find greater social approval of abortion among their working peers. Conversely, women who work outside the home are also more likely to gain exposure to information about efficient contraception, and the increased autonomy that is associated with employment may increase a woman's willingness to take an active role in planning her fertility. As with education, then, the effect of women's employment on the practice of induced abortion is likely to vary according to contraceptive availability (and consequently, to vary over time).

In sum, we view abortion as an indicator of women's autonomy. Socioeconomic and cultural characteristics that promote female empowerment are expected to increase the likelihood of abortion, except when these same characteristics encourage the use of contraception (which would avert the need for abortion). On the other hand, those factors and conditions that emphasize traditional gender role divisions are unlikely to provide women with the freedom to exercise complete control over their reproductive behavior, and will, therefore, discourage the practice of abortion.

Sources of Data

Data for this study were drawn from two national surveys of the fertility of married women in Israel: the 1974-1975 Israel Fertility Survey and the 1987-1988 Study of Fertility and Family Formation. These are the only two nationally representative surveys of the reproductive behavior of married Jewish women in Israel. While the Central Bureau of Statistics gathers monthly data on pregnancy terminations, this information does not permit us to determine the full range of variables affecting abortion rates in Israel. The 1974-1975 and 1987-1988 surveys provide us with the unique opportunity to assess how the impact of a wide range of socioeconomic and cultural determinants of abortion has changed over time among Jewish women in Israel.

The 1974-1975 Israel Fertility Survey was administered to a random sample of Israel's urban Jewish population—persons living in cities of 30,000 or more (Goldscheider and Friedlander 1981). Only currently married Jewish women, in their first marriage and below age fifty-five, were eligible for inclusion in the survey. The sampling frame followed the model employed by the Central Bureau of Statistics of Israel for its sample surveys: a list of dwelling units was selected from the municipal housing lists and systematic samples of units were drawn in proportion to population size (Goldscheider and Friedlander 1980). The fieldwork began in April 1974 and was completed in early 1975. The response rate was 89 percent and a total of 3,250 interviews were completed. Interviews were conducted face-to-face by trained female interviewers and the quality of the data is considered quite high.

The 1987-1988 Study of Fertility and Family Formation was conducted from August 1987 to November 1988. This survey was part of a larger project financed by the Israeli Government and conducted chiefly by the Ministry of Labor and Social Welfare. The 1987-1988 Study of Fertility and Family Formation consisted of three components: 1) a comprehensive study of Jewish fertility; 2) an investigation of Moslem fertility; and 3) a study of fertility on the kibbutzim. This analysis is limited to the first group, namely, to Jewish women living in areas with populations of 5,000 or greater. According to the 1983 census, the overwhelming majority of married women (89.5 percent) lived in such localities (Keysar et al. 1992).

The 1987-1988 study was based on a nationally representative sample of currently married Jewish women (ages 22-39) who lived in Israel at the time of the survey. The national sampling design relied on names obtained from the

Israel Population Register, which provided the survey team with information on the age, marital status, religion, and area of residence of the women (Kupinsky 1992). Some divorced and widowed women, persons residing abroad and other ineligible persons were excluded at the interviewing stage. In a few cases, address corrections were found in the files of the National Insurance Institute (Keysar et al. 1992). Although the original goal was to interview 2,500 women, only 2,452 were actually eligible because a number of the women in the sampling frame (2,770 women) had changed their marital status, moved to small towns, or emigrated. The overall response rate was 71.4 percent (1751/2452). If we exclude those who could not be located, the survey's response rate climbs to 84 percent (16 percent refusal rate).

The twelve-to-fourteen-year time lapse between the 1974-1975 and 1987-1988 surveys allows for the possibility of overlap in the cohorts represented in the two studies. Although the surveys did not interview the same women, it is important to note that the cohort of women aged thirty-four to thirty-nine in 1987-1988 was also represented in the 1974-1975 survey.

While we cannot determine the precise characteristics of non-respondents, researchers have reported that for both surveys (1974-1975 and 1987-1988), the majority of women who refused to participate were very religious (ultra-Orthodox) (Keysar et al. 1992; Lawton 1988). The exclusion of these women is likely to result in estimates that overestimate the extent to which Israeli women relied on induced abortion.

Methods

This analysis examines the practice of induced abortion in Israel in 1974-1975 and 1987-1988. We begin by presenting two-way cross-tabulations that look at abortion by ethnicity for both time periods. Student's t-test is used to determine whether the likelihood of having had an abortion changed significantly between 1974-1975 and 1987-1987 among a variety of ethno-immigrant and religious groups. This is followed by bivariate logit models that estimate the likelihood of having ever had an induced abortion according to a variety of socioeconomic and cultural determinants. To ensure comparability, we have attempted to construct equivalent measures of the independent variables from the two data sets. Both surveys have been restricted to women aged 22-39 in their first marriage.

Variables in Analysis

The dependent variable indicates whether the respondent ever had an abortion. Ideally we would like to assess respondents' behavior during their years of greatest abortion risk (the peak reproductive years). One limitation of our study is that we lack full information on the timing of the abortions. More specifically, the 1974-1975 survey gathered data only on the pregnancy interval in which the women obtained their abortions (e.g., before first birth, between second and third birth, etc.). Another potential weakness is that many of our predictors vary over the life course but were measured only once. While there are limitations associated with using current measures of religiosity and socioeconomic status to predict the prior use of abortion, past and present measures of these predictors are likely to be highly correlated.

The use of current socioeconomic indicators for the women and their spouses may be appropriate, however, since abortion is widely practiced among married women in Israel (Goldscheider 1996), unlike in most other countries. Up through the early 1990s, nearly 60 percent of applications for abortions in Israel came from married women (Central Bureau of Statistics 1993). The overwhelming majority of women who reported prior abortions in 1987-1988 had their first abortion in the same year that they married (7.5 percent) or some time after marriage (80.1 percent).

Frequency distributions for the categorical independent variables, with accompanying abortion rates (the proportion of women in each category who had obtained an induced abortion), are presented in table 10.2. Our models also include two continuous measures not shown in table 10.2: 1) respondent's age (measured in years) and 2) household income [from the previous month, measured in 100-lirot (1974-1975) and 100-shekelim (1987-1988) intervals]. Tests for multi-collinearity revealed no serious problems among the variables selected for inclusion in the analysis.

Findings

Abortion Rates in Israel

Table 10.3 shows the results of t-tests assessing whether rates of abortion changed significantly over the course of time for selected ethno-immigrant groups. In 1974-1975, approximately 23 percent of married Jewish women in the sample reported having had at least one induced abortion (see table 10.3.). This figure is higher than the estimates provided in a 1959-1960 maternity survey that showed that approximately 10 percent of Jewish Israeli women had obtained an induced abortion (Bachi 1970; Bachi and Matras 1962). The authors of these earlier studies acknowledge the selectivity of their sample, which was restricted to childbearing women (maternity cases). Although the extent of bias is likely to be greatest for older women, these studies probably underestimate the overall incidence of induced abortion in Israel since the practice of abortion is inversely related to the likelihood of inclusion in the sample.

Our 1974-1975 results show that foreign-born women of all ethnic origins were more likely to report having had an abortion than their native-born counterparts. Within the younger population (ages 22-30), the highest abortion rates were found among women born in Africa or Asia. Among older women (ages

31-39), however, those born in Eastern Europe, Africa, and Western Europe/America were most likely to report having had an abortion. Overall, our 1974-1975 results show only minor ethnic differences in the proportion of women reporting having had at least one abortion.

Abortion rates among Israeli Jewish women declined from 1974-1975 to 1987-1988. (This difference was statistically significant at the 0.10 level.) In 1987-1988, only 20.7 percent of women aged 22-39 reported having obtained an induced abortion (see table 10.3.). The decline was even greater among younger women (ages 22-30) from Africa and Asia. This may be attributed to a number of factors including increasing duration of residence in Israel and greater adoption of efficient contraception. In 1974-1975, the average time in Israel among young, foreign-born African women in our sample was seventeen years; in 1987-1988, it was twenty-four years. Thus, foreign-born African women in 1987-1988 had gained greater exposure to the pro-natalist, anti-abortion social norms prevalent in Israel. These differential rates of abortion may also reflect changes in the ethnic composition of immigrants from each continent of origin. For example, Iraqi Jews comprised a disproportionate share (38 percent) of young, foreign-born Asian immigrants in 1974-1975. By 1987-1988, however, there were no Iraqi women in the young, foreign-born category, and Iranian women comprised the largest single group of young, foreign-born Asian women in the sample.

In accordance with the secularization thesis, one might anticipate that declining levels of religious observance (an accompaniment of socioeconomic modernization) would render abortion more common among all Jews. Our results measuring changes in rates of abortion according to religiosity (table 10.4) do not support this conclusion, however. While secular and Orthodox women were no more (or less) likely to report having had an abortion in 1987-1988 than in 1974-1975, women self-defined as "religious/traditional" were significantly less likely to report having had an abortion in the more recent survey. While overall there has been an increase in the proportion of Jews who self-identify in the lesser observant categories (for example, 48 percent of couples were secular in 1974-1975 versus 56 percent in 1987-1988), rates of abortion have remained constant (or declined) within each of the religious groups. This finding suggests that observant Jews continue to uphold strong anti-abortion norms.

Israel's abortion rates during the 1980s were comparable to those of the other Western countries. (See figure 10.3.) During the 1980s, the Total Legal Abortion Rate (TLAR) for Israel (0.9 in 1982) was similar to that of the United States (0.9 in 1982 and 0.8 in 1987), although a lower percentage of Israeli pregnancies ended in abortion (13.5 percent versus 29.7 percent) (Frejka 1985; Henshaw 1990). It is also the case that fertility rates in Israel are higher than in other developed nations, and an unplanned or unwanted pregnancy is more likely to be carried to term in Israel than in other Western countries (Sabatello 1990). [Overall it is estimated that approximately one in three pregnancies ends

Table 10.3
Prior Induced Abortion, by Navity, Ethnicity, and Age, 1974-75 and 1987-88

	Place of Birth									Total
	Israel					E. Eur	W. Eur[a]	Asia	Africa	
	Father born in									
	E. Eur	W. Eur	Asia	Africa	Israel					
1974–75										
Total all ages	290	84	128	24	86	214	122	341	267	1567
% had abortion	20.0	17.9	18.8	12.5	19.8	26.6	22.1	23.5	29.2	23.0
1987–88										
Total all ages	357	61	343	232	130	161	68	88	234	1683
% had abortion	19.9	16.4	16.6	19.4	16.2	32.9	30.9	23.9	20.5	20.7
Change	–0.1	–1.5	–2.2	6.9	–3.6	6.3	8.8	0.4	–8.7*	–2.3
1974-75										
Total 22–30	150	45	81	23	42	116	76	144	120	806
% had abortion	12.7	8.9	13.6	8.7	19.0	18.1	15.8	19.4	25.0	16.9
1987–88										
Total 22–30	132	24	186	168	67	44	27	23	78	754
% had abortion	12.9	16.7	16.1	13.1	11.9	22.7	11.1	8.7	14.1	14.3
Change	0.2	7.8	2.5	4.4	–7.1	4.6	–4.7	–10.7*	–10.9*	–2.6*
1974–75										
Total 31–39	140	39	47	1	44	98	46	197	147	761
% had abortion	27.9	28.2	27.7	100.0	20.5	36.7	32.6	26.4	32.7	29.2
1987–88										
Total 31–39	225	37	157	64	63	117	41	65	156	929
% had abortion	24.0	16.2	17.2	35.9	20.6	36.8	43.9	29.2	23.7	25.8
Change	–3.9	–12.0	–10.5	–64.1	0.1	0.1	11.3	2.8	–9.0	–3.4

[a] W. Eur = Western Europe/America.

One-tailed t-tests were conducted to determine if significant differences existed between 1974–75 and 1987–88.

***$p < .001$ **$p < .01$ *$p < .05$

Sources: 1974–75 Israel Fertility Survey, 1987–88 Study of Fertility and Family Formation.

in an abortion worldwide (Henshaw 1987).] While 30 percent of the women in our 1987-1988 sample are of Eastern European ethnicity, Israel's abortion rates remain far behind those of the Eastern European countries. Israel is similar to the Eastern European countries in that a high proportion of abortions occur among married women, however (Central Bureau of Statistics 1993).

Compared with 1974-1975, our 1987-1988 results reveal a wider range of ethnic variation in the practice of abortion. Women born in Eastern Europe and the other Western countries exhibited abortion rates considerably higher than those of African, Asian, and Israeli-born women. Of all the ethnic groups, native-born Israeli women were least likely to have reported prior use of abortion.

Multivariate Models

Tables 10.5 and 10.6 show the results of our logistic models examining prior use of abortion. Table 10.5 includes all the women in our sample, while table 10.6 is restricted to the Israeli-born population. In both 1974-1975 and 1987-1988, Israeli-born women were the least likely to report having had an abortion, and the differences between Eastern European-born women (our reference category) and Israeli-born women were statistically significantly in both time periods. The decreased likelihood for native-born Israeli women to report prior use of abortion is probably related to the fact that Israeli society is more "child-oriented" than a variety of countries and a relatively high percentage of the Israeli population objects to abortion on religious or nationalistic grounds (Sabatello 1990). This finding may also indicate an increasing tendency for native-born Israeli women to make use of more efficient methods of contraception, thus avoiding the need for abortion.

It is possible that some of the foreign-born women had abortions prior to their arrival in Israel, but unfortunately the 1974-1975 data do not allow us to

Table 10.4
Prior Induced Abortion by Religiousity, 1974-75 and 1987-88

	1974–75	1987–88	Difference
Total Secular	748	937	
% had abortion	25.8	25.6	–0.2
Total Religious	693	675	
% had abortion	23.2	15.6	–7.6***
Total Orthodox	121	71	
% had abortion	4.1	4.2	0.1

One-tailed t-tests were conducted to determine if significant differences existed between 1974–75 and 1987–88.

***p < .001 **p < .01 *p < .05

Figure 10.3
Abortion Rates in Selected Countries, 1987

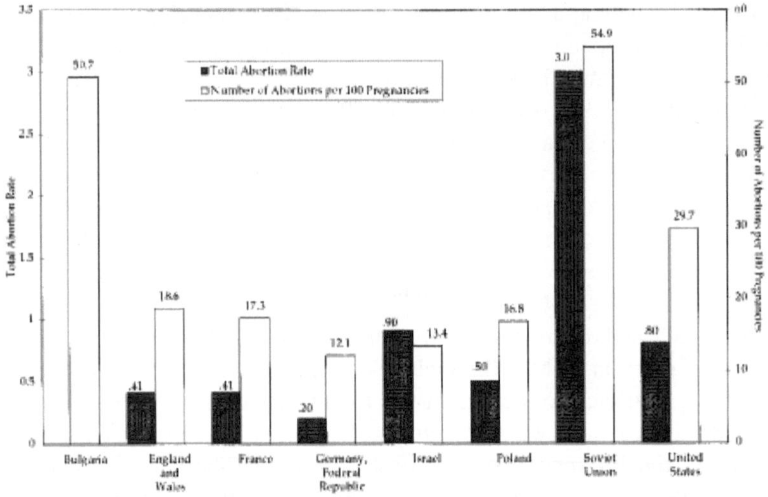

Note: The abortion data for France, the German Federal Republic, Israel, Poland and the Soviet Union are incomplete (Henshaw, 1990). The Total Abortion Rate was not available for Bulgaria for this period. Israel's Total Abortion Rate is taken from 1982 and refers to legal abortions only (Frejka, 1985). Sabatello (1992) estimated the 1988 Total Abortion Rate of the Soviet Union as approximately 3.0. With the exception of the Total Abortion Rates for Israel and the Soviet Union, the data for this table are adapted from Henshaw (1990) and refer to 1987.

determine where all the foreign-born women had their abortions. The 1987-1988 data reveal, however, that less than 1 percent of the abortions reported among foreign-born women in our sample occurred prior to their arrival in Israel.

In order to identify more specific patterns of ethnic variation in rates of abortion, we further classified native-born Israeli women according to ethnic ancestry (birthplace of father). This practice maintains continuity with previous demographic studies of ethnicity in Israel as well as with official government statistics. Among women born in Israel, inter-ethnic marriages among parents (defined by the ethnic categories shown above) constituted fewer than 25 percent of all marriages in each of our samples. We also ran our models separately defining ethnic ancestry for native-born Israeli women according to the birthplace of the respondent's mother. Both models yielded similar results, and ethnic ancestry among native-born Israeli women was not significantly related to the prior use of abortion in either 1974-1975 or 1987-1988. This finding suggests that as the proportion of the Israeli population that is native-born increases, ethnic differences in abortion rates may diminish. At the same time, any growth in the foreign-born population, especially those born in Eastern Europe, may accentuate ethnic differences in abortion rates.

Table 10.5
Parameter Estimates of the Odds of Having Had an Abortion in 1974-75 and 1987-88 among Jewish Women in Israel (Standard Errors are in Parentheses)

	1974–75						1987–88					
Variable	Abort. vs. no Abort.	SE	Odds Ratio	Abort. vs. no Abort.	SE	Odds Ratio	Abort. vs. no Abort.	SE	Odds Ratio	Abort. vs. no Abort	SE	Odds Ratio
Nativity												
Eastern Europe	—	—	—	—	—	—	—	—	—	—	—	—
Western Europe	-0.24	(0.27)	0.78	-0.13	(0.31)	0.88	-0.09	(0.31)	0.91	0.05	(0.35)	1.05
Africa	0.13	(0.21)	1.14	0.21	(0.26)	1.23	-0.64**	(0.23)	0.53	-0.48	(0.27)	0.62
Asia	-0.17	(0.20)	0.84	-0.19	(0.25)	0.82	-0.45	(0.30)	0.64	-0.38	(0.33)	0.68
Israel	-0.43*	(0.19)	0.65	-0.43*	(0.21)	0.65	-0.79***	(0.18)	0.45	-0.61**	(0.21)	0.54
Religiosity												
Secular				—	—	—				—	—	—
Religious				-0.34*	(0.16)	0.71				-0.57***	(0.15)	0.56
Orthodox				-2.27***	(0.49)	0.10				-1.24*	(0.63)	0.29
Income				-0.00	(0.01)	1.00				0.02	(0.01)	0.02
Education of wife												
0–8 years				—	—	—				—	—	—
9–12 years				-0.10	(0.18)	0.91				-0.17	(0.23)	0.84
13 + years				-0.52*	(0.24)	0.59				-0.67*	(0.26)	0.51
Wife's work history												
Never worked				—	—	—				—	—	—
Worked				0.52*	(0.22)	1.68				0.13	(0.23)	1.13
Prior use of contraception												
Did not use modern methods				—	—	—				—	—	—
Used modern methods				1.03***	(0.15)	2.80				0.77***	(0.18)	2.15
Age of wife				0.08***	(0.02)	1.08				0.07***	(0.02)	1.07
Parity												
0 children				-1.81***	(0.49)	0.16				-1.24*	(0.62)	0.29
1–2 children				-0.49**	(0.17)	0.62				-0.09	(0.16)	0.92
3 + children				—	—	—				—	—	—
Chi-Square		12.57			177.43			21.97			119.60	
n		1556			1339			1674			1517	

***p < 0.001 **p < 0.01 *p < 0.05

While previous studies of reproductive behavior in Israel have pointed to the declining significance of ethnicity for understanding variation in the practice of contraception (Okun 1997; Wilder 2000) and fertility (Friedlander and Feldmann, see chapter 2), our results indicate that nativity (continent of birth) remains important for understanding variation in the practice of induced abortion. We showed earlier that young, foreign-born women from Africa and Asia have become significantly less likely to report prior use of abortion over time

Table 10.6
Parameter Estimates of the Odds of Having Had an Abortion in 1974-75 and 1987-88 among Israeli-born Jewish Women in Israel

	1974–75						1987–88					
Variable	Abort. vs. no Abort.	SE	Odds Ratio	Abort. vs. no Abort.	SE	Odds Ratio	Abort. vs. no Abort.	SE	Odds Ratio	Abort. vs. no Abort	SE	Odds Ratio
Ethnicity												
Eastern European	—	—	—	—	—	—	—	—	—	—	—	—
Western European	-0.14	(0.32)	0.87	-0.07	(0.36)	0.93	-0.24	(0.37)	0.79	-0.54	(0.44)	0.58
African	-0.56	(0.63)	0.57	0.13	(0.72)	1.14	-0.03	(0.21)	0.97	-0.04	(0.26)	0.96
Asian	-0.08	(0.27)	0.92	0.16	(0.35)	1.17	-0.22	(0.20)	0.80	-0.23	(0.23)	0.80
Israeli	-0.01	(0.31)	0.99	0.04	(0.37)	1.04	-0.25	(0.27)	0.78	-0.26	(0.29)	0.77
Religiosity												
Secular				—	—	—				—	—	—
Religious				-0.65*	(0.27)	0.52				-0.51**	(0.20)	0.60
Orthodox				-2.66*	(1.06)	0.07				-0.88	(0.77)	0.42
Income				-0.03*	(0.01)	0.97				0.00	(0.01)	1.00
Education of wife												
0–8 years				—	—	—				—	—	—
9–12 years				-0.10	(0.39)	0.91				-0.40	(0.33)	0.67
13 + years				-0.07	(0.44)	0.93				-0.80*	(0.37)	0.45
Wife's work history												
Never worked				—	—	—				—	—	—
Worked				0.72	(0.57)	2.05				-0.17	(0.28)	0.84
Prior use of contraception												
Did not use modern methods				—	—	—				—	—	—
Used modern methods				0.84**	(0.26)	2.32				0.85***	(0.25)	2.35
Age of wife				0.11***	(0.03)	1.12				0.06**	(0.02)	1.07
Parity												
0 children				-1.27	(0.68)	0.28				-0.42	(0.65)	0.66
1–2 children				-0.55	(0.28)	0.58				0.09	(0.21)	1.10
3 + children				—	—	—				—	—	—
Chi-Square		1.02			69.31			1.99			51.01	
n		612			534			1123			1005	

***p < 0.001 **p < 0.01 *p < 0.05

(1974-1975 vs. 1987-1988). No parallel trend has emerged among foreign-born European women, however. Although some Afro-Asian Jews (especially Iranians and Ethiopians) came to Israel between 1974-1975 and 1987-1988 (Schmelz et al. 1990), the overwhelming majority arrived during Israel's early years of statehood. As a consequence, the 1987-1988 foreign-born Afro-Asian population has had considerable exposure to the pro-natalist, anti-abortion social norms pervasive in Israel. While many Eastern European Jews also arrived during the early period of statehood, there was a sizable proportion who arrived between 1969 and 1975 (Schmelz et al. 1990). The average length of time spent in Israel among the foreign-born Eastern European women in our sample was identical in both 1974-75 and 1987-1988 (seventeen years). Unlike the Afro-Asian Jewish population, the Eastern European Jewish population has been heavily replenished by new arrivals, many of who are likely to have liberal attitudes toward abortion. This demographic trend may explain the continued importance of nativity for understanding variation in rates of abortion.

Of all the socioeconomic and cultural predictors in our models, religiosity emerged as the most significant determinant of the practice of abortion (see table 10.5). Compared to secular women, religious and Orthodox women were far less likely to have had an induced abortion. This finding confirms earlier research and supports our hypothesis that there is a greater stigma associated with abortion among more observant Jews. It is also possible that observant Jews are underreporting the true extent to which they make use of abortion, as Schmelz (1989) has suggested.

Although household income was not significantly related to prior termination of a pregnancy, our logistic results point to the growing importance of women's education for understanding variation in the practice of induced abortion. In both time periods, women who had post-secondary schooling were significantly less likely to have experienced an abortion than those with fewer than nine years of formal education. Interestingly, however, among the native-born Israeli population, the effect of education was significant only in 1987-1988 (see table 10.6.). This latter finding suggests that education may exert a more powerful effect in inhibiting the practice of abortion when efficient methods of contraception are more readily available. The increased effect of education may also reflect changes in the schools' curricula that have become more open to family planning education. For example, during the 1980s sexual education was effectively popularized through voluntary organizations (such as the Israeli Family Planning Association) and public health agencies (Sabatello 1995). Meanwhile, the inverse association between education and the practice of induced abortion is consistent with recent research showing that educated Israeli women are more likely to make use of efficient birth control techniques (Okun 1997; Wilder 2000).

Female employment was positively related to the prior use of abortion in 1974-1975 although this effect was not statistically significant in 1987-1988 (see table 10.5.). In the earlier time period, the odds of having had an abortion were approximately 1.7 times higher for women who had worked than for those who had never worked. Abortion was illegal in Israel both before and during the 1974-1975 period, and it is likely that working women gained information and knowledge about abortion services through workplace interaction. As abortion became legal and more widely accessible, however, it seems that employment outside the home was no longer as important for entry into the social networks which directed women toward these services. It is also possible that employment outside the home became more closely associated with reliance on efficient contraception. Further research in this area is warranted.

Age was positively associated with the practice of abortion in both 1974-1975 and 1987-1988. This finding reflects the increased duration of exposure to the risk of incurring an unwanted pregnancy. Moreover, older women are more likely to have grown up at a time when contraception was less readily available and abortion was more often treated as a primary method of birth control. The link between age and abortion may also reflect older women's inexperience with modern birth control techniques. Among Israeli Jews, older women are less likely to have used efficient methods of birth control such as the pill (Wilder 2000).

Parity was also positively associated with the practice of abortion in both time periods. The positive association between parity and abortion implies that the procedure has been used not only for spacing births, but for stopping (avoiding further births once fertility goals are met). With increasing parity, women are more likely to have achieved their desired family size and are more strongly motivated to rely on abortion to prevent additional births. In both time periods, women with no children were the least likely to report prior use of abortion.

Interrelations between Contraceptive Use and Abortion

Many of the women who reported prior use of abortion in the 1974-1975 survey obtained their abortions during the 1960s. At that time there was very limited access to contraception, and it was not until the late 1960s that the pill first became available in Israel (Okun 1997). Although a wide range of contraceptive methods was available in Israel during the early 1970s, access to modern contraception required consultation and regular examination by a physician. This was generally only available on a private basis (Friedlander 1973; Friedlander and Goldscheider 1979). Throughout the 1970s, however, there was a growing tendency to disseminate knowledge of family planning through the large network of health institutions that were in continuous contact with the population (Bachi 1977). Even though problems with dissemination and access continued into the mid-1980s (Friedlander and Goldscheider 1984), efforts to increase the use of contraceptives were largely successful. Our data show that fewer than half (43.9 percent) of married women aged twenty-two to thirty-nine had ever used efficient contraception in 1974-1975 whereas by 1987-1988 the overwhelming majority (72.3 percent) had.

It is interesting to note that in both 1974-1975 and 1987-1988, prior use of efficient contraception was positively associated with prior use of abortion. In both time periods women who reported prior use of modern methods of contraception were over twice as likely to report having had an abortion as those who had never used efficient techniques. These findings parallel earlier research by

Slonim-Nevo (1988) who investigated the contraceptive practices of seventy-two women who underwent abortions. She found that the majority of Israeli women who sought abortions had used modern contraceptives previously, but not before their most recent pregnancy. Slonim-Nevo found that the interruption in contraception use resulted from adverse side effects of the contraceptives and from instability in partner relationships.

The 1987-1988 Fertility Survey provides us with an opportunity to explore whether women who reported abortions had used contraception prior to the termination of their pregnancies. Our findings (table 10.7) show that the use of modem methods is far more common after the first abortion. While less than 53 percent of aborting women used modem contraception before their first abortion, over 85 percent used modem methods afterward. Likewise, the percentage using no method declined from 18.4 percent to 4.0 percent. These results indicate that many women in our sample made use of modem methods of birth control only after their abortions. Although socio-demographic factors may partially account for the increasing adoption of contraception observed at the time of the survey (e.g., age, parity, etc.), the experience of having terminated a pregnancy—especially the physical and psychological stress—may well encourage the use of efficient contraception. Moreover, the process of obtaining an abortion may provide an introduction to the formal healthcare sector. By law, women receiving abortions (with the exception of abortions permitted for medical reasons) must be referred to family planning and contraceptive counseling services (Sabatello 1995), where they may learn about contraceptive methods previously unavailable to them.

Table 10.7
Prior Use of Contraception Before and After Abortion, Among Respondents Who Had an Abortion

	Lifetime Contraceptive Use Prior to Abortion[a]	Lifetime Contraceptive Use at the Time of the 1987–1988 Fertility Survey
Method(s) Used:		
No Method	18.4	4.0
Traditional[b]	28.7	10.9
Modern	52.9	85.1

n = 348

[a]Lifetime contraceptive use measures contraception used at first intercourse and the primary method used in any interpregnancy interval. For lifetime contraceptive at the time of the 1987–88 Fertility Survey, the measure also incorporates current contraceptive use. If respondent had more than one abortion, lifetime contraception use was measured prior to the first abortion.

[b]Traditional methods include one or more of the following: condom, rhythm, spermicides, and withdrawal. Modern methods include one or more of the following: diaphragm, cervical cap, pill, and IUD. These latter methods are female-controlled and necessitate a visit to a physician's office. If a respondent reported prior use of both traditional and modern methods of fertility control, she was categorized as having used modern methods.

Conclusions and Implications

Whereas 23 percent of married women of childbearing age reported prior use of abortion in 1974-1975, only 21 percent reported prior use of abortion in 1987-1988. Given all the changes that have occurred in Israel over the past few decades, it is remarkable that the percentage of Israeli women who report having had an abortion has not declined even further. Most notably, Israel has experienced a "contraceptive revolution" (Wilder 2000) that might be expected to significantly reduce the extent to which Israeli women rely on induced abortion. It is also possible that the 1974-1975 figure underestimates the true extent to which Israeli women relied on induced abortion, since the procedure was illegal at the time of the survey and women may have been reluctant to admit having had an abortion.

Meanwhile, our findings indicate that the likelihood that Israeli women reported prior use of abortion was significantly lower in 1987-1988 than in 1974-1975, net of a variety of socioeconomic and cultural variables.[1] Young foreign-born women from Africa and Asia were less likely to report prior use of abortion in the later time period, possibly owing to the adoption of efficient contraception. It is also likely that older women are becoming less likely to make use of abortion. Since our analysis is based on lifetime abortion practices, however, it is probable that many of the older women in our 1987-1988 sample had their abortions when they were younger (and prior to the widespread availability of contraception). Data from the Central Bureau of Statistics reveal that rates of abortion have declined slightly from the 1980s to the 1990s. Further research should be undertaken to determine whether attitudes governing the practice of induced abortion have also changed over time.

A number of factors are likely related to the decline in rates of abortion in Israel. One possible explanation is the growth of efficient contraception and its adoption by Israeli women. While our findings showed that Israeli women who had used efficient contraception were more likely to have obtained abortions than those who had never used modem birth control techniques, further analysis of the 1987-1988 Survey revealed that many of these women made use of efficient contraception only *after* their abortions. Prior to their abortions, nearly half of the women reported that they had used either no birth control or inefficient methods. It would be interesting to ascertain whether the experience of having had an abortion encourages women to make use of efficient contraception.

Our analysis revealed that foreign-born Eastern European women were considerably more likely to report prior use of abortion than other nativity groups. With the recent influx of Eastern European Jews (many of whom are secular), differences in rates of abortion by nativity may have become even more marked since the 1987-1988 survey. The results of this study indicate that Israeli-born women are less likely to make use of abortion than their foreign-born counterparts. Our findings point to the need to incorporate information about contraception and family planning into existing programs of immigrant absorption. Efforts to inform new arrivals about the wide range of contraceptive services available in Israel may help ward off potential increases in abortion rates.

In both surveys, reliance on induced abortion was lowest among native-born Israelis. This finding most likely represents an increased tendency toward the adoption of efficient methods of contraception among native-born Israeli women, but it may also reflect the influence of an Israeli social climate less favorable to abortion. Moreover, ethnic differences in rates of abortion among the native-born population were not statistically significant. As previously noted, the religious and political establishment is anti-abortion. This was perhaps most clearly evident in 1979 when a Knesset member established links between the practice of abortion in Israel and Hitler's murder of several million Jews in the gas chambers (Yishai 1993). To the extent that the native-born population increases, reliance on induced abortion may further decline.

Religiosity emerged as the most significant determinant of induced abortion in Israel. The effect of religiosity in inhibiting the practice of abortion was marked in both 1974-1975 and 1987-1988. Religious women were significantly less likely to report having had an abortion in the later time period, possibly owing to greater adherence to pro-natalist religious norms. While it is likely that observant women, like others, also experience unanticipated pregnancies, the social ban on the practice of abortion and a pro-natalist ideology discourage these women from obtaining abortions. Further changes in levels of religious observance among the population of Israel have important implications for abortion rates. The link between religiosity and abortion (higher rates of abortion among secular Jews) may also reflect a greater tendency to report abortion among non-observant women.

Our analysis has provided important insights into the ways in which key socioeconomic and cultural variables shape the practice of induced abortion. Over the course of socioeconomic development, some determinants lose their explanatory power whereas others become increasingly important for understanding variation in the practice of abortion. In the earlier stages of the development process, higher levels of socioeconomic achievement among women may have actually promoted reliance on abortion. Our findings from 1974-1975, for example, showed that women who had worked were considerably more likely than others to have had an induced abortion. While educational attainment was not significantly related to the prior use of abortion among native-born Israeli women in 1974-1975, by the late 1980s abortion was much less common among highly educated women. This finding implies that policies that promote female education in order to reduce rates of reliance on induced abortion may be more effective if school curricula emphasizing sexual education or alternative methods of birth control are more widely available.

While our analysis suggests that the state of Israel might further reduce abortion rates by encouraging heightened levels of religious observance, a more desirable public policy would also promote women's reproductive autonomy and socioeconomic well-being. Previous research in Israel has shown that variables such as education and economic status are positively associated with the use of efficient contraception (Okun 1997; Wilder 2000). Meanwhile, religiosity is inversely associated with the use of birth control. While both heightened levels of religiosity and socioeconomic well-being are inversely associated with the use of abortion, efforts to advance the position of women in Israeli society may be better served by promoting socioeconomic advancement.

Although it is imperative that abortion remains safe and legal in Israel, it is preferable that women make use of efficient methods of contraception to limit births. Our results show that women's education is very effective in reducing rates of reliance on induced abortion. The experience of abortion may be psychologically traumatic for women. Meanwhile, the increased control that results from the ability to plan one's fertility via contraception may enhance women's psychological well-being. If the Israeli government takes a more active role in promoting women's socioeconomic position and encouraging the use of efficient contraception, abortion rates are likely to further decline. This same policy might also help safeguard women's reproductive autonomy.

Note

1. In separate models (not shown) we also examined whether the likelihood of having had an abortion changed significantly over time, net of the key socioeconomic, cultural and demographic variables presented here. Income was expressed in z-scores (to maintain comparability) and an additional variable was introduced for survey year. Our results showed that women were approximately 30 percent less likely to report having had an abortion in 1987-1988 than in 1974-1975. Due to statistical concerns about combining data from two differently sampled surveys, however, these results should be seen as speculative rather than definitive.

References

"Abortion in Israel." 1978. *People* 5: 43-44.

Bachi, R. 1970. "Abortion in Israel." In R. E. Hall (ed.), *Abortion in a Changing World,* vol. 1, 274-283. New York: Columbia University Press.

Bachi, R. 1977. *The Population of Israel.* Jerusalem: Scientific Translations International Ltd.

Bachi, R., and J. Matras. 1962. "Contraception and induced abortion among Jewish maternity cases in Israel." *Milbank Memorial Fund Quarterly* 40: 207-229.

Biale, R. 1995. *Women and Jewish Law.* New York: Schocken.

Blake, J. 1971. "Abortion and public opinion: The 1960-1970 decade." *Science* 171: 540-549.

Central Bureau of Statistics. 1983. *Statistical Abstract of Israel, 1983.* Jerusalem: Central Bureau of Statistics.

Central Bureau of Statistics. 1984. *Statistical Abstract of Israel, 1984.* Jerusalem: Central Bureau of Statistics.

Central Bureau of Statistics. 1986. *Statistical Abstract of Israel, 1986.* Jerusalem: Central Bureau of Statistics.

Central Bureau of Statistics. 1987. *Statistical Abstract of Israel, 1987.* Jerusalem: Central Bureau of Statistics.

Central Bureau of Statistics. 1990. *Statistical Abstract of Israel, 1990.* Jerusalem: Central Bureau of Statistics.

Central Bureau of Statistics. 1991. *Statistical Abstract of Israel, 1991*. Jerusalem: Central Bureau of Statistics.

Central Bureau of Statistics. 1993. *Demographic Characteristics of Women Applying for Interruption of Pregnancy in Israel 1991* (Reprint from *Supplement to the Monthly Bulletin of Statistics* no. 11, 1993). Jerusalem: Central Bureau of Statistics.

Central Bureau of Statistics. 1995. *Statistical Abstract of Israel, 1995*. Jerusalem: Central Bureau of Statistics.

Central Bureau of Statistics. 1998. *Statistical Abstract of Israel, 1998*. Jerusalem: Central Bureau of Statistics.

Feldman, D. M. 1975. *Marital Relations, Birth Control, and Abortion in Jewish Law*. New York: Schocken.

Feldman, D. M. 1984. *Jewish Views on Abortion*. New York: William Petschek National Jewish Family Center.

Frejka, T. 1985. "Induced abortion and fertility." *Family Planning Perspectives* 17: 230-234.

Friedlander, D. 1973. "Family planning in Israel: Irrationality and ignorance." *Journal of Marriage and the Family* 35: 117-124.

Friedlander, D., and C. Goldscheider. 1979. *The Population of Israel*. New York: Columbia University Press.

Friedlander, D., and C. Goldscheider. 1984. "Israel's population: The challenge of pluralism." *Population Bulletin* 39 (2): 3-39.

Gober, P. 1994. "Why abortion rates vary: A geographical examination of the supply and demand for abortion services in the United States in 1988." *Annals of the Association of American Geographers* 84: 230-250.

Golan, G. 1987. "Movement toward equality for women in Israel." *Tikkun* 2: 19-21.

Goldscheider, C. 1995. "Ethnicity and nation-building in Israel: The importance of demographic factors." In C. Goldscheider (ed.), *Population and Social Change in Israel*, 1-38. Boulder, CO: Westview.

Goldscheider, C. 1996. *Israel's Changing Society: Population, Ethnicity, and Development*. Boulder, CO: Westview.

Goldscheider, C., and D. Friedlander. 1980. "Fertility expectations, desires and ideals among Jewish women in Israel." In U. O. Schmelz, P. Glikson and S. DellaPergola (eds.), *Papers in Jewish Demography* 1977, 301-314. Jerusalem: Institute of Contemporary Jewry, Hebrew University of Jerusalem.

Goldscheider, C., and D. Friedlander. 1981. "Patterns of Jewish fertility in Israel: A review and some hypotheses." In P. Ritterband (ed.), *Modern Jewish Fertility*, 232-254. Leiden: E.J. Brill.

Henshaw, S. 1987. "Induced abortion: A worldwide perspective." *International Family Planning Perspectives* 13: 12-16.

Henshaw, S. 1990. "Induced abortion: A world review, 1990." *Family Planning Perspectives* 22: 76-89.

Humphries, J. 1980. "The socio-economic determinants of recourse to legal abortion." *Women's Studies International Quarterly* 3: 277-393.

Keysar, A., E. Sabatello, I. Ziegler, R. Shtarkshall, S. Kupinsky, R. Zur and E. Peritz. 1992. "Fertility patterns in the Jewish population of Israel." In E. Peritz and M. Baras (eds), *Studies in The Fertility of Israel*, 21-57. Jerusalem: Hebrew University of Jerusalem.

Kupinsky, S. 1992. "Jewish fertility patterns: Norms, differentials, and policy implications." In C. Goldscheider (ed.), *Population and Social Change in Israel*, 149-176. Boulder, CO: Westview Press.

Lawton, L. 1988. "The impact of religious commitment on fertility among Israeli Jews." *PSTC Working Paper Series* No. 88-05. Providence: Population Studies and Training Center, Brown.

Margolies, I. R. 1970. "A reform rabbi's view." In R. E. Hall (ed.), *Abortion in a Changing World*, 30-33. New York: Columbia University Press.
Matras, J., and C. Auerbach. 1962. "On rationalization of family formation in Israel." *Milbank Memorial Fund Quarterly* 40: 453-480.
Nigem, E., and M. H. Nagi. 1988. "Fertility patterns and differences in Israel." *Biology and Society* 5: 119-126.
Notzer, N., D. Levran, S. Mashiach and S. Soffer. 1984. "Effect of religiosity on sex attitudes, experience, and contraception among university students." *Journal of Sex and Marital Therapy* 10: 57-62.
Okun, B. 1997. "Family planning in the Jewish population of Israel: Correlates of withdrawal use." *Studies in Family Planning* 28: 215-227.
Osborne, S. A. 1997. "Bill sparks abortion controversy." *Christianity Today* 41: 60.
Population Crisis Committee. 1991. *Access to Affordable Contraception* [chart]. Washington, DC: Population Crisis Committee.
Powell-Griner, E., and K. Trent. 1987. "Sociodemographic determinants of abortion in the United States." *Demography* 24: 553-561.
Rahman, A., L. Katzive and S. K. Henshaw. 1998. "A global review of laws on induced abortion, 1985-1997." *International Family Planning Perspectives* 24: 56-64.
Sabatello, E. F. 1990. "Estimates of illegal abortion in Israel, 1980-1983." *Israel Journal of Medical Science* 26: 204-209.
Sabatello, E. F. 1992. "Estimates of demand for abortion among Soviet immigrants in Israel." *Studies in Family Planning* 23: 267-273.
Sabatello, E. F. 1995. "Continuity and change in reproductive and abortion patterns of Soviet immigrants in Israel." *Social Science and Medicine* 40: 117-124.
Sabatello, E. F., and N. Yaffe. 1988. "Israel." In P. Sachdev (ed.), *International Handbook on Abortion*, 263-278. New York: Greenwood Press.
Schiff, G. S. 1981. "The politics of fertility policy in Israel." In P. Ritterband (ed.), *Modern Jewish Fertility*, 255-278. Leiden: E. J. Brill.
Schmelz, U. O. 1989. "Religiosity and fertility among the Jews of Jerusalem." In U.O. Schmelz and S. DellaPergola (eds.), *Papers in Jewish Demography 1989*, 157-185. Jerusalem: Institute of Contemporary Jewry, Hebrew University of Jerusalem.
Schmelz, U. O., S. DellaPergola and U. Avner. 1990. *Ethnic Differences among Israeli Jews: A New Look.* Jerusalem: Hebrew University of Jerusalem.
Silber, T. J. 1980. "Abortion: A Jewish view." *Journal of Religion and Health* 19: 231-239.
Slater, P. E., D. Weiner and A. M. Davies. 1978. "Requests for abortion and outcomes of pregnancy in Jerusalem, Israel." *Journal of Reproductive Medicine* 21: 279-283.
Slonim-Nevo, V. 1988. "Abortions among Jewish women after interruption in contraceptive use." *Health and Social Work* 3: 137-144.
Tietze, C. 1983. *Induced Abortion: A World Review.* New York: Population Council.
van der Tak, J. 1974. *Abortion, Fertility and Changing Legislation: An International Review.* Lexington, MA: Lexington Books.
Wilder, E. I. 2000. "The contraceptive revolution in Israel: Changing family planning practices among ethnoimmigrant groups." *Social Science Research* 29: 70-91.
Yaffe, N. 1976. *Family Planning in Israel.* Jerusalem: Hebrew University (in Hebrew).
Yishai, Y. 1978. "Abortion in Israel: Social demand and political responses." *Policy Studies Journal* 7: 270-289.
Yishai, Y. 1993. "The hidden agenda: Abortion politics in Israel." *Journal of Social Policy* 22: 193-212.

Part 3

Mortality

11

Old-Age Mortality in Israel: Analysis of Variation and Change

Dov Friedlander, Jona Schellekens and Refaela Sharashov Cohen

Inequalities in longevity across population subgroups characterize every society. This study analyzes such differentials in life expectancy and cause-specific death rates among the elderly Jewish population in Israel. It covers a period of five years around the 1983 census, with comparisons to a similar period around the 1972 census. The analysis is restricted to the Jewish population because the socio-economic and cultural characteristics, as well as the quality of data, differ greatly between the Jewish and the Arab populations. Indeed, the quality of vital records as well as census data of the Arab population is problematic and raises difficulties both in analysis and in interpretation.

The units of analysis in this study are defined by geographic divisions based on census statistical areas. We show that old-age mortality levels are subject to very significant differences among subpopulations in geographic units, whether these are towns and cities, or smaller divisions. It is also shown that inequality across geographic units in life expectancy tended to increase between the early 1970s and the early 1980s. Our major aim is to analyze and explain old-age mortality differences among such population units, with respect to socioeconomic and culture explanatory variables. Israel has extensive welfare programs including comprehensive and highly subsidized health schemes, covering almost the entire range of medical services. Nevertheless, there are differences in life expectancies across localities of up to eight years at age sixty-five. Differences across the smaller divisions are even larger. How can such variations, under conditions of extensive welfare and health programs, be explained? A major hypothesis is that variations among population units in economic and social status, ethnicity, religiosity, and proximity to leading specialized medical centers, as well as some other characteristics, are associated among the elderly with cause-specific death rates and therefore with life expectancies.

Previous Studies

The interrelationship between mortality levels and socio-economic variables is not a new research issue. Ecological interrelationships between socio-economic variables and mortality had already been studied in the nineteenth century, for example in London, as well as in some other regions and countries (Antonovsky 1967). Several ecological analyses of mortality differentials for more recent periods can be traced in the literature. Notable were a series of projects undertaken at the University of Chicago focusing on ecological relationships in the Chicago area between 1930 and 1960. More modem studies, using ecological relationships to analyze mortality patterns, have been conducted for the United States (Silver 1972), Japan (Sakai 1986) and some other countries. The most important common finding of these studies is the existence of socio-economic status differences in mortality. Indeed, some studies with historical perspectives indicate that socio-economic status tends to increase in importance over time as an explanation of life expectancy differentials (Preston and van de Walle 1978; Friedlander et al. 1985; Mosk and Johansson 1986). The analysis presented here is distinct in that it deals specifically with old-age mortality, and in that it employs a relatively large number of explanatory variables. Additionally, the analyses are based on a large number of units with relatively small populations, probably smaller than most studies of its kind.

Previous research on life expectancy levels and their socio-economic determinants in Israel is very limited. Several studies of differential mortality undertaken in the 1960s and 1970s dealt mainly with the effects of ethnicity and duration in Israel as potential explanations (Muhsam 1966; Peritz et al. 1973). Anson (1988) analyzed standardized death rates for about seventy localities in Israel. He discovered significant differences and established interrelationships with welfare variables.

An important long-term project undertaken by the Unit for the Study of Health Services, at the Chaim Sheba Medical Center, Tel Aviv University, deals with different aspects of infant mortality among localities in Israel. Significant socio-economic and ethnic differences in infant mortality rates were discovered (Barell, Wax, and Ruder 1988). Another study by this unit focused on adult mortality differences among the metropolitan areas of Tel Aviv (Lusky, Gurvitz, and Barell1992).

In a very detailed individual level study, Peritz and his associates measured the impact of birthplace (Europe, Middle Eastern countries in Asia, North Africa, and Israel), controlling for duration in the country. Their most interesting finding concerns the convergence patterns of mortality levels of recent migrants from these different origins with those who migrated earlier. In a follow up study (Peritz et al. 1983), comparisons among these different groups were made to document the changing patterns of differentials in cause-specific mortality levels. It was shown that during 1969-1973 differences in cause-specific mortality levels still prevailed. This finding is most relevant to the present study. We analyze cause-specific death rates by ethnicity among geographic units for 1972 and 1983. One of our objectives is to ascertain whether there are still significant ethnic effects after socio-economic status variables are controlled for.

Immigration, Socio-Economic Differentiation and Mortality Trends

Life expectancy at age sixty-five increased by one-and-a-half years between the early 1970s and the early 1980s and by another year during the 1980s, while it was almost constant during the two decades before 1970. Hence, while there has been a strong and continuous decline in overall mortality since the massive immigration in the late 1940s and early 1950s, the decline in old age mortality is a recent phenomenon. This raises an important analytic question. Under what conditions and circumstances are current life expectancies at age sixty-five high, and under what conditions are they likely to increase rapidly? It will be shown that socio-economic status, ethnicity and religiosity are key variables explaining both the variation and the change in life expectancy.

Israel is a country of immigration with ethnic and socio-economic diversity. Its Jewish population has grown and developed mainly as a result of extensive wave-like immigration during the present century. The "mass immigration" wave following the foundation of the state in 1948 was most conspicuous in its enormous volume. It was not only variation in the volume of immigration but also the changing ethnic composition of immigrants over time that shaped Israel's socio-economic structure. Up to the foundation of the State in 1948, immigrants came predominantly from European countries. This group of veterans and their Israeli-born descendants now form a major part of Israel's higher-status population. Israel's ethnic structure changed radically with the wave of mass immigration when increasing proportions of immigrants came from African or Asian countries, a tendency which became even more pronounced during 1952-1967. Another feature of the immigration waves was that the immigration from Asian and from African countries was not equally distributed over time either. While immigration from Asian countries was concentrated in the early years of statehood, immigration from North African countries was spread over a longer period—up to 1967. Subsequently, it was again European migration that dominated. While origin or ethnicity indicates the initial socio-economic and demographic characteristics at time of immigration, duration in Israel represents exposure to the new conditions in Israel. Hence, immigration patterns have created an extremely heterogeneous society. Indeed, Israel's Jewish population is differentiated not only by ethnicity, but also by socio-economic status levels. The historical patterns of immigration, particularly origins and time of arrival, have contributed towards a long-term association between ethnicity and socio-economic status. Considering immigrants from European, Asian, and African origins as well as their respective descendants, their status levels from high to low can be ranked in that order (see Eisenstadt, Lissak, and Nahon 1993). Many studies have demonstrated the existence of differentiation, in many social and demographic aspects, by both ethnicity and length of stay in Israel. The studies of differential mortality by Peritz and his associates (1973, 1983) have, indeed, shown that life expectancy at various adult ages was differentiated by these two factors. It has been demonstrated in these studies that Israeli-born (with no regard to their parents' origin) had the highest life expectancies, followed by Asian and by European-born, while African-born had significantly lower life expectancies. Although these differences tended to diminish over time, even in very recent years immigrants of African origins show higher mortality at adult ages compared with other ethnic groups (e.g., Central Bureau of Statistics 1992: 149). However, because ethnicity and socio-economic status levels are so tightly interrelated, a question of major importance is whether ethnic differences in mortality still persist after controlling for socioeconomic status. The analysis in this paper attempts to answer this question.

Data and Variables

Units of Analysis

This study employs geographic aggregated data from the 1972 and the 1983 censuses and death registration data for five years centered on these Census years to explain variation in old-age mortality levels at each period. The basic geographic divisions consist of standard statistical areas defined by the Central Bureau of Statistics. These range mostly between population sizes of several hundred and a few thousand and are the smallest areas for which census returns as well as death statistics can be manipulated. However, our analysis is based on aggregates of these standard statistical areas—small local areas—whenever the population sizes of standard statistical areas are small. In all, some 580 small local areas are used in the analyses of life expectancies. These units range mostly between 2,500 and 7,000. The analysis of cause-specific mortality rates forced us to use larger aggregates, that is, localities, because of data limitations. There are sixty-five units in these analyses, ranging mostly between 10,000 and 90,000. Some more details on the aggregation procedures are discussed in Appendix A.

Both vital registration records and census data, for the Jewish population, are considered to be of high quality. No burial can take place unless a death certificate has been signed by an authorized official. Both place of residence and place of death are registered, which is of particular importance in the analysis of old age mortality.

Age Structures

Many of the population aged sixty-five and over are former immigrants who arrived in Israel with the mass immigration of 1948-1951. Their current reported ages as well as their age at death still depends, to a large extent, on the ages immigrants reported at arrival. There was a suspicion that among migrants from Asian and African countries, ages were overstated, which is a well-known problem in age statistics (see Carrier and Farrag 1959). One implication would be that life tables as well as cause-specific death rates based on such age structures could produce biased estimates at the older ages. Appendix B discusses the ways in which age structures have been examined to detect such possible age overstatements. The conclusion is that serious age overstatement among these populations is unlikely.

Dependent Variables

The major dependent variable in this study is life expectancy at age sixty-five, e_{65}. Additional dependent variables are cause-specific (and for wider age groups age-standardized) death rates at age sixty-five and over, using five major cause-of-death categories:

$M_{in,x}$: The age-standardized or age-specific death rate of infectious diseases.
$M_{hc,x}$: The age-standardized or age-specific death rate of heart and circulatory diseases, excluding cerebrovascular diseases.
$M_{cva,x}$: The age-standardized or age-specific death rates of cerebrovascular diseases.
$M_{ca,x}$: The age-standardized or age-specific death rate of all cancer diseases.
$M_{ot,x}$: The age-standardized or age specific death rate of all other causes.
These dependent variables are analysed with respect to several explanatory variables.

Explanatory Variables

The explanatory variables in the analyses are: economic status; social status measured in terms of educational attainment; ethnicity; religiosity; proximity to locations with specialized medical services; loneliness in terms of marital status; industry and employment status. Some of these variables can be defined in alternative ways. For example, social status is represented by the proportion of the population with at least nine years of formal education among the population aged sixty and over. This variable is preferred to the proportion with at least thirteen years of education, which is used in many studies, because the general educational levels of these older population cohorts are relatively low. The explanatory variables are defined below.

EC_{90}: Proportion of all wage earners in the geographic unit whose earnings are within the upper decile range of the national income distribution. This is the economic status variable.

$ED_{9,60}$: Proportion with at least nine years of formal education among the population aged sixty years and over. This is considered as the social status variable.

ETAF: Proportion born in North African countries or their Israeli-born children, in the total population of the geographic unit. This is considered as the African ethnicity variable.

REL: Proportion of the total adult population who voted for religious political parties during the general elections of 1984. Three major religious parties participated in these elections. Two are ultra-religious parties, one dominated by people of European ethnicity, the "Agudah," and the other dominated by people of Asian-African ethnicity, the "Shas" party. The third, the "National Religious Party," is a more modem religious party, has no clear ethnic identification, and is nationalistic. Altogether they formed over 15 percent of the total electorate in 1983. The percentage of all three religious parties in a geographic unit is taken as the religiosity variable.

PROX: Proximity to locations with major specialized medical centers. This is the road distance from the geographic unit to the nearest of the three major cities in the country: Haifa, Tel-Aviv and Jerusalem.

LON_{65}: The "loneliness" variable, calculated as the ratio of the number of never-married and divorced persons to the total number of persons in the 65-74 age-group. The widow category is not included in this variable, neither in the nominator nor in the denominator, to eliminate the representation of a mortality element on both sides of the regression equation. As the widow and widower subgroups are so important in the old-age population, their inevitable omission from the analysis is a shortcoming.

IND: Proportion of the male labor force engaged in industry. It is considered as a rough proxy for the exposure to pollution.

WLF_{55} and MLF_{55}: Proportion of women or men participating in the labor force in the 55-64 age group.

The Inequality in Old-Age Mortality

Variations in life expectancy at infancy or at age sixty-five among populations in geographic units are high, regardless of the kind of geographic divisions that are considered. Differentiation and inequality are present among small local areas or localities. Moreover, the inequality in life expectancy increased during the period 1972 to 1983. While in the present section we illustrate the inter-locality inequality in life expectancies, in a following section we attempt to provide explanation and interpretation.

We begin our examination of life expectancies with some comparisons. Whereas the 1972 life expectancy at age sixty-five was 13.4 for males and 14.5 for females in the country as a whole, localities range between 10.6 and 16.5 for males, and between 10.7 and 17.0 for females. In 1983 life expectancy at age sixty-five was 14.5 for males and 15.3 for females in the country as a whole, while localities range between 11.5 and 18.0 for males, and between 11.5 and 20.8 for females. While life expectancy at birth in 1972 was nearly seventy-two years for the entire Jewish population of Israel, individual localities range between sixty-eight and seventy-six years. In 1983 life expectancy at birth was seventy-five years for the entire population, while individual localities range between sixty-nine and eighty-one years.

Table 11.1 suggests that localities of low socio-economic status, particularly "new towns" that were established to settle new immigrants after the early 1950s, have much lower life expectancies than average in 1983 (see the upper section in this table). Table 11.1 also suggests that almost all localities with high life expectancies, such as Hod Hasharon or Raanana, were established before independence and are characterized by high economic status. An illustration of differences in life expectancies at age sixty-five (for males) between localities of low and of high socio-economic levels, may be taken as between Dimona, a low socio-economic status locality, and Raanana, a high socio-economic status locality. Life expectancy at age sixty-five in Dimona was 12.5 years in 1983, with lower and upper 95 percent confidence limits of 10.7 and 14.2 respectively. In comparison, life expectancy at sixty-five for males in Raanana was 17.6 years, with lower and upper confidence limits of 15.6 and 19.5 years respectively. Similar patterns, though less extreme, can be found for 1972. Such differences in longevity are recorded among many units. These are explained and interpreted in a following section. Table 11.1 also presents standardized death

Table 11.1
Life Expectancies and Standardized Death rates from Heart and Circulatory Diseases: Selected Localities, 1983

Locality	Life expectancy at age 65		Life expectancy at birth		Standardized death rate at age 65-79 from heart and circulatory diseases	
	Males	Females	Males	Females	Males	Females
			Localities of low socio-economic status			
Dimona	12.5	13.1	69.2	72.4	29.9	31.6
Tirat Karmel	12.8	12.7	69.8	72.9	29.1	30.5
Kiryat Malachi	13.0	13.4	72.2	72.7	23.2	28.8
Kiryat Shmona	13.6	14.4	69.4	73.0	21.2	22.1
Ramla	13.8	14.6	70.8	75.0	26.4	24.8
Or Yehuda	13.9	15.0	70.5	75.8	25.7	19.5
Bet Shemesh	14.1	14.2	70.6	73.2	32.7	27.4
			Localities of high socio-economic status			
Rehovot	15.8	17.3	74.8	77.5	19.3	14.5
Givatayim	16.1	18.1	75.4	78.6	18.1	12.7
Ramat Gan	16.1	17.7	74.7	78.3	19.1	13.8
Ramat Hasharon	16.2	15.9	74.7	76.5	23.3	20.6
Kiryat Ono	16.4	16.5	74.9	77.3	16.0	12.9
Hod Hasharon	16.8	22.9	73.9	81.4	20.9	13.6
Raanana	17.6	20.8	77.3	80.8	18.9	18.3

rates at ages 65-79 from heart and circulatory diseases. Like life expectancies, these death rates are much lower for high-status localities than for those of low socio-economic status presented in the upper part of table 11.1.

If life expectancies of smaller units, such as the small local areas, are compared, the range between extreme life expectancies either at age sixty-five or at birth is much larger, although significance declines. Comparison of these smaller areas shows large variations among different neighborhoods in larger cities. For example, while a large number of neighborhoods in Tel-Aviv are ranked at the top in their life expectancies, there are quite a few neighborhoods ranked at the bottom.

Table 11.2 presents several parameters describing the amount of differentiation among localities in life expectancies at age sixty-five for both 1972 and for 1983. The table shows that along with the overall increase in life expectancies between 1972 and 1983, there was an increase in inequality among localities. This is clearly seen from comparisons of the standard deviations, the quartile deviations and the various ranges shown for 1972 and 1983. Moreover, the table shows that in the lower range of life expectancies the increase in life expectancies between 1972 and 1983 was small. In the upper range of life expectancies, on the other hand, the increase between 1972 and 1983 was quite large. This pattern is particularly conspicuous for females relative to males. For example, while the lower quartile of life expectancy at age sixty-five increased from 12.68 in 1972 to 13.54 in 1983 for males, these values are 13.86 and 13.82 for females. On the other hand, the upper quartile for males is 14.20 in 1972 and 15.40 in 1983 and for females 15.38 and 16.54.

Three observations are suggested by the tables. First, socio-economic differ-

Table 11.2
Means, Standard Deviations and Percentiles of Life Expectancy at Age 65 (e65) by Sex, 1983 and 1972

	Both sexes		Males		Females	
Year	1983	1972	1983	1972	1983	1972
Mean ($\bar{x}$)	14.83	13.96	14.45	13.44	15.30	14.54
Standard deviation(s)	1.44	1.02	1.42	1.11	1.86	1.30
$\bar{x}$ - 2.5 s	11.23	11.41	10.90	10.66	10.65	11.29
$\bar{x}$ + 2.5 s	18.43	16.51	18.20	16.22	19.95	17.79
Minimum value	11.50	11.44	11.50	10.55	11.48	10.66
Maximum value	19.26	15.55	18.04	16.50	20.82	16.85
Range	7.76	4.11	6.54	5.95	9.34	6.19
Median	14.79	14.11	14.44	13.62	15.22	14.57
Lower quartile (Q_1)	13.95	13.20	13.54	12.68	13.82	13.86
Upper quartile (Q_3)	15.92	14.73	15.40	14.20	16.54	15.38
Interquartile range	1.97	1.53	1.86	1.57	2.72	1.52
Lower decile (P10)	12.90	12.56	12.56	11.90	13.18	12.57
Upper decile (P90)	16.62	15.28	16.29	14.67	17.70	16.35
(P90) - (P10)	3.72	2.72	3.73	2.77	4.52	3.78

entiation in life expectancies appears to be substantial. Second, among localities of low socio-economic status (and therefore relatively low life expectancies), there was little increase in life expectancy between 1972 and 1983, while large increases were experienced in localities of relatively high socio-economic status levels, which were already characterized by relatively high life expectancies. This means that socio-economic inequality in life expectancies, which was already alarmingly large in the early 1970s, has further increased up to the early 1980s. Third, the pattern of increasing inequality in life expectancy among localities, was more conspicuous for women than for men. While the first and the second observations are subject to analysis in the present article, the third will be analyzed in a forthcoming paper.

Can we be sure that our seemingly large socio-economic life-expectation differentials are not simply a consequence of different degrees of death under-registration, of misreporting of locality of residence or other such errors? Could misreporting account for errors that would increase mortality differentials among the localities? There can, of course, be no certainty about the precision of any vital registration system. However, Israel's census data are considered reasonably accurate by international standards, and the possibility of a significant effect of age misreporting by Asian or African migrants has been shown to be minimal (see the section on data and Appendix B). As for the death registration system, it should be noted that no burial can take place without registration, independent of the type of locality. Place of residence, not place of death, is recorded so that the effect of major hospitals being located mostly in large places is unlikely to be serious. We have also attempted to make comparisons of inter-locality differential mortality with other studies of geographic variations. However, no study dealing with such small divisions as those employed in this study could be found in the literature. One study for France uses "small" divisions of two million on average, half of Israel's total Jewish population, while another study, for Spain, used divisions of similar size. For these divisions, the differences in life expectancies were around four years (Higueras Arnal 1991; Chauvire 1991; Thumerelle 1991). When we aggregate Israel's population into ten divisions with mean populations of about 400,000, we also have smaller differences of about five years. Allowing for the smaller size of our divisions, the mortality inequalities we find might exist in many other countries.

Table 11.3 illustrates old-age mortality differentials for several explanatory variables, for 1972 and for 1983. It presents selected characteristics for aggregated units characterized by lower and upper quartiles of life expectancy, both at birth and at age sixty-five. Whereas among the low life-expectancy areas the mean percentages of high income (i.e., EC_{90}) were between 6.0 and 7.0, these percentages for high life-expectancy areas were over twelve. Likewise, the table shows that areas of high life expectancies are characterized by large percentages of higher education, large percentages of the labor force in high-status occupations, and high levels of women's participation in the labor force.

Table 11.3
Means Values of Selected Socio-Economic Variables for Aggregated Populations Belonging to Quartile Ranges in Life Expectancies, 1983 and 1972

Socio-economic variables	All areas	Areas within quartile range of e_0		Areas within quartile range of e_{65}	
		Lower quartile (1)	Upper quartile (2)	Lower quartile (3)	Upper quartile (4)
				1983	
Mean percentage income within Israel upper decile	10.4	5.7	14.1	6.3	13.4
Mean percentage with 13+ years of formal education at 25-34 age group	36.5	23.8	48.4	22.7	46.6
Mean percentage with 9+ years of formal education at 60-69 age group	42.4	28.8	54.3	28.3	52.8
Mean percentage males with high status occupations	26.2	17.8	33.3	17.6	32.5
Mean percentage women in labour force at age 55-64	31.7	25.5	38.6	24.8	37.2
Mean percentage born in Africa	9.3	14.9	5.4	15.7	6.0
				1972	
Mean percentage income within Israel upper decile	10.2	8.6	12.3	7.4	12.2
Mean percentage with 13+ years of formal education at 25-34 age group	19.8	12.3	27.0	11.0	27.0
Mean percentage with 9+ years of formal education at 60-69 age group	28.9	17.3	37.6	15.7	37.8
Mean percentage males with high status occupations	17.2	11.3	23.1	10.9	23.0
Mean percentage women in labour force at age 55-64	20.6	19.0	21.7	16.3	22.1

Religiosity is a complex variable: its effect on life expectancy cannot be seen clearly through these bivariate illustrations and it is excluded from this table. However, the multivariate analyses show that its effect on life expectancy is very significant.

It can be concluded that socio-economic status, ethnicity, and old-age participation in the labor force, as well as some other variables, reveal associations with old-age mortality. However, these associations are not controlled by other explanatory variables and are reexamined through multivariate analyses.

The Framework

The framework for the analyses is illustrated in figure 11.1. Primarily, the focus of interest is on the relationship between life expectancy at age sixty-five—the dependent variable—and socio-cultural explanatory variables. The effects of these explanatory variables on old-age mortality may be assumed to operate through intermediate variables, mainly "behavioral." Food consumption and diets, the amount of smoking, exercise, the rational use of medical facilities, are just a few examples of such variables. Another category of intermediate

Figure 11.1
Interrelationships among the Major Variables

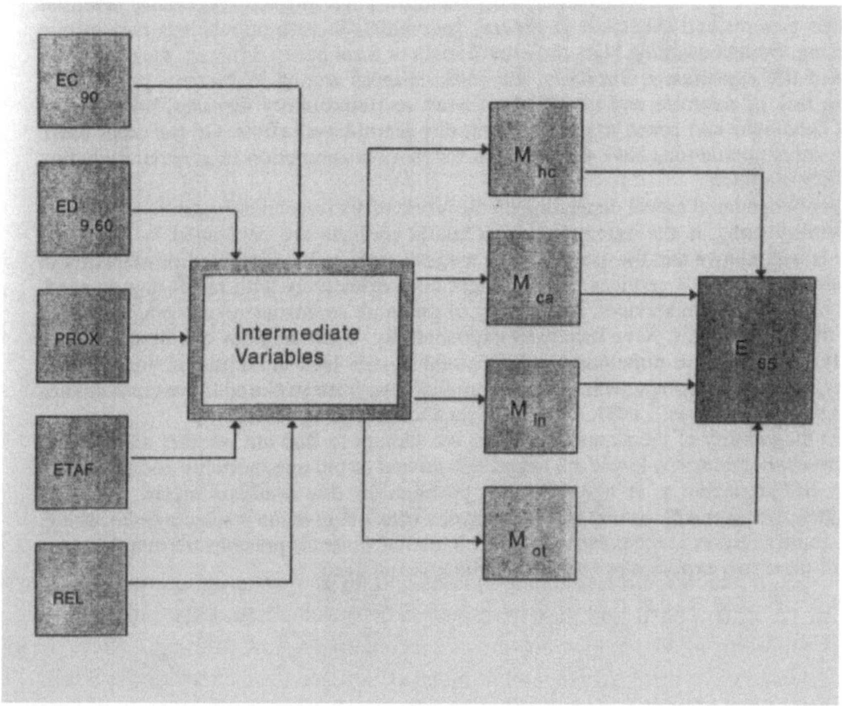

variables is biological factors, which might intervene, for instance, between ethnicity and mortality. Hence, the socio-economic and culture variables affect, through behavior characteristics, the cause-specific death rates that in turn determine old-age life expectancies.

While we do have data to express the more important socio-cultural variables, the cause specific death rate variables and life expectancy at the older ages, we have no information on the intermediate behavior or biological variables. Hence, the empirical analyses of the interrelationships cannot include explicitly the intermediate variables of the system proposed above. These have been included in figure 11.1 just in order to present our analysis in a proper perspective.

Old-age Mortality Variations: Hypotheses and Explanation

We now attempt to evaluate hypotheses concerning the interrelationships between old-age mortality and the explanatory variables in the system described. Some of these hypotheses are based on previous studies mentioned above. Additionally, in formulating our hypotheses we make use of findings in various socio-demographic studies of Israel's population. Such studies have consistently shown significant interrelationships of demographic processes, not only with socio-economic status, but also with culture variables such as ethnicity and religiosity (e.g., Friedlander and Feldmann, see chapter 2).

Do variables such as socio-economic status, ethnicity, and religiosity affect cause-specific mortality and life expectancy at the older ages? The analyses in tables 11.4 and 11.5 present t-statistics of multiple regression coefficients, and multiple correlation coefficients (R^2) for 1983 and 1972 respectively, for both males and females. Each line in these tables contains the coefficients of one equation relating to an age group within a cause-of-death category.

A brief glance at these tables provides a summary of their detailed content. There is a high concentration of significant effects on old-age mortality involving a small number of explanatory variables. These include economic and social status, ethnicity and religiosity, which are strongly related to death rates from heart and circulatory and from cerebrovascular diseases. All other explanatory variables are of much less importance in their explanatory power. The mortality patterns related to each explanatory variable are evaluated for 1983, with comparisons to 1972.

The Effects of Economic and Social Status Levels

High educational levels in a population may increase consciousness regarding healthier consumption patterns and behavior in general. Individuals in such populations may refrain from smoking, from consuming high-cholesterol food, or from heavy drinking; the result may be increased life expectancy. Similarly, the consciousness among high-status populations concerning lack of exercise and its effect on heart and circulatory diseases, may lead to change in behavior and hence to reduced mortality from these causes. On the other hand, such high-status populations have the potential for more consumption in general, including unhealthy consumption.

Another behavioral aspect depending on the levels of socio-economic status, which may affect mortality rates, is the extent to which health services are consumed in a rational manner. It is well known that the use of private medical services has increased substantially in recent years, as the public services can no longer cope effectively with increasing demand. The costs of these private services, particularly of the more sophisticated procedures, which are often used at old ages, have increased exponentially. Such services can be used more extensively by high-status populations which could in turn lead to additional years of life expectancy. Such relationships with overall mortality have been explored in previous studies (McMichael 1985; Pagnanelli 1991; Powell-Griner and Rosenberg 1991).

To test the validity of the status hypothesis we attempt to find out whether and to what extent socio-economic status levels are negatively related to old-age mortality and positively related to life expectancy at age sixty-five. One problem in this analysis arises from the interdependence between economic and social status that is in some instances quite strong. Indeed, in some analyses in the present study such interdependence prevents the simultaneous inclusion of these two explanatory variables in the same analysis.

Considering first the 1983 patterns, we find that status variables have significant explanatory power in the analysis of death rates from heart and circulatory diseases, from cerebrovascular and all other causes, for both males and females (see tables 11.4-11.5). More specifically, for both the 65-79 and the eighty and over age groups, the economic status and the social-status variables affect these death rates negatively. Moreover, there is a negative effect of economic or social status on male death rates from cancer at the 70-74 age group, which however is not highly significant; and there are significant effects of status on death rates from all "other causes." Finally, our analysis shows that the effect of economic status is significant and positive in the equation of life expectancy at age sixty-five for males, while for females, both the economic and the social-status variables are significant. Hence, there is strong evidence to support the hypothesis that economic and social-status levels are negatively associated with death rates at the older ages and positively associated with life expectancies at age sixty-five. The interrelationship between status and death rates from heart and circulatory diseases is of particular importance since this category by itself accounts for about half of old age mortality: the status inequalities in society play an important role in its mortality patterns.

Comparison to 1972 shows some similarity, particularly in the effects of status on death rates from heart and circulatory as well as from cerebrovascular diseases. It can be seen however that status was not as dominant in explaining death rates and life expectancy in 1972 as it was in 1983. Tables 11.4 and 11.5 suggest that during the period 1972-1983 there was a shift in the explanation of death rates and life expectancy from ethnicity to socio-economic status.

The Effect of Ethnicity on Old-Age Mortality

The ethnic composition of a community may affect death rates and life expectancy even when other major variables, particularly socio-economic status, are controlled; ethnicity may have an impact on survivorship through various intermediate biological and behavioral variables. For example, genetic factors associated with the susceptibility to some diseases may be associated with ethnicity. Ethnicity may imply cultural characteristics connected with diets, and other activities or modes of behavior, which may be related directly or indirectly to the risk of mortality from specific causes. Some evidence to the effect of ethnicity on mortality can be found in the literature (e.g., Keith and Smith 1988; Powles 1989).

It was stated in a previous section that micro-level analyses of ethnic differences in mortality have been undertaken in the past, although socio-economic

Table 11.4a

t-Statistic of Tegressions of Various Explanatory Variables on Cause Standardized Death Rates and Life Expectancy at Age 65, Males 1983[a]

Dependent variables: life expectancy and causes of death by age		Explanatory variables								
		Economic status	Social status (education)	Ethnicity (Africa)	Religiosity	Labour participation	Proximity	Loneliness	Industry	R^2
Life expectancy at age 65		3.993***		-4.022***	4.606***					0.588
Heart and circulatory	65-69			2.167***	-2.581***					0.133
	70-74	-1.631*			-3.915***					0.192
	75-79			2.521***	-2.302***					0.138
	80 +[b]	-2.942***	Not in model		-3.065***				1.730**	0.292
	65-79[b]	-2.203***			-4.165***					0.219
	65+[b]	-3.776***			-4.720***					0.301
Cerebro-vascular	65-69	-2.431***								0.083
	70-74		-1.914**			-3.209***		-1.550*		0.412
	75-79		-2.649***	1.959**						0.332
	80 +[b]		-1.656***	2.281***		Not in model		3.735***		0.376
	65-79[b]		-3.099***			-2.039***			2.064***	0.517
	65+[b]		-2.332***	3.210***					2.413***	0.565
Cancer	65-69			1.916**	-2.111***					0.100
	70-74	-1.541*			-2.736***					0.109
	75-79									c
	80 +[b]									c
	65-79[b]				-2.735***				2.171***	0.162
	65+[b]		Not in model		-2.727***				1.764**	0.143
Infectious	65-79[b]			1.609*	-1.477*	-1.965**	Not in model		Not in model	0.203
Others	65-79[b]		-2.436***	4.638***		-1.998***				0.674

[a] Significance: ***=5%; **=10%; * =15% [b] Standardized [c] No equation

Table 11.4b

t-Statistic of Regressions of Various Explanatory Variables on Cause Standardized Death Rates and Life Expentancy at Age 65, Males 1972[a]

Dependent variables: life expectancy and causes of death by age		Explanatory variables								
		Economic status	Social status (education)	Ethnicity (Africa)	Religiosity	Labour participation	Proximity	Loneliness	Industry	R^2
Life expectancy at age 65			1.715**	-5.973***						0.658
Heart and circulatory	65-69				-2.367***				1.468*	0.113
	70-74	Not in model			-2.213***					0.078
	75-79		-1.801***							0.052
	80 +[b]									c
	65-79[b]			1.843**	-2.621***					0.130
	65+[b]	Not in model		2.363***	-2.647***					0.156
Cerebro-vascular	65-69			3.578***						0.179
	70-74	-2.246***	Not in model	3.373***	-1.672**					0.306
	75-79			1.688**						0.046
	80 +[b]		-2.319***			Not in model		1.914**		0.117
	65-79[b]			5.279***						0.322
	65+[b]			5.747***						0.364
Cancer	65-69									c
	70-74				-1.745**	Not in model				0.049
	75-79									c
	80 +[b]									c
	65-79[b]				-2.720***					0.113
	65+[b]				-2.150***					0.074
Infectious	65-79[b]	-2.138***								0.071
Others	65-79[b]		-3.664***		-1.931**	-3.131***				0.421

[a] Significance: ***=5%; **=10%; *=15% [b] Standardized [c] No equation

Table 11.5a
t-Statistic of Regressions of Various Explanatory Variables on Cause Standardized Death rates and Life Expentancy at Age 65, Females 1983[a]

Dependent variables: life expectancy and causes of death by age		Explanatory variables: Economic status	Social status (education)	Ethnicity (Africa)	Religiosity	Labour participation	Proximity	Loneliness	Industry	R^2
Life expectancy at age 65		2.511***	2.596***	-2.232***	4.078***					0.629
Heart and circulatory	65-69			4.390***	-1.525*					0.241
	70-74	-1.828**	-1.791**	1.528*	-2.110***					0.438
	75-79		-4.275***							0.220
	80+[b]	-4.219***			-3.197***					0.248
	65-79[b]		-3.402***	1.932**	-1.643*					0.418
	65+[b]	-2.349***	-2.173***		-2.412***			-1.468*		0.424
Cerebro-vascular	65-69		-2.065***			-1.493*	1.791**			0.334
	70-74			5.262***					2.078***	0.463
	75-79	Not in model	-2.936***	2.075***	-2.278***					0.391
	80+[b]		-2.373***	2.650***	-1.634*					0.385
	65-79[b]		-2.302***	3.531***	-1.693*	-1.762*		-1.544*		0.594
	65+[b]		-2.589***	3.284***	-2.329***	-1.516*				0.565
Cancer	65-69				-1.921**	3.585***				0.245
	70-74				-2.171***					0.067
	75-79			-2.114***	-2.029***					0.136
	80+[b]									c
	65-79[b]									c
	65+[b]				-3.537***	1.885**	-1.724**			0.301
Infectious	65-79[b]		-1.561*			1.958*	2.138***			0.364
Others	65-79[b]	-3.324***		2.345***			2.605***	-1.512*		0.642

[a] Significance: ***=5%; **=10%; *=15% [b] Standardized [c] No equation

Table 11.5b
t-Statistic of Regressions of Various Explanatory Variables on Cause Standardized Death Rates and Life Expentancy at Age 65, Females 1972[a]

Dependent variables: life expectancy and causes of death by age		Explanatory variables: Economic status	Social status (education)	Ethnicity (Africa)	Religiosity	Labour participation	Proximity	Loneliness	Industry	R^2
Life expectancy at age 65			2.424***	-4.295***						0.573
Heart and circulatory	65-69		Not in model	4.229***		Not in model		-2.258***		0.354
	70-74			2.649***		Not in model				0.111
	75-79		-1.679***							0.048
	80+[b]									c
	65-79[b]			3.341***				-2.233***		0.282
	65+[b]			3.259***				-2.245***		0.276
Cerebro-vascular	65-69			5.098***		-1.485*				0.463
	70-74	-1.930***		4.982***						0.434
	75-79		-2.595***					-1.790***		0.219
	80+[b]			2.216***						0.080
	65-79[b]		-2.701***	3.652***						0.535
	65+[b]		-2.824***	4.167***						0.581
Cancer	65-69									c
	70-74			-1.802***						0.054
	75-79									c
	80+[b]									c
	65-79[b]									c
	65+[b]									c
Infectious	65-79[b]	-2.387***				Not in model				0.094
Others	65-79[b]	-2.204***		4.025***				-1.925**	Not in model	0.453

[a] Significance: ***=5%; **=10%; *=15% [b] Standardized [c] No equation

variables could not be controlled (Peritz et al. 1973, 1983). The analyses have shown that North African ethnicity is negatively related with survivorship at most ages; on the other hand, Asian ethnicity has no such effect. Our analytic question is whether, and to what extent, these ethnicity variables affect old-age mortality, when socio-economic variables are controlled. The regressions for 1983 in tables 11.4 and 11.5 show that African ethnicity affects life expectancy negatively through significantly higher death rates from heart and circulatory diseases, and in particular from cerebrovascular and "other" causes at the oldest age groups, for both males and females. As mentioned earlier, the association of African ethnicity with mortality from cerebrovascular diseases was hypothesized to have a genetic explanation, but the present study cannot contribute towards its validation.

Tables 11.4 and 11.5 present similar regression coefficients for 1972. It has been argued that ethnicity, as defined by Asian, African or European origin, has been a major determinant of mortality, as well as of other demographic processes, since the early 1950s. However, with the increased exposure of Asian and African immigrants to Israeli society the importance of ethnicity as a determinant of mortality has declined. In particular, evidence from several sources has shown that the negative impact of Asian origin on life expectancy has decreased significantly since the early 1950s, and our analysis shows that it was virtually eliminated by the early 1970s. In contrast, the negative association between African origin and life expectancy has remained, although a decline is noticeable during the 1970s, while status and religiosity variables became increasingly influential. Hence, as was found by Peritz and colleagues (1973; 1983) ethnicity still has a significant independent effect on old-age mortality. Our data are insufficient for further interpretation of these results.

The Effect of Religiosity on Old-age Mortality

Is religiosity likely to affect survivorship at the older ages, when social and economic status variables are controlled? The existence of such an effect has been established among Jews in the United States (Idler and Kasl 1992). A negative relationship between religiosity and the incidence of myocardial infarction has been observed in Israel (Snyder et al. 1978). The interrelationship between religiosity and survivorship operates through intermediate behavioral variables. Religiosity involves behavior and life style, which include a variety of familial as well as community activities, particularly at the older ages. Frequent visits to the synagogue for various religious activities, work with communal mutual aid organizations, and other voluntary activities may be assumed to provide purpose and moral strength at old age, which may contribute to higher life expectancies. While such extra-familial activities are more frequent for males, females' activity is more concentrated around the wider family and the household. It would indeed be interesting to find out whether the positive effect of community activities, such as can be found among religious groups, on life expectancy, is valid in general, when other variables are controlled. Unfortunately, this cannot be done in the present study.

The relationship between religiosity and life expectancy at the older ages is somewhat complex. On the one hand, it is inversely related with both economic and educational levels, which in turn are positively related with life expectancy. On the other hand, religiosity levels are positively related with life expectancy, through life-style characteristics, which we are unable to measure (see also the section on recursive models).

It can be seen in tables 11.4 and 11.5 that, for males, the religiosity variable is consistently negative, particularly for heart and circulatory diseases, but also for cancer and infectious diseases. Among females, religiosity also affects negatively the death rates from heart and circulatory diseases and from cancer; however, unlike the regression for males, religiosity also affects negatively the death rates from cerebrovascular diseases. Moreover, religiosity has the highest t value in the life expectancy equation (at age sixty-five) for both males and females.

Can we find similar religiosity effects on old-age mortality in 1972? These tables provide comparisons to 1983, and suggest that such effect was not as systematic for males, and was not significant at all for females. However, we cannot offer an interpretation to the change in this effect during the period 1972-1983. Nevertheless, by the evidence of the data presented, we accept the religiosity hypothesis and consider its interrelationship as one of the more interesting observations in this study.

Old-age Mortality and Other Variables

We are left with the remaining three variables, loneliness (defined in terms of marital status), industry and participation in the labor force. We deal with all these three variables in this section because their interrelationships with old-age mortality are less consistent than the variables in the previous hypotheses.

The loneliness hypothesis has been considered in previous studies. It has been repeatedly observed that non-married persons, that is, those of single, divorced, or widowed status, have higher probabilities of dying compared with the married. Part of the explanation is "selectivity" while part is "protective" (Spiegelman 1968: 91-92; Hu and Goldman 1990; Powell-Griner and Rosenberg 1991).

Our aggregate level analyses in tables 11.4 and 11.5 suggest that the hypothesis that life expectancy at age sixty-five is negatively related with this variable, is not supported for males at either period; however, the loneliness variable for females shows some consistent relationships with mortality. But a more appropriate individual-level analysis published recently, which is partly consistent with our findings, shows that unmarried persons are disadvantaged in life expectancy in Israel in general: particularly widowers (Eisenbach 1994).

Another hypothesis is concerned with the relationship of old-age mortality, particularly from cancer, with the industry variable. A positive relationship should be expected. Table 11.4 suggests that such expected relationships are significant for males and only in some cause-of-death and age categories. For example, the industry variable has a significant positive effect on the male death rate from cancer at the 65-79 age group, which is consistent with expectation. The industry variable also affects the death rate from heart and circulatory diseases at the 80-and-over age group, and the death rate from cerebrovascular diseases. This interrelationship seems to be a new phenomenon, as we do not find it for 1972; it may reflect an increase over time in environment problems.

Our last hypothesis is concerned with the rate of old-age participation in the labor force. This variable was considered to represent a proxy for extra-familial activity at the older ages, but has also an income effect. It is hypothesized to have a positive effect on life expectancy and negative effects on cause-specific death rates. It has in addition a qualification that healthier people tend to be more active economically. Table 11.4 suggests that this variable is negatively related with the death rate from cerebrovascular diseases among both sexes, and from infectious and "other" diseases at the 65-79 age group for males, while its other coefficients are positive and contrary to the hypothesis. We must conclude, therefore, that this hypothesis has little support in this study.

Another hypothesis that was considered at the early stages of this project is concerned with the geographic proximity of place of residence to major units of specialized medical services. The three major cities in the country offer such specialized medical services: the distance from each locality to the closest of these cities was considered as a proxy variable for the accessibility of the population to such medical services. Controlling for status and ethnicity variables is of critical importance in testing this hypothesis because these explanatory variables tend to be associated with distance from the three major cities.

We expected strong positive relationships between proximity and the cause-specific death rates, particularly heart diseases for which distance and time are critical. However, our analysis shows that the effect of proximity was insignificant whenever status and ethnicity were controlled.

The Increase in Life Expectancy 1972-1983: Different Patterns

In the discussion concerning the inequality in old-age mortality (see table 11.2), it was suggested that an increase in inter-locality differentiation in life expectancy at age sixty-five occurred in the period 1972-1983. In particular, localities with relatively low life expectancies in 1972 seemed to have experienced only slight increases in life expectancies, if any, particularly among women. Table 11.6 provides the interpretation for that pattern. It shows unequivocally that when other variables are controlled, the increase in life expectancy 1972-1983 is inversely related with its initial level and with African ethnicity, while it is positively related with status and religiosity. Hence, localities with small proportions of high income earners or with high proportions of population of African ethnicity, experienced small increases in life expectancy during 1972-1983, despite being located at the lower part of the 1972 life expectancy distribution. Almost all these localities are new towns, as shown in the lower part of table 11.2. This pattern explains the increase in the inequality in life expectancy during that period.

The Analysis of Life Expectancy at Age Sixty-Five through a Recursive Model

We now propose to explore more complex interrelationships, through a system of structural equations using recursive models. Such models may provide a clearer interpretation of the interrelationship structure among the dependent and the explanatory variables. They enable the distinction between direct and indirect effects of the explanatory variables on the dependent variable, life expectancy, under the assumptions specified below. For example, the observation that the population of African ethnicity has experienced higher mortality levels for many years, was interpreted in terms of a possible ethnic-genetic factor (see tables 11.3-11.5; Peritz et al. 1973, 1983). On the other hand, it has also been shown that socio-economic status has a dominant negative effect on life-expectancy levels. The analytic question we pose is whether, and to what extent, the higher "African mortality" is related to the direct ethnic effect, or to the lower level of socio-economic status among this ethnic group: the indirect effect.

These models are estimated under the assumption that the variables in the system can be arranged hierarchically in terms of their causal priorities. This assumption implies that ethnicity and religiosity may affect all other variables in the system, but these cannot affect ethnicity and religiosity. Education may affect life expectancy, but this cannot affect education, or other variables in the system. In addition, it is assumed that the error terms of the equations are uncorrelated. These assumptions allow the estimation of the regression coefficients of the proposed model through ordinary least square methods (e.g., Wonnacott and Wonnacott 1970; Blalock 1971; Johnston 1987). Since the present analysis does not use information on cause of death it is possible to use thc 600 smaller units.

Table 11.6
T-Statistic of Regressions Coefficients of Various Explanatory Variables on Differences in Life Expentancies 1972-1983, at Age 65

Explanatory variables	Males		Females	
	t	Significance	t	Significance
Initial life expectancy e_{65}, 1972	-4.261	.0001	-2.958	.0047
Religiosity	+2.665	.0103	+3.343	.0016
African ethnicity	-1.919	.0605	-2.190	.0330
Social status (education levels)	+2.508	.0153	+1.776	.0819
R^2	0.325		0.316	

The following structural equations are estimated under these assumptions, and describe the hypothesized interrelationship system between life expectancy at age sixty-five and the explanatory variables among men and women:

$$ED_{9.60} = A_{ed} + B_{ed.et}ETAF + B_{ed.re}REL + e_{ed}$$

$$E_{65} = A_e + B_{e.et}\ ETAF + B_{e.re}\ REL + B_{e.ed}ED_{9.60} + B_{e.lo}LON_{70} + e_e$$

where A_{ed}, $B_{ed.et}$, $B_{ed.re}$, and e_{ed}, denote the constant term, the regression coefficients of ethnicity and of religiosity, and the residual error term, respectively, of the education dependent variable $ED_{9.60}$. A_e, $B_{e.et}$, $B_{e.re}$, $B_{e.ed}$, $B_{e.lo}$, and e_e denote the constant term, the regression coefficients of ethnicity religiosity and of loneliness, and the residual error term, respectively, of the life-expectancy dependent variable at age sixty-five, E_{65}. ETAF, REL, $ED_{9.60}$, and LON_{70} are the explanatory variables of these equations as defined above. The structural equations for women are similar.

Figures 11.2 and 11.3 show the main results of these analyses for men and women respectively. The numerical values above each arrow in these figures represent the t statistics of the appropriate regression coefficient.

Beginning with the analysis for men, it can be seen that African ethnicity affects life expectancy both directly, and indirectly. The indirect effect of African ethnicity on life expectancy operates through the educational level: social status. African ethnicity affects the social status variable negatively, and social status affects life expectancy positively. African ethnicity has, therefore, a negative indirect effect on life expectancy through the status variable. Furthermore, the direct effect of African ethnicity on life expectancy is also negative. This is the ethnicity effect discussed in an earlier section, which might be genetic, as hypothesized in a previous study (Peritz et al. 1973, 1983), or behavioral, or both. The structural equations enable the calculation of the relative strength of the direct and the indirect effects of African ethnicity. For example, a difference of ten percent in African ethnicity between localities implies a difference of about ten months in life expectancy at age sixty-five. About eight and a half months of these are due to the direct effect.

As for the religiosity variable for men, its indirect effect on life expectancy is negative, but quite small. This may be referred to as the socio-economic effect of religiosity on life expectancy at age sixty-five. However, the direct effect of religiosity on life expectancy is positive. This may be interpreted as the religious "life-style" effect that has been discussed above. Again, the relative strength of the direct and the indirect effects of religiosity can be calculated. For example, a difference of 10 percent in religiosity between localities implies a difference of about two and a half months in life expectancy at age sixty-five. While the direct effect is positive and amounts to almost three months, the indirect effect is negative and small.

Figure 11.3 presents the regression coefficients of the recursive model for women. Again, both the indirect (socio-economic) and the direct ethnicity effects are negative. Religiosity, on the other hand, has an indirect negative effect

Figure 11.2
Recursive Model: Male Life Expectancy at Age Sixty-Five (*T* Statistic for Variables in Structural Equations Shown above Arrows)

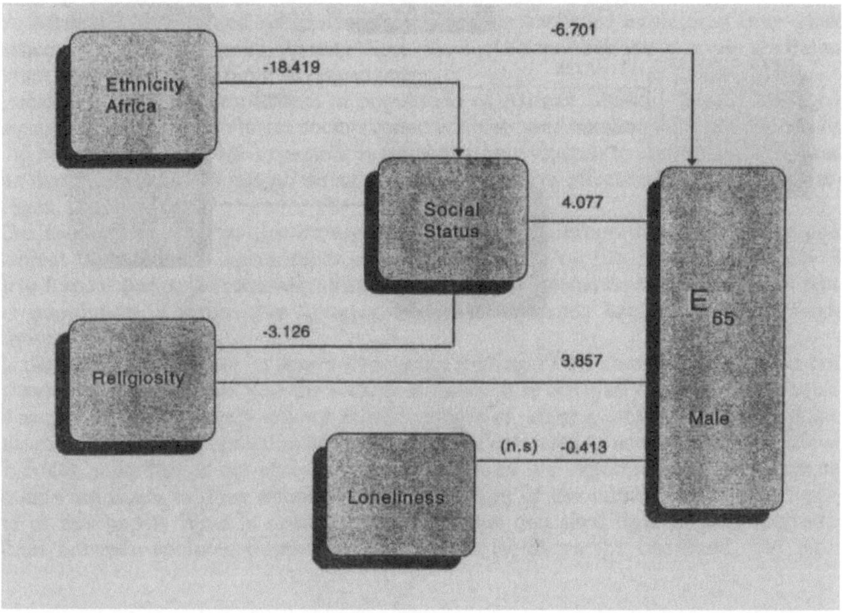

on life expectancy through education, and a positive direct effect. In contrast with the analysis for men, the indirect effects of both ethnicity and religiosity are stronger than the direct effects. For example, a difference of ten percent in African ethnicity between localities implies a difference of about fourteen months in life expectancy at age sixty-five. About nine months of these are due to the indirect (socio-economic) effect. A difference of ten percent in religiosity between localities implies a difference of one month in life expectancy at age sixty-five. This difference is the result of a negative indirect effect of two months and a positive direct effect of one month. One interpretation for the strong negative socio-economic effect of ethnicity on women's life expectancy may be a low level of consciousness regarding their health condition. The finding of a strong indirect socioeconomic effect of religiosity on women's life expectancy is consistent with the hypothesis that women benefit less than men from the advantages of a religious lifestyle.

Summary and Conclusion

The decline in old-age mortality is a new demographic process. Indeed, up to the 1970s there was hardly any increase in life expectancy at age sixty-five in the country as a whole. Old-age mortality data for other developed countries show a similar pattern.

Figure 11.3
Recursive Model: Female Life Expectancy at Age Sixty-Five (*T* Statistic for Variables in Structural Equations Shown above Arrows)

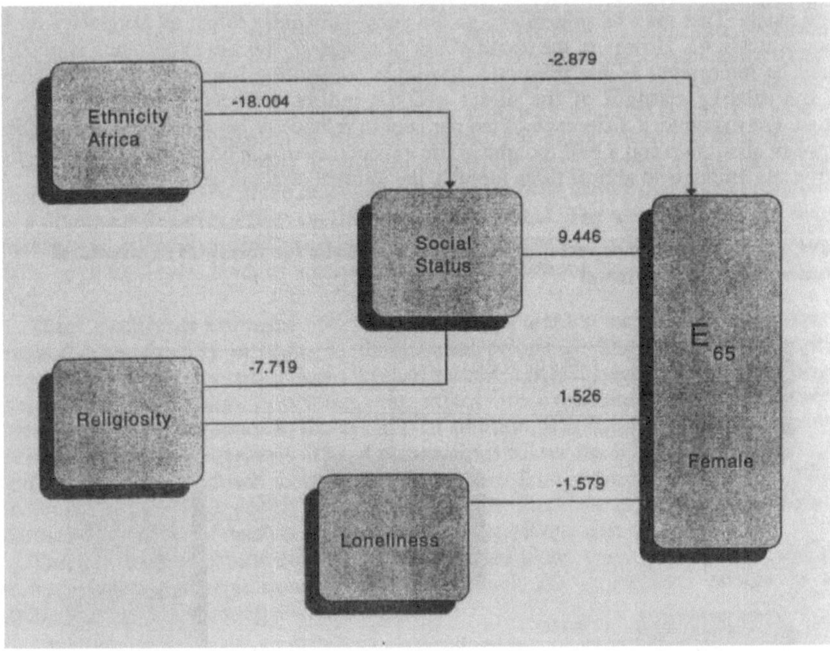

Our analysis has documented very large differences among geographic areas in both overall and old-age mortality levels. These mortality inequalities, across subpopulations in a country with highly subsidized health services, with relatively small numbers of homeless or hungry, led us to attempt to explain inter-locality variations in cause-specific death rates and life expectancies at age sixty-five.

A comparison of old-age mortality from the early 1970s to the early 1980s shows an overall increase in life expectancy. However, while life expectancy increases in localities characterized by high status levels, mostly with high initial life expectancies, were relatively large, increases for localities with low socio-economic status, mostly with relatively low initial life expectancies, were small. Hence, the socio-economic inequality in longevity increased during that period in general, even more strongly among women.

Death rates from heart and circulatory diseases account for about half of old-age mortality. Our analysis suggests that large proportions of people with high socio-economic status, high proportions of religious people and low proportions of population of African ethnicity are associated with low death rates from these diseases. Contrary to expectations, close proximity to major medical centers was not found to be a significant determinant of low mortality levels from heart and circulatory diseases, when socio-economic status and ethnicity are controlled.

Cancer makes a much smaller contribution to old-age mortality, less than 20 percent, and its explanation, in general, is not as good as for heart and circulatory diseases. Indeed, the analysis for women, in particular, provided poor explanation. However, for men, high levels of socio-economic status and large proportions of religious people are associated with low rates of cancer mortality, while high proportions of the labor force in industries are associated with high cancer mortality in localities.

Hence, viewing the overall patterns of our results, we can confirm that socio-economic status, African ethnicity and religiosity are the major variables explaining inter-locality differences in old-age mortality. Among these, the socio-economic status levels are the most important, especially at the more advanced ages.

Localities with high proportions of population of African ethnicity have relatively low life expectancies both due to lower socio-economic levels, and because this ethnic group has a specific negative effect on life expectancy, genetic or behavioral. In contrast, it is interesting to note that Asian ethnicity has no direct or indirect negative effect on life expectancy at the older ages.

Our analyses suggest that localities with relatively high proportions of religious people are subject to two forces operating in opposite directions on life expectancy levels. The negative force is due to the relatively lower socio-economic status among the religious section of the population. The positive force is connected with the life style of the religious population.

Is there a lesson that can be drawn from these findings? Can these be a basis for a policy to increase the life expectancy of the society at large? It is obviously impossible to equalize socio-economic status levels among ethnic groups or among other kinds of population subgroups. Equally, the population at large cannot be expected to adopt a religious life style which could, according to our analysis, lead to increased life expectancy. These rather naive statements are made to draw attention to the structure of the initial framework discussed earlier in this paper. What is needed is research that can shed light on the intermediate variables between socio-economic and cultural variables on the one hand, and old-age mortality from the different causes of death, on the other. Indeed, a contribution might be made by a better understanding of the mechanisms under which variables such as ethnicity, the level of social or economic status and the life style of religious people affect the death rates from major causes. This could make it possible to design policies that will lead to increases in overall life expectancies without inconceivable revolutionary changes in the structure of society.

Acknowledgements

This project was sponsored by the Basic Research Foundation of the Israel Academy of Sciences and Humanities, for which the authors are grateful. We are also grateful to the JOINT (JDC) Israel, and the Brookdale Institute of Gerontology and Adult Human Development in Israel, for support in the final stages of this project. We wish to express our appreciation for the skilful assistance provided by Orly Sivan, Carole Feldmann, Yifat Klopstock, and Hagit Weiss. We express our thanks to Barbara Okun for very helpful comments and suggestions.

Appendix A: Constructing Life Tables in Small Local Areas

Estimates of life table functions may be inaccurate for small populations, such as those in statistical areas. Hence, the smaller statistical areas were aggregated. These aggregates are referred to as small local areas.

The full enumeration of both the 1983 and the 1972 Population Censuses provided the mid-year populations by age and sex. The distribution of deaths by age and sex was extracted from vital registration data for five years.

Statistical areas were aggregated into small local areas under the constraint that sub-quarter borders were not crossed, and with a preference for joining areas with similar socioeconomic characteristics. Small settlements such as *kibbutzim* and *moshavim* were aggregated within sub-districts *(nafoth)* by type of settlement.

Using the population data from the full enumeration of the Census and the number of deaths from registration data we computed age-specific mortality rates. We used the Reed-Merrell method of life table construction (Shryock and Siegel 1973:443-444).

Appendix B: The Accuracy of the Reported Age Structure

Birth registration in the State of Israel is considered to be accurate and complete. However, a possible source for deviations from the true age structure of death rates may be the incorrect registration of the age of new immigrants upon their arrival.

Many Israelis were born in countries in Asia and Africa. It is common in less developed countries for the elderly to overstate their ages: consequently, mortality levels may be underestimated among the elderly. The purpose of this appendix is to detect the presence of age-overstatement.

If the real age of a cohort is less than its reported age, we would expect the cohort's mortality level to be relatively low over time. Thus, we should be able to observe a cohort effect on mortality due to the initial age-overstatement; for real cohort effects see for instance Preston and van de Walle (1978); Anderson and Silver (1989); Caselli and Capocaccia (1989).

We assume that the people born in Europe or America tend to report correct ages compared with those born in Africa or Asia. Hence, we used ratios of the age-specific mortality rates for African and Asian Jews relative to those for European and American Jews for each age group above age forty to detect age-overstatement. Our comparison reveals that mortality patterns among Asian men are closest to those of Europeans and Americans, followed by Asian women, African men and African women, in that order.

If age-overstatement were common, we would expect these ratios to decline with age. Ratios for older men and women born in Africa, however, show no such decline. Hence, we found no evidence of age-overstatement among Asian or African Jews. Thus, old-age mortality is unlikely to have been underestimated. The rising ratios of African mortality rates relative to those of Europeans and Americans are consistent with the findings in this chapter regarding the effect of ethnicity.

References

Anderson, Barbara A. and Brian D. Silver. 1989. "Patterns of cohort mortality in the Soviet population." *Population and Development Review* 15: 471-501.

Anson, J. 1988. "Mortality and living conditions: Relative mortality levels and relation to the physical quality of life in urban populations." *Social Science and Medicine* 27: 901-910.

Antonovsky, A. 1967. "Social class, life expectancy and overall mortality." *Milbank Memorial Fund Quarterly* 45: 151-193.

Barell, Vita, Yochanan Wax and Avima Ruder. 1988. "Analysis of geographic differentials in infant mortality rates: The Or Yehuda community." *American Journal of Epidemiology* 128: 218-230.

Blalock, Hubert M. 1971. *Causal Models in the Social Sciences.* London: Macmillan.

Carrier, N. H. and A. M. Farrag. 1959. "The reduction of errors in census populations for statistically underdeveloped countries." *Population Studies* 13: 240-285.

Caselli, Graziella and Riccardo Capocaccia. 1989. "Age, period, cohort and early mortality: An analysis of adult mortality in Italy." *Population Studies* 43: 133-153.

Central Bureau of Statistics. 1992. *Statistical Abstract of Israel* 43. Jerusalem: Central Bureau of Statistics.

Chauvire, Y. 1991. "Les inégalités en matière de mortalité à Paris et dans la petite couronne." *Espaces, Populations, Sociétés* 1991-1: 47-53.

Eisenbach, Zvi. 1994. "Socioeconomic differences in old-age mortality in Israel: An individual-level analysis." In D. Friedlander and Y. Tamir (eds.), *Patterns of Old-Age Mortality in Israel.* Jerusalem: Joint-Brookdale Institute (in Hebrew).

Eisenstadt, S. N., Moshe Lissak and Yaacov Nahon. 1993. *Ethnic Communities in Israel - Socio Economic Status.* Jerusalem: Jerusalem Institute for Israel Studies (in Hebrew).

Friedlander, Dov, Jona Schellekens, Eliahu Ben-Moshe and Ariela Keysar. 1985. "Socioeconomic characteristics and life expectancies in nineteenth century England: A district analysis." *Population Studies* 40: 137-151.

Higueras Arnal, A. 1991. "Mortalité et changement social en Espagne 1975-1988." *Espaces, Populations, Sociétés* 1991-1: 143-150.

Hu, Y., and N. Goldman. 1990. "Mortality differentials by marital status: An international comparison." *Demography* 27: 233-250.

Johnston, J. 1987. *Econometric Methods.* New York: McGraw-Hill International Editions.

Idler, Ellen L. and Stanislav V. Kasl. 1992. "Religion, disability, depression, and the timing of death." *American Journal of Sociology* 97: 1052-1079.

Keith, V. M. and D. P. Smith. 1988. "The current differentials in black and white life expectancy." *Demography* 25: 625-632.

Lusky, Ayala, Rachel Gurvitz and Vita Barell. 1992. "Variation in mortality rates in Tel Aviv region municipalities." Unpublished paper.

McMichael, A. J. 1985. "Social class (as estimated by occupational prestige) and mortality in Australian males in the 1970s." *Community Health Studies* 9: 220-230.

Mosk, Carl, and S. Ryan Johansson. 1986. "Income and mortality: evidence from modern Japan." *Population and Development Review* 12: 415-440.

Muhsam, H. V. 1966. "Mode of life and longevity in Israel." *Jewish Journal of Sociology* 8: 39-48.

Pagnanelli, Floriano. 1991. "Les différences de mortalité en Italie selon certains facteurs socio-économiques: Une synthèse des informations." *Socio-economic Differential Mortality in Industrialized Societies* 7: 82-115.

Peritz, E., F. Dreyfuss, H. S. Halevi, and U. O. Schmelz. 1973. *Mortality of Adult Jews in Israel* 1950-1967. Jerusalem: Central Bureau of Statistics.

Peritz, E., U. Goldbourt, S. Yaari, P. Zadka and U. O. Schmelz. 1983. "An analysis of adult mortality by cause of death among immigrants from several countries." Unpublished research report (in Hebrew).

Powell-Griner, E. and H. M. Rosenberg. 1991. "New data on socio-economic differential mortality in the United States." *Socio-economic Differential Mortality in Industrialized Societies* 7: 182-199.

Powles, J. W. 1989. "The best of both worlds: attempting to explain the persisting low mortality of Greek migrants to Australia." In J. C. Caldwell, S. Findley, P. Caldwell, G. Santow (eds.), *What We Know about Health Transition,* 584-594. Canberra: Australian National University.

Preston, Samuel H., and Etienne van de Walle. 1978. "Urban French mortality in the nineteenth century." *Population Studies* 32: 275-297.

Sakai, Hiromichi. 1986. "A study of the socioeconomic correlates of Japanese life expectancy at 60 years and over." *Journal of Population Problems* 180: 46-51 (in Japanese).

Shryock, Henry S. and Jacob S. Siegel. 1973. *The Methods and Materials of Demography.* Washington DC: Bureau of the Census.

Silver, M. 1972. "An econometric analysis of spatial variations in mortality rates by race and sex." In Victor R. Fuchs (ed.), *Essays in the Economics of Health and Medical Care,* 161-227. New York: Columbia University Press.

Snyder, M., U. Goldbourt, J. H. Medalie, H. N. Neufeld and D. Orono 1978. "A lower incidence of myocardial infarct among religious Jews than among irreligious Jews." *Torah u'Mada* 8: 35-44.

Spiegelman, Mortimer. 1968. *Introduction to Demography.* Cambridge MA: Harvard University Press.

Thumerelle, P.J. 1991. "La mortalité dans le Nord-Pas-de-Calais: Un exemple de la stabilité des modèles régionaux de mortalité." *Espaces, Populations, Sociétés* 1991-1: 55-72.

Wonnacott, R. J. and T. H. Wonnacott. 1970. *Econometrics.* New York: John Wiley.

12

Does Religious Observance Promote Health? Mortality in Secular vs. Religious Kibbutzim in Israel

Jeremy D. Kark, Galia Shemi, Yechiel Friedlander, Oz Martin, Orly Manor, and S. H. Blondheim

Introduction

Awareness of psychosocial and cultural determinants of health is necessary as a renewed balance and integration is sought between organic biomedical and biopsychosocial models of causation (O'Boyle 1993). The possible association of religion and religious observance with health status has long intrigued scholars of diverse disciplines (e.g., Galton 1872). The focal role of religion and its importance in the social and cultural context (as reflected by the persistence and resurgence of religion in human populations) suggest that study of this attribute may provide valuable insights into determinants of health and disease. The question of whether religious belief and practice promote health is unresolved, and the effect may vary according to religion (Kaplan 1976; Jarvis and Northcott 1987). Different denominations have been compared, but few studies have considered the effect of religiousness within a single religious denomination (Kaplan 1976; Levin and Vanderpool 1987). Except for studies of Mormons (Gardner and Lyon 1982) and Seventh-Day Adventists (Phillips et al. 1978) and a recent investigation of Chinese (Phillips et al. 1993) most within-denomination studies have focused on church attendance as the variable expressing the degree of religiousness (Kaplan 1976; Levin and Vanderpool 1987). However, attendance can be influenced by health status and may not be a determinant thereof (Levin and Markides 1986). Investigation of other dimensions or expressions of religion is worthwhile (Kaplan 1976; Levin and Vanderpool 1987).

Several studies in the Jewish population of Israel have pointed to a protective association between religious orthodoxy and coronary heart disease (Snyder et al. 1978; Friedlander et al. 1986). However, comparison across different degrees of observance among Jews in Israel may be confounded by other factors that have been related to morbidity and mortality, such as ethnic group (Central Bureau of Statistics 1991), social class (Susser et al. 1985; Marmot et al. 1991), or the availability of social supports (Berkman and Syme 1979). Our objective was to determine the association between Jewish religious observance and mortality among study populations with maximal similarity in social structure, social support mechanisms, and lifestyle. These similarities, despite religious differences, are found in Israeli kibbutzim.

Most of the kibbutzim (egalitarian collectives) were initially established by and affiliated with political movements that were secular in nature. A small number, representing about 6 percent of the total adult kibbutz population, were established by religiously observant Jews who maintained a homogeneous religious lifestyle in their settlements. Other than this central difference, secular and religious kibbutzim have been highly similar in their social and economic structure and function. Both are cohesive, supportive communities (Spiro 1983; Fishman 1992). The kibbutz population as a whole, relative to the general Israeli Jewish population, is characterized by low mortality (Leviatan and Cohen 1985). The question posed in our study was whether belonging to a religious community provides additional protection.

Methods

Study Design and Population

We undertook a historical prospective study of mortality in secular and religious kibbutzim over a sixteen-year period (January 1. 1970, through December 31, 1985). Eleven religious kibbutzim established before 1965 were pair matched with eleven secular kibbutzim from the labor movement according to the following criteria: same geographic locale, use of the same regional hospital, similar numbers of members forty years of age and older, and dates of establishment as close as possible.

Included in the study were male and female members who were thirty-five years old or older at any time during the follow-up. Residents who were not members were excluded. Based on the population registry of each kibbutz, the population was reconstructed for January 1, 1970. Calculation of duration of exposure in these dynamic cohorts took account of in- and out-migration, achieving the age of thirty-five years, and deaths. The data available for this study included sex, date of birth, entrance into or departure from the kibbutz, and death.

Over the sixteen-year period, the 3,900 individuals included in the follow-up contributed 41,347 person-years of observation, and 268 deaths occurred (table 12.1). There were 16 percent fewer subjects in religious kibbutzim (1,777) than in secular kibbutzim (2,123); this difference was 7 percent in aggregated years of exposure (19,879 person-years in religious kibbutzim and 21,468 person-years in secular kibbutzim). The members of religious kibbutzim were younger; 8.9 percent of time (in person-years) accrued in those sixty-five years of age and over, in comparison with 16.6 percent in the secular kibbutzim (table 12.1).

Stability of the population above the age of thirty-five years was marked in both types of kibbutz. There was less out-migration in the religious kibbutzim than in the secular kibbutzim, with losses of sixty-three and 162 individuals, respectively, over the sixteen-year follow-up. Of those who left religious kibbutzim, 75 percent did so before they were fifty years old; the corresponding figure for secular kibbutzim was 80 percent. Only twenty new members fifty years old or older joined the kibbutzim during the study period.

Information on Deaths

Data sources to ascertain deaths were: 1) individual kibbutz population registers, which were verified and supplemented by records of primary care providers; 2) central population files of the religious and labor kibbutz movements; and 3) kibbutz burial and remembrance committees. Two hundred sixty-eight deaths were recorded, sixty-nine in religious kibbutzim and 199 in secular kibbutzim. Members who left the kibbutz movement were not followed up for subsequent mortality.

Information on underlying cause of each death, as routinely coded between 1970 and 1985, was obtained from the Israel Central Bureau of Statistics. In addition, copies of death certificates were retrieved and recoded according to the *International Classification of Diseases* (9th edition) (ICD-9) by a trained nosologist unaware of the study hypothesis or religious affiliations. Obvious discrepancies between the two sources were checked, and Central Bureau of Statistics codes were preferred unless unavailable (seven deaths) or clearly in error. In seven cases in which cause of death was coded as unknown (all out-of-hospital deaths), and in five cases with missing information for both sources, kibbutz clinic data were used to determine cause of death.

Statistical Analysis

Sex-specific mortality rates were calculated by the person-time method, based on months of exposure. Time was counted from entry into the study until death, out-migration, or conclusion of the study. Direct age adjustment (using five-year age groups) was performed to account for differences in the age structure of the kibbutzim. Kaplan-Meier survival analysis was applied to birth cohorts (Kaplan and Meier, 1958), and mortality in religious vs.. secular populations

Table 12.1
Person-Years of Exposure (PY) and Number of Deaths in Israeli Religious and Secular Kibbutz Members Aged 35 and Older, by Age Group, 1970 through 1985

		Age Group, y											
		35–44		45–54		55–64		65–74		75+		Total	
	Type of Kibbutz	PY	No. Deaths	PY	No. Deaths	PY	No. Deaths	PY	No. Deaths	PY	No. Deaths	PY	No. Deaths
Men	Religious	3628	1	3085	10	2588	20	910	18	73	2	10 284	51
	Secular	3730	9	2634	10	2568	37	1520	46	262	20	10 713	122
Women	Religious	3379	1	3143	4	2291	6	713	6	69	1	9 595	18
	Secular	3716	6	2615	7	2644	24	1528	27	252	13	10 755	77
Both	Religious	7006	2	6228	14	4878	26	1623	24	143	3	19 879	69
	Secular	7446	15	5249	17	5212	61	3048	73	514	33	21 468	199

Note: There were 924 men and 853 women on religious kibbutzim and 1072 men and 1051 women on secular kibbutzim (a total of 1996 men with 20 997 PY and 1904 women with 20 350 PY follow-up and grand total of 3900 members with 41 347 PY follow-up). PY accrued within age groups at any time during follow-up, and number of deaths refers to those that occurred in the person-time in each age group. Small differences between the sum of the age-specific PY of exposure and the totals shown are due to rounding errors.

was compared by the log rank test. Cox proportional hazards analysis, with age introduced as a continuous variable, was used to incorporate the matched design of the study by summarization across the eleven paired strata (Cox 1972; Kalbfleisch and Prentice 1980). The effect of the method of sampling (by cluster) was evaluated. This effect was shown to be negligible and was disregarded in the analyses presented (a description of the statistical assessment of the cluster sampling is available from the authors).

Results

For each sex, there was a substantial excess rate of death for members of secular kibbutzim relative to members of religious kibbutzim (table 12.2). The age-adjusted rate ratios were 1.76 (95 percent confidence interval [CI] = 1.26, 2.46) in men, 2.72 (95 percent CI = 1.60, 4.62) in women, and 1.98 (95 percent CI = 1.50, 2.62) in the sex-pooled data. The association was generally consistent across ten-year age groups. The age-adjusted mortality rates for religious kibbutzim were 5.67 (SE = 0.82) per 1,000 person-years for men and 2.33 (SE = 0.57) per 1,000 person-years for women. For secular kibbutzim, the rates were 9.96 (SE = 0.91) per 1,000 person-years for men and 6.34 (SE = 0.72) per 1,000 person-years for women.

Cox proportional hazards analyses confirmed these findings: the rate ratios were 1.67 (95 percent CI = 1.17, 2.39; $P < .01$) for men, 2.67 (95 percent CI = 1.55, 4.60; $P < .001$) for women, and 1.93 (95 percent CI = 1.44, 2.59; $P < .0001$) for the total population (controlling for sex). The apparently stronger protective effect of religiousness in women than in men, tested by introduction of a term for interaction into the Cox model, was associated with a P value of .088.

In light of a secular (time) trend toward reduced mortality in Israel during the study period (Central Bureau of Statistics 1991), the follow-up was subdivided into three periods: 1970 through 1975 (sixty-two deaths, 12,822 person-years). 1976 through 1980 (eighty deaths, 12,901 person-years), and 1981 through 1985 (126 deaths, 15,624 person-years). Excess mortality in the secular kibbutzim was apparent in each period in both sexes (table 12.2).

The time trend in mortality, the younger age of the religious kibbutz population, and the person-time method of analysis used could have produced an apparent excess in secular kibbutz mortality as a result of a possible cohort effect. This possibility was further explored by Kaplan-Meier survival analysis of the mortality experience of ten-year birth cohorts during our study period (1970 through 1985). Excess mortality at the end of follow-up was apparent in secular kibbutzim in all cohorts except the youngest (those born between 1940 and 1950; there were only seven deaths in this cohort) (table 12.3). Even in this age group, a comparison of the observed and the expected mortality over the entire follow-up (as assessed by the log rank test) showed a slight excess in secular kibbutzim (mortality ratio = 1.1).

Table 12.2
Age-Adjusted Rate Ratios and 95% Confidence Intervals of Mortality from All Causes: Secular vs. Religious Kibbutzim, 1970 through 1985

Period	Rate Ratio (95% Confidence Interval)		
	Men	Women	Total
1970–1975	1.85 (1.33, 2.58)	3.84 (2.24, 6.58)	2.16 (1.33, 3.50)
1976–1980	1.56 (1.07, 2.27)	5.80 (3.22, 10.45)	2.18 (1.59, 2.99)
1981–1985	1.74 (1.06, 2.86)	1.99 (1.01, 3.90)	1.80 (1.21, 2.68)
1970–1985	1.76 (1.26, 2.46)	2.72 (1.60, 4.62)	1.98 (1.50, 2.62)

Table 12.3
Survival Probabilities and Relative Risk of Death in Secular vs Religious Kibbutzim between 1970 and 1985 for 10-Year Birth Cohorts Born between 1900 and 1950: Kaplan—Meier Analysis

Birth Cohort	Secular Kibbutzim			Religious Kibbutzim			Relative Risk	P^a
	No. Subjects	No. Deaths	Probability of Survival (SE)	No. Subjects	No. Deaths	Probability of Survival (SE)		
1900–1909	130	61	.518 (.044)	35	12	.657 (.080)	1.4	.21
1910–1919	381	77	.793 (.021)	252	29	.883 (.020)	1.77	.003
1920–1929	344	35	.891 (.017)	427	21	.950 (.011)	2.18	.002
1930–1939	434	15	.960 (.010)	410	4	.987 (.007)	3.08	.007
1940–1950	822	4	.991 (.005)	653	3	.952 (.042)	0.19	.88
1900–1950	2111	192[b]		1777	69[b]		1.89	<.0001

Note. Twelve members of secular kibbutzim born before 1900 were excluded.
[a]From log rank test.
[b]Expected numbers of deaths were 155.3 in secular kibbutzim and 105.7 in religious kibbutzim (χ^2 = 23.01; $P < .00001$). Division into 5-year birth cohorts provided similar results, with expected numbers of deaths of 156.3 in secular kibbutzim and 104.7 in religious kibbutzim (χ^2 = 22.01; $P < .00001$; relative risk = 1.86).

The underlying cause of death was categorized into the following groups: all circulatory conditions (ICD-9 codes 390 through 459), of which 73 percent were coronary heart disease (ICD-9 codes 410 through 414); all neoplasms (ICD-9 codes 140 through 239); all external causes (comprising road accidents, all other accidents, and suicide); and all other causes taken together (table 12.4). These four categories, respectively, accounted for 117 (44 percent), eighty-three (31 percent), twenty-two (8 percent), and forty-six (17 percent) of the 268 deaths. The main contribution of this cause-specific analysis is in demonstrating the overall consistency of the association across major diagnostic categories. For each cause of death, when men and women were grouped together, those in secular kibbutzim exhibited significantly higher overall rates than those in religious kibbutzim. The rate ratios ranged from 1.7 to more than four across the different diagnostic groups, an excess evident in each sex in most diagnostic groups (table 12.4).

Discussion

Summary of Findings

There was a distinctly lower mortality rate in religious kibbutzim than in secular kibbutzim that was evident in both sexes, evident at all ages, and consistent throughout the sixteen-year period of observation. The lower mortality persisted, with remarkable overall consistency, across the major categories of underlying cause of death. The magnitude of the protective effect associated with membership in a religious kibbutz is exemplified by ablation of the usual female mortality advantage: secular women did not live longer than religious men.

Possible Biases

The possibility that confounding by socio-demographic variables could explain the findings seems remote. Selected socio-demographic data are available

Table 12.4
Age-Adjusted Cause-Specific Mortality Rates (per 1000 Person-Years) and Rate Ratios, 1970 through 1985

Cause of Death (ICD-9 Codes)	Gender	Secular Kibbutzim No. Deaths	Secular Kibbutzim Rate	Religious Kibbutzim No. Deaths	Religious Kibbutzim Rate	Rate Ratio	95% Confidence Interval
Coronary heart disease (410–414)	Men	45	3.8	14	1.6	2.40	1.30, 4.42
	Women	19	1.4	7	1.1	1.31	0.54, 3.18
	Both	64	2.6	21	1.3	1.93	1.16, 3.20
All circulatory conditions (390–459)	Men	60	4.8	22	2.6	1.88	1.14, 3.10
	Women	27	2.0	8	1.2	1.73	0.77, 3.89
	Both	87	3.4	30	1.9	1.78	1.16, 2.73
Neoplasms (140–239)	Men	27	2.4	18	2.0	1.16	0.63, 2.14
	Women	30	2.6	8	0.9	3.05	1.37, 6.78
	Both	57	2.5	26	1.5	1.67	1.04, 2.69
External causes[a]	Men	13	1.25	4	0.36	3.47	1.13, 10.64
	Women	5	0.47	0	0.00	. . .	. . .
	Both	18	0.86	4	0.18	4.78	1.62, 14.13
All other causes	Men	22	1.63	7	0.76	2.14	0.90, 5.06
	Women	15	1.18	2	0.32	3.69	0.84, 16.19
	Both	37	1.4	9	0.55	2.54	1.21, 5.33

[a]Road accidents, work accidents, other accidents, suicide.

from a subsequent separate cross-sectional study we conducted in 1991 on an age-stratified sample of men and women thirty-five to sixty-four years of age in five of the religious and five of the matched secular kibbutzim initially studied. A total of 460 people participated (a response rate of 79 percent) (unpublished data) (table 12.5).

Ethnic origin is associated in Israel with differential mortality (Central Bureau of Statistics 1991). However, members of the kibbutzim studied were overwhelmingly of European origin (table 12.5). Educational level was almost identical between the kibbutz types (table 12.5). Occupation and standard of living were very similar in religious and secular kibbutzim, although personal consumption of goods in the religious kibbutzim tended to be lower (Fishman 1993). The economic structure and advanced technology of the kibbutzim were almost identical. Hence, social class differences, an important determinant of health (Susser et al. 1985; Marmot et al. 1991), cannot explain the findings. Duration of membership in the kibbutz, another potential confounding variable, did not affect the strength of the association when included in the multivariable Cox survival models.

Absence of social supports has been repeatedly shown to be associated with elevated mortality (Berkman and Syme 1979; Blazer 1982). One of the possible explanations for a protective effect of being religious is the benefit derived from support by the group (Kaplan 1976; Jarvis and Northcott 1987; Levin and Vanderpool 1987). However, kibbutz society in general is characterized by

Table 12.5
Sociodemographic Characteristics of Members of Five Secular and Five Religious Kibbutzim, 1991

	Secular Kibbutzim		Religious Kibbutzim	
	Women	Men	Women	Men
No.	120	99	120	116
Country of origin of father, %				
Europe	79	78	88	92
Israel	9	11	3	4
Asia/Africa	12	11	9	4
No. of children	3.3	3.3	4.4	4.6
Schooling, y	11.4	11.2	11.2	11.2
Higher education, %	57	55	55	55
Marital status, %				
Married	79	88	91	98
Divorced	13	1	3	0
Religiousness, %				
Orthodox	1	0	90	94
Nonobservant	90	98	1	0

Note. Members were 35–64 years of age when studied. Equal numbers of men and women were invited to participate. Five members with missing data were excluded.

strongly structured support mechanisms consisting of both formal and informal networks (Spiro 1983; Fishman 1992; Levitan and Cohen 1985; Anson et al. 1990). Indeed, perceived and instrumental social supports assessed in the cross-sectional study we conducted in 1991 in ten of the kibbutzim were similar in the religious and secular individuals (unpublished data). Provision, quality, and accessibility of primary care services, also possible determinants of mortality, were equally high in each kibbutz, and the geographic proximity and use of the same secondary and tertiary care facilities ensured equality of access.

The possibility of bias in completeness of ascertaining all deaths is small. Considerable effort was expended in obtaining complete mortality data and in cross checking alternative sources of information. As for underlying cause of death, differences in the quality of certification—in hospitals, in other medical institutions, or in deaths occurring in the community—are unlikely. Similar proportions of religious and secular deaths occurred in hospitals, and the same regional hospital served each matched pair of kibbutzim. Also, it is most unlikely that bias occurred in coding underlying causes of death because reclassification by a nosologist unaware of the study hypothesis produced nearly identical results.

Selection bias requires consideration. Might there have been differences in the health characteristics of those who established, joined, or left religious vs.. secular kibbutzim that could have led to such substantial differences in subsequent mortality? Such a "healthy worker effect" (McMichael 1976) or "healthy migrant effect" (Marmot et al. 1984) probably operated within both types of kibbutz. However, it is difficult to conceive of a reasonable mechanism whereby this could differentially affect religious and secular kibbutzim. There is no evidence that religious kibbutzim were more stringent in the health criteria used in selecting founding members and new members, and neither type of kibbutz had a policy of dismissing unhealthy members. Indeed, in both types of kibbutz hardiness was required for similarly strenuous physical labor and the difficult living conditions, particularly in the early years. Furthermore, the small number of members who left either type of kibbutz during the sixteen-year study period (3.5 percent of religious and 7.6 percent of secular members) reflects the stability of the population. The low overall mortality of kibbutzim (Leviatan and Cohen 1985) suggests that differential out-migration of healthy members since establishment of the kibbutzim, leaving a more disease-prone residue, is an improbable explanation. While the selection argument cannot be totally discounted, it is unlikely that differential forces of selection at various ages and time periods were operative between the two kibbutz movements or, if present, could have been of a sufficient magnitude to produce the effects we documented.

Mortality Differences and Characteristics of Religious vs.. Secular Kibbutzim

We compared two societies living in almost identical cohesive communal settlements with the same kibbutz ideology of equality and sharing in production and in fulfilling needs. Those residing in secular kibbutzim are almost all agnostic or nonreligious, whereas almost all of those residing in religious kibbutzim are religiously orthodox and observant (table 12.5).

Conventional Risk Factors

Differences in the more traditional risk factors such as diet, smoking, obesity, alcohol intake, exercise, and exposure to accidents might play a role. Information on these factors, some of which may be viewed as potential intervening variables in a causal pathway rather than as confounders (i.e., they are determined by religious practices), was not available at the onset of this historical prospective study. For example, travel is forbidden on the Sabbath and on certain holidays. Furthermore, other studies have shown intakes of saturated fatty acid and total fat to be moderately lower among religiously orthodox urban dwellers (Snyder et al. 1978; Friedlander et al. 1985) and intake of fish greater (Kark, J. D. et al., unpublished data, 1987-89 and 1989-91). Much of the difference in fat intake was attributed to the *kashrut* ritual of milk products and meat not being consumed at the same meal. However, there are no proscriptions against use of alcohol, coffee, tea, and tobacco (except the latter, which is not permitted on the Sabbath and some holidays) and no encouragement of exercise, in contrast with Mormons and Seventh-Day Adventists (Gardner and Lyon 1982; Beeson et al. 1989).

In urban populations in Israel, blood cholesterol concentrations and the prevalence of cigarette smoking have been shown to be lower in those who are religiously orthodox (Snyder et al. 1978; Friedlander et al. 1985). However, levels of blood pressure, exercise, and adiposity have been shown to be similar in the two groups (Snyder et al. 1978; Friedlander et al. 1985).

Conventional risk factors for mortality were compared in the cross-sectional study of 1991. Blood pressure and body mass index were similar between the kibbutz groups. Plasma cholesterol was higher in the secular kibbutzim (by 16 mg/dl in women and 6 mg/dl in men), and high-density lipoprotein cholesterol and triglyceride were higher in secular women (by 3 mg/dl and 14 mg/dl, respectively). Religious men and women reported a diagnosis of diabetes (9 percent and 6 percent, respectively) more frequently than secular men and women (3 percent and 2 percent, respectively). Smoking was more frequent in secular kibbutzim, in which 19 percent of men and 18 percent of women smoked regularly (vs.. 12 percent and 6 percent, respectively, in religious kibbutzim). Differences were greater in terms of individuals ever having smoked regularly (56 percent vs. 42 percent for men and 48 percent vs. 14 percent for women).

As a means of assessing the potential effect of risk factor differences, logistic regression coefficients for these variables were derived from three separate mortality studies of the Israeli population, two involving men and one involving both men and women (the Israel Ischemic Heart Disease Study [Goldbourt and

Kark 1982]; the Kiryat Hayovel Community Health Study Mortality follow-up [Kark, J.D, Karle, JD, Yofin, J., Epstein, L., Abramson, J. H., unpublished data 1969-71 through 1993]; and the Jerusalem Lipid Research Clinic Study mortality follow-up [Kark, J.D., Friedlander, Y. and Stein, Y., unpublished data 1969-79 through 1988]). These coefficients were applied to the thirty-five- to sixty-four-year-old kibbutz members studied in 1991. Estimates of the relative risk of mortality in secular vs.. religious kibbutzim reflecting the risk factor differences were on the order of 1.0 to 1.2. Assuming that these risk factor differences measured in 1991 reflected those that prevailed during the incidence study between 1970 and 1985, other explanations for the protective effect associated with living on a religious kibbutz should be sought.

Amelioration of Stress

A cogent explanation for the salutary effect of living on a religious kibbutz would need to relate to a pervasive protectivity evident for all main causes of death (see table 12.4). A major possibility is that such a social environment induces less stress, enhances host resistance, and promotes overall well-being and a positive health status, consistent with the hypotheses proposed by Cassel (1976), and Antonovsky (1987). In line with this concept is a previous finding that although orthodox Jewish men reported more "problems," they were less worried by them (Snyder et al. 1978).

Possible components of stress reduction include the following:

1. An overall coherent world view (Levin and Vanderpool 1987) and sense of belonging (over and above that peculiar to the kibbutz) that could promote emotional well-being.

2. A relaxation response (Benson 1975) induced by frequent prayer. However, this pertains almost exclusively to orthodox men, who pray together up to three times daily, but not to orthodox women. They usually attend prayers only on the Sabbath (if at all) as well as holidays, but are apparently protected from premature morbidity as much as the men, if not more so. The communal aspects of prayer may be important (see component 6).

3. Belief in the Almighty and religious heteronomy. The authority setting normative behavior in the orthodox religious is derived from an external divine source, whereas secular autonomy determines that the source is within people (Fishman 1993).

4. Repetitive ritualistic behaviors based on the religious law that governs many aspects of a carefully regulated life, resulting in less ambivalence and exposure to stress (orthodox certainty and determinism vs. secular ambiguity and doubt). Strict observance of the Sabbath and festivals dedicated to rest and prayer may also contribute to stress reduction.

5. Highly stable marital bonding in the religious kibbutzim. The kibbutz is a close-knit, family-oriented society, but the divorce rate was eleven-fold higher

in secular than in religious kibbutzim (Kaffman et al. 1986). Between 1974 and 1984, there were only ten divorces in all seventeen religious kibbutzim in Israel (0.7 percent of the 1381 married couples). Our cross-sectional study of 1991 confirmed these differences (table 12.5). There is very strong social pressure in religious kibbutzim against dissolution of marriage, with preservation of the family a top priority. Marital expectations appear to be lower with regard to satisfaction of individual needs, with fewer prior illusions and consequently less disillusionment (Kaffman et al. 1986). The birth rate is higher (as seen also in table 12.5), which may in itself be protective for certain cancers in women. The traditional attitudes toward marriage and the family are similar to those prevailing among Mormons (West et al. 1980), another population characterized by low mortality. However, differences in mortality between single, divorced, and married individuals evident in the general population (Central Bureau of Statistics 1991), cannot explain more than a small fraction of our study findings.

6. A sense of well-being deriving from living in a cohesive religious community. Although social supports are substantial in secular kibbutzim, participating in a religious collective may reinforce the shared attributes of the secular socialistic collective and provide additional support. In this regard, daily and Sabbath communal prayer enhances the feeling of collective solidarity (Fishman 1993). In a cross-sectional study of a religious kibbutz and a secular kibbutz, recent stressful life events were associated with adverse health status among members of the nonreligious, but not the religious, kibbutz (Anson et al. 1990). Anson and coworkers (1990) invoked Durkheim (1951; 1961) in their investigation of the possible protection and enhanced ability to cope with stress afforded by collective attributes of religion rather than by individual religiosity. Durkheim showed that religions with better social integration provided greater protection against suicide. This was confirmed by Pescosolido and Georgianna, who inferred that religious networks provide additional social support and guidance at times of personal crisis, reducing the risk of suicide (Pescosolido and Georgianna 1989). Our findings for suicide are consistent in this regard; five members of secular kibbutzim committed suicide vs. one in a religious kibbutz.

Conclusions

The breadth of the protective effect, encompassing all major causes of death, and its strength, reflected in the elimination of the sex difference in mortality between religious men and secular women, are remarkable.

Our study suggests that even when the increasingly recognized and powerful effects of socioeconomic differences on the health of populations (Susser et al. 1985; Marmot et al. 1991; Pappas et al. 1993), are removed and a high level of health is attained (as in an egalitarian utopian society such as the kibbutz), profound influences of the social environment on health may remain. Understanding how this embracing protective effect of religious observance is actually mediated could provide valuable etiologic insights.

Acknowledgments

This research was supported in part by a grant from the E. and H. Low family, New York. We thank Bryna Shatenstein, PhD, for reviewing the coding of death certificates in this study.

References

Anson, O., S. Carmel, D. Y. Bonneh, A. Levenson and B. Maoz. (1990. "Recent life events, religiosity, and health: An individual or collective effect." *Human Relations* 43: 1051-1066.

Antonovsky, A. 1987. *Unraveling the Mystery of Health.* San Francisco, CA: Jossey-Bass.

Benson, H. 1975. *The Relaxation Response.* New York: Morrow.

Beeson, W. L., P. K. Mills, R. L. Phillips, M. Andress and G. E. Fraser. 1989. "Chronic disease among Seventh-day Adventists, a low-risk group." *Cancer* 64: 570-581.

Berkman, L. F., and S. L. Syme. 1979. "Social networks, host resistance and mortality: A nine-year follow-up study of Alameda County residents." *American Journal of Epidemiology* 109: 186-204.

Blazer, D. G. 1982. "Social support and mortality in an elderly community population." *American Journal of Epidemiology* 115: 684-694.

Cassel, J. 1976. "The contribution of the social environment to host resistance." *American Journal of Epidemiology* 104: 107-123.

Central Bureau of Statistics. 1991. *Statistical Abstract of Israel 1991.* Jerusalem: Central Bureau of Statistics.

Cox, D. R. 1972. "Regression models and life tables." *Journal of the Royal Statistical Society* 34: 187-220.

Durkheim, E. 1951. *Suicide.* New York: The Free Press.

Durkheim, E. 1961. *The Elementary Form of Religious Life.* New York: Collier Books.

Fishman, A. 1992. *Judaism and Modernism on the Religious Kibbutz.* Cambridge: Cambridge University Press.

Fishman, A. 1993. "Religion and economic success in Hakibbutz Hadati." *Cathedra* 68: 126-139 (in Hebrew).

Friedlander, Y., J. D. Kark, N. A. Kaufmann and Y. Stein. 1985. "Coronary heart disease risk factors among religious groupings in a Jewish population sample in Jerusalem." *American Journal of Clinical Nutrition* 42: 511-521.

Friedlander, Y., J. D. Kark and Y. Stein. 1986. "Religious orthodoxy and myocardial infarction in Jerusalem – a case control study." *International Journal of Cardiology* 10: 33-41.

Galton, F. 1872. "Statistical inquiries into the efficacy of prayer." *Fortnightly Review* 12: 125-135.

Gardner, J. W., and J. L. Lyon. 1982. "Cancer in Utah Mormon men by lay priesthood level." *American Journal of Epidemiology* 116: 243-257.

Goldbourt, U., and J. D. Kark. 1982. "The epidemiology of coronary heart disease in the ethnically and culturally diverse population of Israel." *Israeli Journal of Medical Sciences* 18: 1077-1097.

Jarvis, G. K., and H. C. Northcott. 1987. "Religion and differences in morbidity and mortality." *Social Science and Medicine* 25: 813-824.

Kaffman, M., S. Shoham, M. Palgi and M. Rosner. 1986. "Divorce in the kibbutz: Past and present." *Contemporary Family Therapy* 8: 301-315.

Kalbfleisch, J. D., and R. L. Prentice. 1980. *The Statistical Analysis of Failure Time Data.* New York: John Wiley & Sons.
Kaplan, B. H. 1976. "A note on religious beliefs and coronary heart disease." *Journal of the South Carolina Medical Association* 76 (supplement): 60-64.
Kaplan, E. L., and P. Meier. 1958. "Nonparametric estimation from incomplete observations." *Journal of the American Statistical Association* 53: 457-481.
Levin, J. S., and K. S. Markides. 1986. "Religious attendance and subjective health." *Journal for the Scientific Study of Religion* 25: 31-40.
Levin, J. S., and H. Y. Vanderpool. 1987. "Is frequent religious attendance really conducive to better health? Toward an epidemiology of religion." *Social Science and Medicine* 24: 589-600.
Leviatan, U., and J. Cohen. 1985. "Gender differences in life expectancy among kibbutz members." *Social Science and Medicine* 21: 545-551.
Marmot, M. G., A. M. Adelstein and L. Bulusu. 1984. "Lessons from the study of immigrant mortality." *Lancet* 1 (8392): 1455-1457.
Marmot, M. J., G. D. Smith, S. Stansfeld, C. Patel, F. North, J. Head, I. White, E. Brunner and A. Feeney. 1991. "Health inequalities among British civil servants: the Whitehall II study." *Lancet* 337 (8754): 1387--1393.
McMichael, A. J. 1976. "Standardized mortality ratios and the 'healthy worker effect': Scratching beneath the surface." *Journal of Occupational Medicine* 18: 165-168.
O'Boyle, C. A. 1993. "Diseases with passion." *Lancet* 342 (8880): 1126-1127.
Pappas, G., S. Queen, W. Hadden and G. Fisher. 1993. "The increasing disparity in mortality between socioeconomic groups in the United States, 1960 and 1986." *The New England Journal of Medicine*, 329: 103-109.
Pescosolido, B. A., and S. Georgianna. 1989. "Durkheim, suicide, and religion: Toward a network theory of suicide." *American Sociological Review* 54: 33- 48.
Phillips, D. P., T. E. Ruth and L. M. Wagner. 1993. "Psychology and survival." *Lancet* 342 (8880): 1142-1145.
Phillips, R. L., F. R. Lemon, W. L. Beeson and J. W. Kuzma. 1978. "Coronary heart disease mortality among Seventh-day Adventists with differing dietary habits: A preliminary report." *American Journal of Clinical Nutrition* 31 (supplement): S191-S198.
Snyder, M., U. Goldbourt, J. B. Medalie, H. N. Neufeld and D. Oron. 1978. "A lower incidence of myocardial infarction among religious Jews than among irreligious Jews." *Torah u'Mada* 8: 35-44.
Spiro, M. E. 1983. "Introduction: thirty years of kibbutz research." In E. Krausz (ed.), *The Sociology of the Kibbutz.* New Brunswick, NJ: Transaction Books.
Susser, M. W., W. Watson and K. Hopper. 1985. *Sociology in Medicine*, 3rd ed. New York: Oxford University Press.
West, O. W, J. L. Lyon and J. W. Gardner. 1980. "Cancer risk factors: An analysis of Utah Mormons and non-Mormons." *Journal of the National Cancer Institute* 65: 1083-1095.

13

Death Rests a While: Holy Day and Sabbath Effects on Jewish Mortality in Israel

Jon Anson and Ofra Anson

The assumption of an association between religion, religiosity, and well-being is as old as social philosophy (Levin and Schiller 1987). "Observe and hear all these words which I command thee, that it may go well with thee, and with thy children after thee for ever, when thou doest that which is good and right in the sight of the Lord thy God" (Deut. XII:28). In most recent research, a positive, although weak, association has been found between religiosity, mainly measured by church attendance, and physical and mental well-being (Witter, Stock, Okun, and Haring 1985; Levin and Vanderpool 1987). The association between religion, religiosity and mortality, however, has received less attention until recently (Zuckerman, Kasl, and Ostfeld 1984; Jarvis and Norcott 1987; Kark, Shemi, Friedlander, Martin, Manor, and Blondheim, see chapter 12; Strawbridge Cohen, Shema, and Kaplan 1997; Oman and Reed 1998; Hummer, Roger, Nam, and Ellison 1999; Koenig et al. 1999). The purpose of this study is to investigate the patterns of daily mortality among the Jewish population of Israel before and after religious holy days and the weekly Sabbath.

Much of the sociological research in this field, explicitly or implicitly, has drawn its conceptual framework from Durkheim's discussion of religion as a social institution enhancing social integration and regulation (Durkheim 1886, 1915). The integrative function of religion has most often been studied, treating religious participation as a source of social support which offers comfort, guidance, and help especially at times of crisis (Pescosolido and Georgianna 1989; Idler 1987; Idler and Kasl 1992). The accumulating evidence, that it is the collective aspect of religion (rather than individual devotion or praying), that enhances well-being and coping, has further supported this line of argument (Ellison 1991; Anson, Carmel, Levenson, Maoz, and Bonneh 1990; Anson, Carmel, Levenson, Bonneh, and Maoz 1993; Krause and Van Tran 1989; Sherkat and Reed 1992). Others have focused on Durkheim's perception of religion as one of the three main institutions of social control. This body of research has concentrated on the function of religion as regulating daily life and, thus, health-related behavior such as fertility, substance consumption, and dietary intake (Jarvis and Norcott 1987; Troyer 1988; Anson, Carmel, Levenson, Maoz, and Bonneh 1991). The results indeed suggest that religious communities and sects conduct a healthier life-style and generally enjoy better health and lower mortality from behavior-related causes (e.g., malignancies). However, predicted disease-specific effects of religious prohibitions have not always been found. The religious dietary prohibitions do not always decrease mortality from stomach and colon-rectal cancer, nor is adherence to religiously prescribed fertility behavior necessarily associated with lower mortality from neoplasms of the breast (Troyer 1988). Indeed, the social role of religious taboos is not to promote a healthier life-style, but rather to distinguish the sacred from the profane, to help individuals maintain their spiritual purity and to avoid possible contamination (Nisbet 1975).

Yet, there is more to religious involvement than social support and regulation of daily behavior. Several recent longitudinal studies and survival analyses have shown that a religious life style can promote health and prolong life above and beyond the effect of social ties, social support, and health behavior (Kark et al. 1996; Strawbridge et al. 1997; Oman and Reed 1998; Hummer et al. 1999; Koenig et al. 1999). In these studies, religious participation was indeed associated with a healthier life style, stable social relationships and support, all positively associated with survivorship. However, religious involvement had an added value of its own: lower mortality among those who frequently attended religious services was observed, even after controlling for a broad range of possible confounding, intervening variables, such as baseline health, health risks, and social support. This effect of religious commitment and intensive involvement was found whether the unit of analysis focused on individual adults of different ages (frequent church attendance) or on the community (religious kibbutzim). The authors of these studies raised several hypothesis to explain their findings, none of which, however, relate to the possible effect of religious rituals performed collectively.

While the implications of the integrative and regulative functions of religion for well-being have been studied extensively, the role of rites and ceremonies, so central to Durkheim's theory of religion, has rarely been explored (Idler and Kasl 1992). Yet, for Durkheim, the only mechanism for social integration and regulation is collective action, when individuals get together and act conjointly (1915: 418). On religious holy days "... (men's) thoughts are centered upon their common beliefs, their common traditions, the memory of their ancestors, the collective idea of which they are the incarnation; in a word, upon social things" (1915: 348-349). Not only social integration is re-created through rites. "The individual soul is regenerated, too, by being dipped again in the sources from which its life came; consequently, it feels itself stronger, more fully master of itself, less dependent on physical necessities" (1915: 349). According to Durkheim (1919), participation in religious life, that is, in rites, ceremonies, and festivities, provides the individual with internal forces to deal with daily experiences and the difficulties they entail. According to this view, such participation is the mainspring of the internal coping resources that are so central to current medical sociological discourse (Thoits 1995). It can thus be hypothesized that religious collective actions, such as holy days, will affect well-being, disease onset, and survival.

The *conscience collective* and sentiments, however, have to be maintained, and religious holy days, which revive social integration, are periodically repeated (Durkheim 1897, book 2, chapter 2). On the individual level, the recurring festivals not only regenerate one's internal strength, but give meaning to the passage of time.

> (Time) is an abstract and impersonal frame which surrounds . . . all of humanity. And ... these indispensable guidelines, in relation to which all things are temporally located, are taken from social life. The divisions into days, weeks, months, years etc. correspond to the periodical recurrence of rites, feasts, and public ceremonies (1915: 10).

Holy days, then, present a meaningful time-table (Roth 1963), definable "end-points," or goals to aspire to before death. Indeed, folk narratives as well as anecdotal evidence allude to the possibility that individuals are able to prolong life and delay death until a meaningful ceremony has been performed, affairs settled, or a significant event has taken place (Kubler-Ross 1969, 1975).

Past Research

To the best of our knowledge, only six studies have explored the association between religious holy days and the timing of death. Phillips and Feldman (1973) were the first to investigate this association by studying September mortality rates in New York City from 1921 to 1969, and in Budapest from 1875 to 1915. Over 20 percent of the population in both cities was Jewish, and a decline in mortality was found during September in the years that *Yom Kippur* fell between September 28 and October 3 (the Jewish calendar is based on a year of twelve lunar months, or 355 days, with a periodic adjustment of an extra month seven times in nineteen years to maintain synchronization with the solar calendar. The Gregorian date of the festivals thus varies from year to year).

Phillips and King (1988) studied the pattern of mortality changes before and after Passover in California from 1966 to 1984. They used surnames to define religious affiliation, and they compared the timing of death of decedents with unambiguous Jewish surnames, with that of decedents with ambiguous Jewish surnames, Japanese and Chinese surnames, Blacks, and Jewish infants. For males with unambiguous Jewish names, they observed a death-dip (i.e. decline in mortality) a week before Passover, followed by a death-peak (i.e. mortality increase) a week after the holiday. The dip-peak pattern was particularly noticeable in years when the ceremonial meal (the *Seder)* fell on a weekend, and was concentrated in deaths caused by heart, cerebro-vascular, and malignant diseases. No such pattern was observed for Jewish women, and the authors suggested that men, whose symbolic part during the principal rite of Passover is greater than that of women, postponed death until after the holiday, especially when it coincided with the weekend, enabling the family to be gathered for the celebration.

A similar death dip-peak pattern was found for Chinese women aged seventy-five and over, around the Harvest Moon Festival (Phillips and Smith 1990). Using the California data described above, they reported a decline in mortality a week before the festival, and an increase a week after it. The pattern again was stronger for deaths caused by heart, cerebro-vascular, and malignant diseases. While the authors do not present the rationale for restricting the analysis to this one specific age-sex group, it can be assumed that during the period leading up to the festival, when the traditional ceremonial meal is prepared, elderly Chinese women have a critical role, guiding and supervising younger women's work.

Idler and Kasl (1992) looked at mortality around religious holy days among subjects of the Yale Health and Aging Project. The data included self-reported religious affiliation and frequency of service attendance, but included only 1,037 deaths, which forced the authors to search for the holy-day effect one month before and one month after a holy day. Among the Jews, there was a clear dip-peak pattern for men, and for synagogue attendees (also mostly men) around *Yom Kippur* and Passover, but an opposite, peak-dip pattern, for women. For all groups of Christians—men, women, Catholics, White Protestants, Black Protestants, the more and the less observant—there were fewer deaths in the month before than in the month after Christmas. This was similar to the findings reported by Harrison and Kroll (1985-1986) basing themselves on obituaries in the *New York Times* and on the timing of death of eminent Americans.

However, Idler, and Kasl also reported a similar, but weaker, pattern for Jews around Christmas. Although they do not discuss this further, we suggest that this derives from the social meaning of Christmas, and the collective activity around it, which is not specifically related to the religious observance of Christmas. For anyone living in a Christian country, Christmas imposes itself as a social fact around which both inter-personal and communal life must structure itself.

Thus a clear pattern emerges of a dip in the number of deaths before, and a peak after, religious holidays among a variety of groups in the United States, with one exception: Jewish women, for whom a consistent, even if not statistically significant, pattern in the *opposite direction* has been observed, with a peak before the holy day, and a dip after. This exception led Anson and Anson

(1997) to suggest that the nature of women's roles in the ritual preparations leading up to major holy days creates what Durkheim (1897) termed an *altruistic* situation, one in which "the ego is not its own property, where it is blended with something not itself, where the goal of conduct is exterior to itself, that is, in one of the groups in which it participates" (p. 221). The enhanced solidarity associated with anticipation of the holiday, combined with the social responsibility for transforming the profane household into a place of spiritual purity for the observance of the festive rites, creates a situation in which commitment to the group and its demands is so strong that it overrides commitment to the self, even to the point of self-sacrifice. Studying the mortality patterns of Muslims over a ten year period, they found the expected, peak-dip pattern for Muslim women, whose role in religious holy days resembles that of Jewish women, around two of the three major Muslim holidays, and a dip-peak pattern for men before and after one of the these three holy days.

The Plan of Research

The present study seeks to replicate and expand the above analyses, by examining mortality around Jewish holy days among Jews in Israel. The use of Israeli data to search for patterns of Jewish mortality around holy days in Israel has certain advantages over previous research. First, an overwhelming majority of the population of Israel (over 80 percent) is Jewish, a majority feeling which is amplified by the official designation of Israel as a Jewish State, and by the residential and social segregation of Jews and Arabs (Horowitz and Lisak 1990; Central Bureau of Statistics 1997). The social distinction between Jews and non-Jews is reproduced in political debate, and in civil rights and duties, such as social benefits and mandatory army service.

Second, national holidays are set according to the Jewish holy days, and Saturday is the national day of rest, so that the Jewish calendar takes on a civil, as well as a religious, connotation. On Saturdays, and on all sabbatical holidays, law prohibits non-essential work. As a consequence, from early afternoon on Friday and on holiday eves, businesses, services and public transportation close down, with very few exceptions. Health services and the defense forces operate with reduced staff, and even entertainment (e.g., restaurants, movie theatres) is available on a lower scale than on profane weekdays. Religious holy days, including the *Sabbath,* thus impose themselves as days of rest, or at least as days set apart from other days, for most of the population, be they religious or secular. In this respect, major Jewish holidays and the *Sabbath* resemble Thanksgiving and Christmas in the United States: national holidays which impose themselves on all the population as a collective, irrespective of their legal status, religious affiliation, or level of religious observance. As we suggested above, it is this attribute of Christmas that may well account for the slight decline in mortality observed among the Jews in the United States (Idler and Kasl 1992).

Other religious holy days, those that do not require a full sabbatical (e.g., *Purim* or *Hanukkah),* are also distinguished from profane life. On these occasions schools are closed, special activities for children are organized by profit and non-profit organizations, many work places are closed and families take the opportunity to travel. Thus, the distinction of the "sacred" holy days from the "profane" daily routine in Israel is socially organized as collective action, irrespective of the level of personal religious devotion or observance.

Furthermore, affairs of personal status, that is marriage and divorce, and all burials, are in the hands of formal religious organizations, enforcing systematic registration of religious affiliation for all citizens, from the birth certificate to the death certificate. Reliable data on deaths, by the religion of the deceased, are available from the national population register, and neither valid identification of religious affiliation nor sample size poses methodological constraints.

On the basis of the above discussion, we hypothesized that: 1) there will be a dip in the number of deaths before, and a peak in the number of deaths after, sabbatical holidays (holy days). At the same time, previous research leads us to expect some gender differences. Pursuing the "altruistic" argument presented by Anson and Anson (1997), it is hypothesized that 2) the expected dip-peak pattern of mortality around the holy days will be weaker for women than for men; 3) for women, a peak-dip pattern of mortality will be observed around Passover, which is distinguished by the massive preparation which women are required to undertake, including extensive cleansing and a thorough transformation of the household into a purified place for celebrating the Exodus.

Method

We studied the incidence of mortality on different days of the week, with particular reference to a possible holy-day effect, before and after the *Sabbath* (Saturday) and all national and religious festivals, as presented in table 13.1. It is to be noted that in the Jewish calendar all days (and hence, the *Sabbath* and all holy days) begin at sundown and continue until the following sundown. Our data, however, assign deaths according to the civil calendar, beginning at midnight and ending the following midnight. The holidays are analyzed as follows:

Rosh Hashanah (New Year): A major sabbatical holiday, the beginning of the High Holiday season lasting almost a month through the end of *Succot.* We contrasted the four days before the holiday with the holiday itself and with the four days after. Although *Rosh Hashana* is celebrated for two days, our analysis focused on the first day to maintain comparability with the analysis of the other holidays, and to balance the number of days between *Rosh Hashana* and *Yom Kippur.*

Yom Kippur (Day of Atonement): A full day of fast, observed by most of the population, and considered the most solemn day of the year. *Yom Kippur* is on the tenth day of the New Year, so there are exactly eight days between *Rosh*

Hashana and *Yom Kippur,* split into four days after the first and four days before the second. We contrasted the time before and after with the day itself.

Succot (Tabernacles): A week-long holiday (eight days) commencing with a sabbatical five days after *Yom Kippur* and ending with a sabbatical on the last day. The intermediate six days are non-sabbatical holidays *(khol hamo'ed)* as discussed above. The four days before *Succot* are thus identical with the four days after *Yom Kippur.*

Hanukkah (Dedication): A minor, non sabbatical holiday celebrated by lighting candles each evening in the home and in public places for eight days. This is a school holiday but no other work holiday.

Purim (Lots): A minor, non sabbatical holiday lasting one day, mainly celebrated by children's fancy dress parties and a school holiday, but no work holiday.

Pesach (Passover): A major, seven-day holiday with a sabbatical on the first and last days and five days of *khol hamo'ed* in between. During the week special dietary restrictions apply, and before the holiday the house must be purified

Table 13.1
Operationalization of Holy-Day Variables

Holy day	Civil month[a]	Abbreviation	Variables	Definition
Rosh Hashana[b] (New Year)	September	RS	BRS	4 days Before
			RS	1 holy day
			ARS	4 days After
Yom Kippur (Day of Atonement)	September	YK	BYK	4 days Before
			YK	1 holy day
			AYK	4 days After
Succot[c] (Tabernacles)	September–October	SUC	SUC1	1st day
			SUC	6 middle days
			SUC2	last day
			ASUC	4 days After
Hanukkah[d] (Dedication)	December	HAN	BHAN	4 days Before
			HAN	8 festive days
			AHAN	4 days After
Purim (Lots)	March	PUR	BPUR	4 days Before
			PUR	1 holy day
			APUR	4 days After
Pesach[e]	April	PAS	BPAS	4 days Before
			PAS1	1st holy day
			PAS	5 middle days
			PAS2	2nd holy day
			APAS	4 days After
Independence day	May	ID	BID	4 days Before
			ID	1 holy day
			AID	4 days After
Shavu'ot[f] (Pentecost)	June	SHV	BSHV	4 days Before
			SHV	1 holy day
			ASHV	4 days After
Fast 9th of Av	August	FAV	BFAV	4 days Before
			FAV	1 holy day
			AFAV	4 days After

[a] The Jewish calendar has 12 lunar months, and is 355 days long, augmented by an extra month in seven times in a 19 year cycle. The civil date of Jewish holidays thus varies over a period of about four weeks, e.g. in 1983 *Rosh Hashana* was celebrated on the 8 September, and in 1986 on 4 October.

[b] The *Rosh Hashana* holiday is 2 days, the analysis focuses on the first day to maintain comparability with the other holidays, and to balance the number of days between *Rosh Hashana* and *Yom Kippur.*

[c] In Israel, *Succot* is celebrated for 8 days, with the first and last days having the status of full sabbatical.

[d] *Hanukkah* is celebrated for eight, non-sabbatical days, with no special status for the first and last days.

[e] In Israel, *Pesach* is celebrated for 7 days, with the first and last days having the status of full sabbatical.

[f] In Israel, *Shavu'ot* is celebrated for one sabbatical day only.

from all trace of non-Pesach foods *(khametz)*. The first evening begins with a big festive meal *(Seder)* generally celebrated within the extended family.

Independence Day: A non-religious, non-sabbatical holiday, preceded by a day of remembrance for soldiers killed in action, followed by national independence celebrations in the evening. Independence day is often celebrated in family and communal picnics.

Shavuot (Pentecost): A one-day, sabbatical holiday, of major religious importance, but of minor importance for the non-religious population.

Fast of the Ninth of Av: A non-sabbatical fast day in remembrance of the destruction of the First and Second Temples, and the expulsion of the Jews from Spain. The day has attained growing civil importance over the past couple of decades, and is now generally a non-work day, particularly in the public sector.

Data

Data were obtained from the Central Bureau of Statistics in Jerusalem, listing every recorded death of Israeli residents over the time period 1 January 1983-31

December 1992. For each death, there were recorded the person's religion (Jewish, Muslim, Christian, Druze, or Other), sex, date of birth and date of death. As daily population counts are not available to compute rates, the analysis was performed using the number of deaths on each day. For the present analysis, we focused on all Jewish deaths for which the date of death was given fully, and for date of birth at least the year was recorded. Missing days of birth were imputed to the fifteenth of the month, if month but no day was recorded, and to July 1 if both day and month were missing. Deaths were broken down into four age groups for analysis, as presented in table 13.2, of which we analyzed the first, third and fourth.

Age groups were chosen as follows:

1. Age group 1 represents the pre-social population who should show no effect for impending holidays, for even though they may be imbued with the excitement around the upcoming feast, the social mechanisms discussed above are not expected to apply. This group is analyzed as a contrast to the main analysis of adult mortality.

2. Age groups 2 includes children, youths and young adults. Age thirty-five is defined as the upper limit to this age group, following Anson's (1992) analysis, in which age thirty-five is identified as the critical turning point in the life table, the age at which young mortality ends and mature mortality begins. This age group is not analyzed both because of the small number of cases and because the major cause of death at these ages is accidental mortality.

3. Age groups 3 and 4 are split at age seventy-five to distinguish the socially active from the older, socially less active, adults. Any such distinction is necessarily arbitrary, and age seventy-five was chosen following Phillip and

Smith's (1990) analysis of elderly Chinese women whom he defined as being aged seventy-five and over. This was also the age that approximately divided the number of male deaths into two equal segments.

Table 13.2
Age Groups for Analysis

Age group	Age range	Mean deaths per day	
		Females	Males
1	0–4	0.92	1.16
2	5–34	0.69	1.47
3	35–74	13.40	17.00
4	75+	18.80	18.20

Time Trends and Seasonal Cycles

Our data refer to the numbers of deaths, not to rates, and we must therefore beware of two long-term patterns that are liable to be reflected in, and to confound, short-term effects. Over time, the population is growing, and the risk of death is declining, though both these processes occur at different rates in the different age groups. However, a secular growth or decline in the number of deaths may appear as a change in mortality after, when compared to that before, the holiday. Similarly, daily numbers of deaths tend to move in cycles, in particular annual cycles but also cycles of the longer and shorter term. Again, the effect of a cycle, and in particular of more than one concurrent cycle, may be to increase mortality over a small time span, and thus either to create an apparent, or to confound a real, holiday-time effect. Previous analysis of data on Muslim deaths in Israel (Anson and Anson 1997) suggests that the effect we have hypothesized is likely to be numerically small, and thus any trend in the data, whether secular or seasonal, is liable to have a confounding effect on the results. We proceeded to remove these effects as follows:

Time trends. We modeled the daily numbers of deaths in each age group as a Poisson process, subject to a linear increase with time in the (logged) numbers of deaths, that is,

$$\ln(\lambda_i) = a_0 + a_1 y_i/365.25 \qquad (1)$$

with a log-likelihood given by:

$$L = -(D_i \ln(\lambda_i) - \lambda_i - \ln(D_i!)) \qquad (2)$$

where λ_i = the modeled number of deaths on day y_i, y_i= the number of days counted from the 1 January 1988, D_i=*the* recorded number of deaths on y_i, a_0 = expected baseline for 1 January 1988, a_1 = secular annual rate of growth.

Seasonal cycles. Any series of numbers may be depicted as the sum of regularly recurring seasonal cycles, defined by their periodicity (the distance from peak to peak) and their amplitude (the maximum departure from the base line on each cycle), and expressed by a series of pairs of sine and cosine curves, as follows,

$$\ln(\lambda_i) = a_1 \sin\frac{2\pi y_i}{a_2} + a_3 \cos\frac{2\pi y_i}{a_2} + b_1 \sin\frac{2\pi y_i}{b_2} + b_3 \cos\frac{2\pi y_i}{b_2} + \ldots \qquad (3)$$

where y_i is the number of days from the beginning of the measured period (1 January 1983), a_2, b_2, etc. define the periodicity, and a_1, a_3; b_1, b_3 etc. are pairs of coefficients defining the amplitude (Chatfield 1989). If there is a truly cyclical pattern to the data, then most points will be associated with just a few cycles which may then be computed and subtracted from the observed data to produce a residual value which over the total time period, is distributed randomly about the center line. Patterned local variation in this series, if any, may then be attributed to particular local events, such as holidays, etc.

Table 13.3 presents these cycles for combined models (1) and (3), for younger and older males and females (ages 35-74, and over seventy-five), giving the mean, baseline (logged) number of deaths, the annual growth rate, and coefficients of the first three major cycles. Preliminary analysis indicated that there was a consistent pattern of an annual cycle, with a periodicity of 365.25 days, and a semi-annual (182.65 days) cycle, and these were set as fixed, with only the sine and cosine coefficients estimated by the model. The third cycle reflected the decline in mortality during the 1980s and its increase in the 1990s following the large wave of immigration from Eastern Europe that began in 1989. The model estimated periodicity for this cycle. For younger men and women, there was no significant secular trend, and the coefficient was set to zero. For this age group the third cycle has a periodicity of 8.3 years for females and 9.3 years for males, reflecting the noted decline and increase over the ten-year period. For older men and women there is a secular increase of almost four percent per year in the number of deaths, and the third cycle is shorter (5.3 years for females, 5.8 years for males), initially compensating for the secular growth, and later merging with it. For the younger age group, 35-74, the secular and cyclical trends account for an eighth to a sixth of the variation in the daily numbers of deaths. For the older ages, seventy-five and over, the secular and seasonal trends account for almost 40 percent of the variation in the daily number of deaths.

Figure 13.1 shows the original data and the fitted curves, for the four groups. The semi-annual cycle (186.62 days) appears to have no special meaning, except that it overlaps exactly the annual trend, thus flattening out the cycle in the summer, and accentuating the peak in the winter. The long term trend for the younger age group, ages 35-74, shows indeed a slight decline from the early to the late 1980s, and then a slight increase in the early 1990s. For the older population, ages seventy-five and over, the number

Table 13.3
Time Trends and Cyclical Coefficiants for Numbers of Death

Coeff.	Group 3: ages 35–74		Group 4: ages 75 and over	
	Females	Males	Females	Males
Base				
a_0	2.59 (0.00469)[a]	2.82 (0.00439)	2.92 (0.00400)	2.88 (0.00424)
a_1	0	0	0.0383 (0.00145)	0.0365 (0.00175)
First cycle 365.25 days				
b_1 (sine)	0.671 (0.00649)	0.0733 (0.00578)	0.0905 (0.00551)	0.817 (0.0.00566)
b_3 (cosine)	0.117 (0.00637)	0.128 (0.00568)	0.181 (0.00542)	0.189 (0.00551)
Second cycle 182.62 days				
c_1 (sine)	0.0261 (0.00641)	0.0334 (0.00570)	0.0657 (0.00543)	0.0665 (0.00554)
c_3 (cosine)	0.0304 (0.00640)	0.0263 (0.00569)	0.0264 (0.00542)	0.0338 (0.00552)
Third cycle				
d_1 (sine)	−0.0445 (0.00705)	−0.0436 (0.00652)	−0.0448 (0.00578)	−0.0405 (0.00600)
d_2 (period)	3060 (179)	3410 (207)	1930 (52.6)	2110 (133)
d_3 (cosine)	−0.0237 (0.00647)	−0.0326 (0.00601)	0.0358 (0.00563)	0.0178 (0.00672)
R^2[b]	12.2%	17.5%	38.2%	38.4%

[a] Values in parentheses are approximate standard errors of the estimate.
[b] R^2 values represent the proportion of the variation in daily numbers of deaths attributable to the secular and cyclical trends.

of deaths increases, then flattens out in the late 1980s, and rises again in the early 1990s. The modeled cycles, as can be seen, follow the rise and fall in the numbers of deaths, leaving a residual distribution that we shall now analyze for the particular effects of the holy days.

Findings

Residuals of the trend and cyclical analysis were analyzed by Analysis of Variance (ANOVA), to consider the patterning of deaths over the week and over the year. In this and in all subsequent tables, the estimates are least-squares deviations from the mean, and for each set of estimates, days of the week and days of the year, the estimates sum to zero. The two null-hypotheses examined were that:

1. Deaths are evenly distributed over the days of the week, with no significant heaping on any on particular day;
2. Deaths are evenly distributed over the year, with no significant heaping before, during or after any holy day.

Tables 13.4 and 13.5 present the results of the data analysis for the younger (35-74) and the older (over seventy-five) men. A statistically significant change in the number of deaths was found only for days of the week, and not for the holy days, indicating that there is a significantly non-uniform distribution of death over the days of the week, but that deaths are uniformly distributed over the days of the year, irrespective of their proximity to holy days. Separate analysis of High Holiday period (four days before *Rosh Hashanah* to four days after *Succot)* and the Pesach period indicated that within these time groups, too, there was no significant deviation from a uniform distribution of deaths. The details in table 13.5 indicate that, for both younger and older men, there is a clear dip-peak pattern at the weekend, with fewer deaths on the *Sabbath* (Saturday), followed by an increase in the number of deaths on Sunday. For the younger men, but not for the older age group, there was also a decline in the number of deaths on Tuesday.

Although the overall effect of the holy days was not statistically significant, three significant changes in average daily mortality were observed when holy days were examined individually: the number of deaths of younger men decreased during the four days before *Hanukkah,* and in the older age group the number of deaths **increased** on the first day of *Pesach* and during the middle days of *Pesach.* These sporadic differences did not follow any consistent pattern, and seem to be randomly distributed.

As expected, the effect of the holy days on daily mortality patterns of women was weaker than for men (tables 13.6 and 13.7). As with the men, the number of deaths of women did not change significantly around the holy days, but a statistically significant overall effect of the days of the week was found only for the younger women (age 35-74). Both age groups showed a decline, or a dip, in the number of deaths on Saturday, but only the younger women showed a decline on Friday, and neither showed a compensating significant increase on Sunday. Instead, there was a significant increase in the number of deaths of younger women on Monday and on Wednesday.

Examined individually, some significant changes in the daily number of deaths over the holy days could be found. First, the mortality of younger women declined **after** *Yom Kippur,* which overlap the four days **before** the first holy day of *Succot,* followed by a considerable, though not statistically significant increase ($_t = 1.78$, $p = 0.075$) **on** the first day of *Succot.* Second, there was a significant **dip** in number of deaths of the younger women on the last day of *Succot* whereas mortality of older women **increased** on the same day. Finally, the number of deaths of older women declined during *Hanukkah.* Again, the changes do not follow a dip-peak or a peak-dip pattern, and show no consistency with other groups. Given the overall non-significant finding for the distribution of deaths around the holy days, and the lack of any theoretically relevant pattern in the significant deviations from the mean, we consider them to be random rather than meaningful holy-day effects.

Contrast: Jewish Children and the Non-Jewish Population

We thus have a clear and consistent weekend (Saturday) dip-peak effect for younger and older men and a similar, but weaker, effect for women. To validate our argument that this timing of death is, at least partly, affected by socially constructed time-tables and endpoints, we analyze the timing of death over the days of the week, for Jewish children aged 0-4, and for non-Jews, aged thirty-five and over. In neither case do we expect to find the weekend dip-peak pattern. Children are less "social beings" than adults (Phillips and King, 1988), their life is far less patterned by the days of the week (even though they may well be aware of changes of mood in the household), and this lack of meaning should be reflected in a uniform distribution of deaths over the days of the week. For the non-Jewish (Arab) population, Saturday will have meaning as the national day of rest, but this will not be accompanied by any religious meaning, and it will be muted by the continuation of other (including commercial) activities. As the days of the week are evenly spread over the year, this analysis has no seasonal component, and secular and seasonal trends have not been removed.

For the Jewish children there is a median of one male and one female death per day over the ten years. Testing against the null hypothesis of an equal number of deaths on each day of the week gives $\chi^2 = 5.11$ with d.f. = 6 and $p=0.53$ for males, and $\chi^2 = 2.13$, d.f. = 6 and $p= 0.91$ for females. Clearly, there are no grounds for rejecting the null hypothesis of an equal number of deaths on each day of the week. For the Arab population, with a median of three male and three female deaths per day, $\chi^2=9.46$ with d.f.=6 and $p=0.15$, for males; and for

Figure 13.1
Raw data and fitted secular and cyclical trends of male and female deaths, ages 35-74 and 75+. (A) Female deaths, ages 35-74. (B) Female deaths, ages 75 and over. (C) Male deaths, ages 35-74. (D) Male deaths, ages 75 and over.

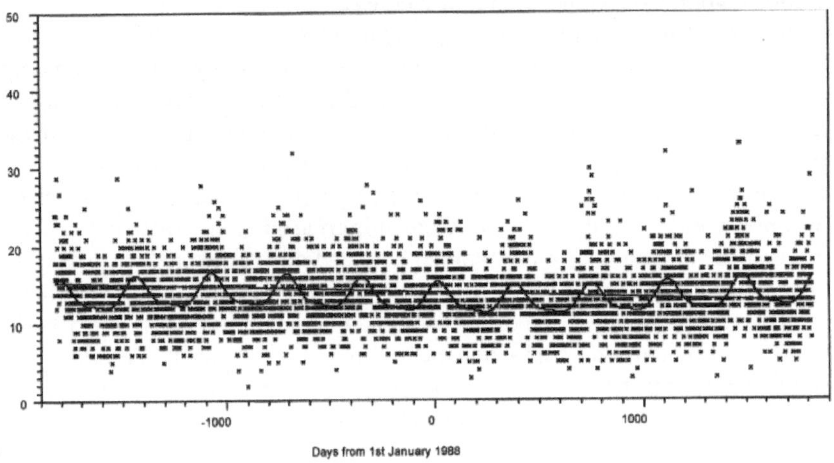

(A)

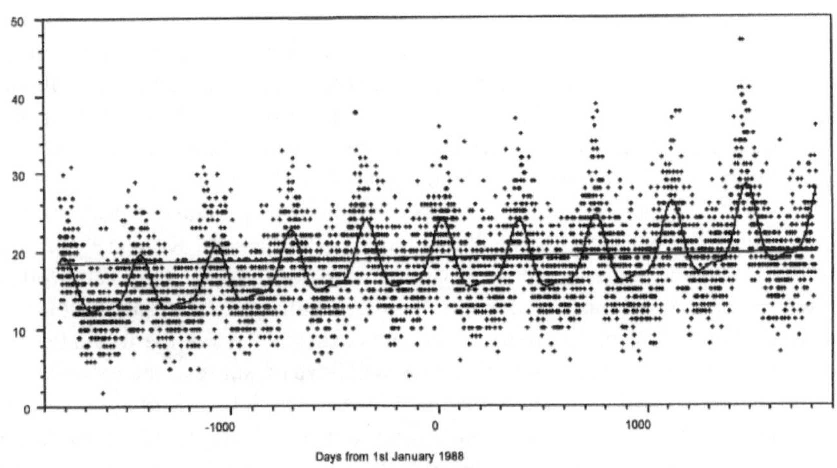

(B)

females χ^2=6.47, d.f.=6 and p=0.37. Here, too, there are no grounds for rejecting the null hypothesis of a uniform distribution of deaths over the week.

Causes of Death

We hypothesized that the social communion of holy days would lead to a delay in mortality, and we have seen that even though there is no specific holiday

Figure 13.1

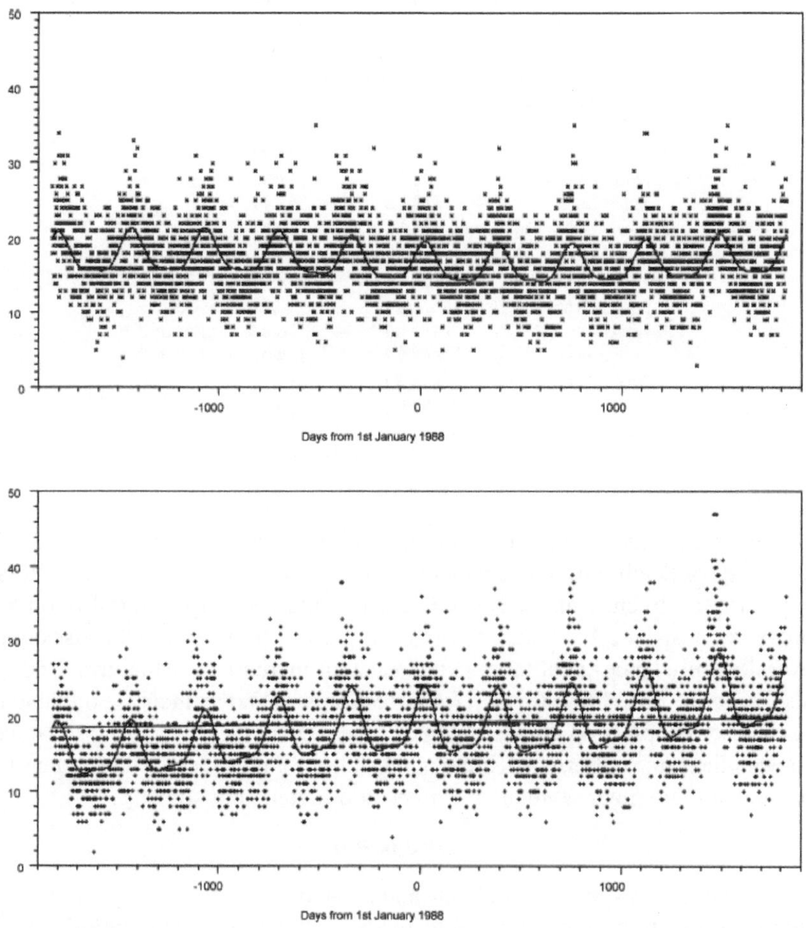

(C)

(D)

effect, there is a very clear weekend effect. For Jewish men, and to lesser extent, for Jewish women, there is a decline in mortality at the weekend (Friday-Saturday) and an increase at the beginning of the week (Sunday-Monday). However, it may yet be argued that this decline derives from a reduction in external risks on the day of rest, rather than from a delay in deaths from internal causes. To consider this possibility, we divided all male and female deaths, at ages over thirty-five, into four cause-specific groups: neoplasms; cardio-vascular; external and other causes, and analyzed the number of deaths by days of the week. Again, the analysis is of the raw data, without correction for trend and cycles (see table 13.8). For men, all causes show a small decline on Friday, a larger decline on Saturday and a rise on Sunday, with significant differences for cerebro-vascular

Table 13.4
ANOVA for Men's Mortality around Weekdays and Holy Days

Source	DF	Sum of squares	Mean square	*F*-ratio
(a) Younger men (35–74)				
Model	36	1221.63	33.93	1.83*[a]
Weekdays	6	802.55	111.03	7.23**
Holy days	30	413.16	555.17	0.74
Error	3617	66,934.36	18.51	
Total	3653	68,156.00		
(b) Older men (75 and over)				
Model	36	1319.06	36.64	1.78*
Weekdays	6	662.22	123.26	5.37**
Holy days	30	683.50	616.32	1.11
Error	3617	74,304.92	20.54	
Total	3653	75,623.99		

[a] $*p < 0.01$; $**p < 0.001$.

and external causes. The weekend dip-peak pattern is thus consistent across all causes of death, internal and external, and is not merely an artifact of lesser exposure to violent causes. For women, too, the decline in mortality on Saturday is consistent, but weaker, across all causes, (only external causes reach overall significance), and there is a consistent increase on Mondays. There is also a decline on Fridays (except for Other Causes) and an increase on Sundays (except for neoplasms). Repeating these analyses for each age group separately showed the same pattern: a decline in mortality for all causes on Saturdays and for men and younger women on Fridays too (details not shown).

Discussion

This study has sought to replicate and expand previous investigations on the timing of death around religious festivals. Following on Durkheim's (1915) perception of religion as a social institution of integration and regulation, these studies suggested that on the one hand, holy days ascribe meaning to the passage of time, and on the other rites, festivals, and ceremonies enhance social integration, support, and a sense of belonging. Consequently, participation in collective action, which characterizes religious holy days, augments internal coping resources and leads to a postponement in mortality, particularly that deriving from degenerative, internal causes.

Research to-date has largely supported this hypothesis, and a decline in mortality before major holy days, followed by an increase soon after it, has been observed in a number of social groups and religious affiliations, with two exceptions: Jewish women in the United States and Muslim women in Israel. We have suggested that the social duties of these women in the ritual

Table 13.5
Mean Daily Mortality of Men around Weekdays and Holy Days

Variable		Younger men (35–74)		Older men (75+)	
		Estimate[a]	t-ratio	Estimate	t-ratio
DAYS	WED	0.13	0.77	−0.11	0.60
	THU	0.22	1.26	0.03	0.17
	FRI	−0.19	−1.09	−0.34	−1.86
	SAT	−0.76	−4.32**[b]	−0.64	−3.45**
	SUN	0.79	4.48**	0.84	4.56**
	MON	0.25	1.43	0.19	1.01
	TUE	−0.44	−2.53*	0.03	0.16
RS	BRS	0.38	0.57	0.04	0.05
	RS	−1.26	−0.96	−1.26	−0.91
	ARS	0.53	0.79	1.11	1.57
YK	BYK	−0.77	−1.15	−0.20	−0.28
	YK	0.17	0.13	1.84	1.33
	AYK	0.06	0.09	−0.00	0.00
SUC	SUC1	1.15	0.87	0.12	0.09
	SUC	0.12	0.23	0.22	0.38
	SUC2	−0.01	−0.01	1.33	0.96
	ASUC	1.26	1.87	−1.00	−1.41
HAN	BHAN	1.19	1.77	0.93	1.31
	HAN	−1.11	−2.32*	−0.37	−0.75
	AHAN	0.11	0.17	−0.43	−0.61
PUR	BPUR	0.42	0.62	−0.84	−1.18
	PUR	0.43	0.33	−0.36	−0.26
	APUR	0.27	0.40	0.55	0.78
PAS	BPAS	0.19	0.28	−0.70	−0.97
	PAS1	−0.94	−0.71	3.13	2.26*
	PAS	−0.01	−0.02	1.36	2.13*
	PAS2	0.61	0.46	−2.20	−1.59
	APAS	−0.33	−0.50	−0.91	−1.28
ID	BID	0.34	0.51	−0.84	−1.18
	ID	−0.13	−0.10	−1.62	−1.17
	AID	−0.85	−1.26	−0.22	−0.31
SHV	BSHV	−0.16	−0.24	0.96	1.35
	SHV	−1.14	−0.87	−1.51	−1.09
	ASHV	0.30	0.45	0.52	0.73
FAV	BFAV	0.57	1.10	−0.23	−0.32
	FAV	−1.31	−1.19	0.51	0.37
	AFAV	−0.20	0.04	0.01	0.01
OTHER		0.05	0.66	0.04	0.51

[a] Estimates are least squares deviations from the Grand Mean. Estimates for the weekdays, and for holy days sum to zero.

[b] $*p < 0.05$; $**p < 0.001$.

Table 13.6
ANOVA for Women's Mortality around Weekdays and Holy Days

Source	DF	Sum of squares	Mean square	F-ratio
(a) Younger women (35–74)				
Model	36	746.27	20.73	1.41*[a]
Weekdays	6	311.02	88.38	3.51**
Holy days	29	445.43	15.36	1.04
Error	36,175	53,281.08	14.73	
Total	3653	54,027.35		
(b) Older women (75 and over)				
Model	36	929.83	25.83	1.11
Weekdays	6	214.91	139.29	1.54
Holy days	29	732.57	696.43	1.05
Error	3617	83,967.08	23.21	
Total	3653	84,896.91		

[a] $*p<0.05$; $**p<0.01$.

preparations of the holy days, the responsibility for transforming the profane household into a sacred place, put them in an 'altruistic' situation (Durkheim 1897). This situation, combined with their absence or, at best, their marginal role in the public ceremonies of the holy days, gives Jewish and Muslim women less opportunity to benefit from the enhancement of internal coping resources through collective action.

We set out to explore patterns of mortality around the holy days among Jews in Israel, where the *Sabbath* on Saturday and all Jewish religious holy days are recognized by civil law, and celebrated as civil as well as religious holidays. Previous research thus led us to expect:

1. A dip in the number of deaths before, and a peak in the number of deaths after, all such holy days;
2. That this dip-peak pattern will be weaker for women than for men; and
3. A peak-dip pattern of mortality for women around *Pesach.*

To test these hypotheses, all deaths from 1983 to 1992 were analyzed, controlling for seasonality and long-term trends. The main finding of these analyses was a consistent decline in mortality on the *Sabbath* (Saturday), for men and women, young and old. This mortality dip was followed by an increase in the number of deaths for men on Sundays and for younger women on Mondays. No such pattern was observed for children under the age of five, or for the non-Jewish population of Israel.

This pattern of reduced mortality on the *Sabbath* could not be attributed to fewer accidental deaths: when deaths were disaggregated by cause, the most

Table 13.7
Mean Daily Mortality of Women around Weekdays and Holy Days

Variable		Younger women (35–74)		Older women (75+)	
		Estimate[a]	*t*-ratio	Estimate	*t*-ratio
DAYS	WED	0.37	2.41*[b]	−0.33	−1.70
	THU	−0.08	−0.50	0.17	0.88
	FRI	−0.26	−1.68	0.23	1.18
	SAT	−0.49	−3.11**	−0.41	−2.09*
	SUN	0.04	0.27	0.19	0.98
	MON	0.38	2.42*	0.14	0.72
	TUE	0.03	0.18	−0.00	−0.00
RS	BRS	0.44	0.73	0.01	0.02
	RS	0.96	0.82	−0.76	−0.52
	ARS	0.45	0.74	0.56	0.75
YK	BYK	0.78	1.30	0.23	0.30
	YK	−0.14	−0.12	1.04	0.71
	AYK	−1.32	−2.20*	−1.03	−1.38
SUC	SUC1	2.09	1.78	−1.76	−1.20
	SUC	−0.54	−1.09	−0.14	−0.22
	SUC2	−2.94	−2.51*	3.26	2.21*
	ASUC	−0.14	−0.23	−0.12	−0.16
HAN	BHAN	−0.27	−0.45	−0.93	−1.23
	HAN	−0.08	−0.43	−1.25	−2.33*
	AHAN	−0.99	−1.65	−0.75	−0.99
PUR	BPUR	−0.29	−0.46	−0.34	−0.45
	PUR	0.93	0.79	−1.48	−1.00
	APUR	0.48	0.81	−0.09	−0.11
PAS	BPAS	0.34	0.56	0.07	0.09
	PAS1	0.39	0.33	2.43	1.65
	PAS	−0.53	−0.99	1.00	1.48
	PAS2	−1.06	−0.90	1.24	0.84
	APAS	−0.14	−0.23	0.62	0.82
ID	BID	0.37	0.63	0.19	0.26
	ID	−0.97	−0.83	−0.13	−0.09
	AID	0.09	0.16	−1.24	−1.64
SHV	BSHV	−0.29	−0.49	0.46	0.61
	SHV	1.80	1.53	−0.12	−0.09
	ASHV	−0.15	−0.25	−0.71	−0.94
FAV	BFAV	0.58	0.96	−0.08	−0.11
	FAV	0.59	0.50	−1.04	−0.71
	AFAV	−0.43	−0.73	0.72	0.96
OTHER		0.01	0.08	0.13	1.41

[a] Estimates are least squares deviations from the Grand Mean. Estimates for the weekdays, and for holy days sum to zero.

[b] $*p<0.05$; $**p<0.01$.

consistent non-uniformity was for cerebro-vascular deaths, particularly for men. Neither could the dip-peak pattern observed be the result of administrative delay in registration: had this been the case, a similar dip-peak pattern would have been observed for children, older women and non-Jews, and the mortality peak for younger women would appear on Sunday rather than on Monday. Moreover, we would expect a dip-peak in mortality around all sabbatical holy days, in particular around *Yom-Kippur,* a day in which all work is reduced to an absolute minimum, including emergency services. We also suggest that this mortality dip did not derive from an absence of work-related stresses, as it was also evident among the older, non-working population.

We suggest that this finding, of a *Sabbath* effect, supports the first hypothesis presented, although no other, consistent, holy day effect was found. If the essence of a holy day is that it is differentiated from the mundane rest of the week, then Saturday in Israel is a holy day *par excellence.* Indeed, by Jewish tradition, the *Sabbath* is the most important festivity in the Jewish year. This interpretation is supported by two previous studies. Cohen (1983), examined changes in the daily number of births in Israel during 1975, and found a consistent dip of about 10 percent in the number of births on Saturday, followed by a peak of 5 percent on Sunday. On other holy days, however, a sporadic, inconsistent effect was found. Also, Phillips and King (1988) reported that the dip-peak pattern in mortality around Passover in California was particularly salient when the holy day coincided with Saturday.

The second hypothesis, of a gendered effect, was also confirmed. The dip-peak pattern of mortality around Saturday is much stronger for men than for women. This pattern was observed for men of both age groups, but only for the younger age group of women. For women aged seventy-five and over, there was a decline in mortality on Saturday, but no observable peak on any other day. Moreover, the F-ratio, reflecting the strength of the deviation from a uniform distribution, is much greater for men than for women: 7.35 and 5.37 for younger and older men respectively, compared with 3.51 and 1.54 for women. It is interesting to contrast these findings with those of recent studies of the effects of Church attendance on mortality and survivorship in the United States, which either showed *no* sex differentiation (Oman and Reed 1998) or a *heightened* effect for women (Strawbridge et al. 1997; Koenig et al. 1999). Without proposing a definitive explanation for these differences, we suggest that the *ritual* demands of women church attendees, and the forms of religious participation, differ little, if at all, from those of men. Unlike Judaism and Islam, Christian practice does not impose on women *ritual* responsibility for the purity of the home, and thus does not create the altruistic condition that offsets the more general dip-peak pattern.

The third hypothesis, which predicted a peak-dip pattern in mortality for women around *Pesach,* was not supported. Nonetheless, the hypothesis that holy days create, at least to some degree, an "altruistic situation" for Jewish women cannot be rejected on the basis of the present analysis. Table 13.7 indicates a clear mortality peak for younger women on Wednesdays, the day on which the preparations for the *Sabbath* begin. This peak is not seen for older women or for men. The majority of the Jewish population in Israel define themselves as orthodox, religious or traditional (Peres and Yuchtman-Yaar 1998), and *Sabbath* observation requires that all food must be prepared before *Sabbath* begins at sunset on Friday. Furthermore, during the period covered by our data, most Israelis worked 6 days a week, from Sunday to Friday early afternoon. For this population, Thursday and Friday are usually devoted to shopping, cleaning and food preparation. The peak in the number of deaths of the younger women on Wednesday could thus reflect the burden of these preparations.

Thus, although this study did not find the previously reported holy day effect around the major holidays, our findings are clearly consistent with this body of research in finding a dip-peak pattern around Saturday, and a differential effect by gender. Only one group in our study did not follow this dip-peak pattern, the elderly women. For this group, the dip in mortality on Saturday was not followed by any peak. We suggest that this finding actually highlights the important role of collective action in generating the holy day effect on the timing of death. Elderly women are far less likely than men of their age to live in the family. In 1989-1991, almost three-quarters (73 percent) of Israeli women aged 75-79 were not married, compared with 17 percent of men of that age; 53 percent of the women of that age lived alone, but only 11 percent of the men (Ministry of Health 1998). These differences increase, of course, with age: by age 85-89, all but 9 percent of the women are not married while 59 percent of

Table 13.8
Daily Mortaility by Causes of Death

	Malignancies	Cardio-vascular	External	All others
(a) Men				
DAYS				
WED	0.02	−0.10	0.16	−0.05
THU	0.21	−0.17	0.09	0.13
FRI	−0.03	−0.22	−0.09	−0.23
SAT	−0.24**[a]	−0.57**	−0.31***	−0.25
SUN	0.17	1.07***	0.07	0.29
MON	0.10	0.05	0.08	0.20
TUE	−0.23*	−0.07	0.01	0.09
Mean *N* of deaths	7.33	16.0	1.84	10.0
Percent of all deaths	(21%)	(45%)	(5%)	(28%)
F (d.f.=6)	2.01	5.24***	6.37***	1.61
(b) Women				
DAYS				
WED	0.20	−0.08	−0.05	−0.02
THU	0.09	−0.17	0.07	0.09
FRI	−0.03	−0.03	−0.01	0.03
SAT	−0.16	−0.37	−0.16***	−0.18
SUN	−0.01	0.14	0.02	0.06
MON	0.01	0.31	0.04	0.17
TUE	−0.11	0.20	0.08	−0.14
Mean *N* of deaths	7.07	14.5	1.32	9.32
Percent of all deaths	(22%)	(45%)	(4%)	(29%)
F (d.f.=6)	0.96	1.18	2.52*	0.56

[a] *$p<0.05$; **$p<0.01$; ***$p<0.001$.

the men are married; only 29 percent of the women in that age group, compared with 61 percent of the men, live with a partner or relative. For many of these women, then, the *Sabbath* is set apart from the mundane daily routine but on the individual, not the social, level.

Conclusion

Deaths occur on Saturdays, of course, just as they do on every other day of the week. Nonetheless, the sacred nature of the *Sabbath,* its being set apart from all the mundane work-days of the week, creates a special situation in which the probability of death is reduced. We have argued that this special nature derives not from what the *Sabbath* is not—a workday—but from what it is: a day of social gathering and family solidarity. In this respect, it would be interesting to see an analysis of the church-attendance data on a *household* level: how does the religious-attendance effect on mortality operate under conditions where only the man, the woman or both partners are regular church attenders.

Perhaps it is the consistency of the *Sabbath* effect that prevents any other holy-day effect from being seen, perhaps it is the regularity of the *Sabbath* that creates the effect, and perhaps it is the universality of the *Sabbath,* across all groups of the Jewish population. Further analysis will need to disaggregate this population into the more and the less religiously observant, in order to consider whether the effect is a civil one, affecting all groups equally, or whether there is an added advantage (as Durkheim's arguments would suggest) to those groups who are religiously observant and for whom the *Sabbath* is not just imposed by civil law, but is an inner imperative.

References

Anson, J. 1992. "The second dimension: A proposed measure of the rectangularity of mortality curves." *Genus* 48: 1-17.

Anson, O., and J. Anson. 1997. "Surviving the holidays: Gender differences in mortality in the context of three Moslem holidays." *Sex Roles* 37: 381-399.

Anson, O., S. Carmel, A. Levenson, D. Y. Bonneh and B. Maoz. 1993. "Coping with recent life events: The interplay of personal and collective resources." *Behavioral Medicine* 18: 159-166.

Anson, O., S. Carmel, A. Levenson, B. Maoz and D. Y. Bonneh. 1990. "Recent life events, religiosity, and health: An individual or collective effect." *Human Relations* 43: 1051-1066.

Anson, O., S. Carmel, A. Levenson, B. Maoz and D. Y. Bonneh. 1991. "Religious community, individual religiosity, and health: A tale of two kibbutzim." *Sociology* 25: 119-132.

Central Bureau of Statistics. 1997. *Statistical Abstract of Israel.* Jerusalem: Central Bureau of Statistics.

Chatfield, C. 1989. *The Analysis of Time Series.* London:Chapman & Hall.

Cohen, A. 1983. "Seasonal daily effect on the number of births in Israel." *Applied Statistics* 32: 228-235.

Durkheim, E. 1886 [1973]. "Review 'Herbert Spencer ecclesiastical institutions: being part of the principles of sociology'." In W. S. F. Pickering, *Durkheim on Religion,* 15-23. London: Routledge & Kegan Paul.

Durkheim, E. 1915. *The Elementary Forms of the Religious Life.* London: George Allen & Unwin.
Durkheim, E. 1897 [1951]. *Suicide.* New York: Free Press.
Durkheim, E. 1919 [1973]. "Contribution to discussion 'Religious sentiments at the present time'." In W. S. F. Pickering, *Durkheim on Religion*, 181-189. London: Routledge & Kegan Paul.
Ellison, C. G. 1991. "Religious involvement and subjective well-being." *Journal of Health and Social Behaviour* 32: 80-99.
Harrison, A. A., and N. E. A. Kroll. 1985-86. "Variations in death rates in the proximity of Christmas: An opponent process interpretation." *Omega* 16: 181-192.
Horowitz, D., and M. Lisak. 1990. *Troubles in Utopia: Israel—an Overloaded Society.* Tel-Aviv: Am Oved (in Hebrew).
Hummer, R. A., R. G. Roger, C. B. Nam and C. G. Ellison. 1999. "Religious involvement and U.S. adult mortality." *Demography* 36: 273-285.
Idler, E. L. 1987. "Religious involvement and the health of the elderly: some hypotheses and an initial test." *Social Forces* 66: 226-238.
Idler, E. L., and S. V. Kasl. 1992. "Religion, disability, depression, and the timing of death. *American Journal of Sociology* 97: 1052-1079.
Jarvis, G. K., and H. C. Norcott. 1987. "Religion and differences in morbidity and mortality." *Social Science and Medicine* 25: 813-824.
Koenig, H. G., J. C. Hays, D. B. Larson, L. K. George, H. J. Cohen, M. E. McCullough, K. G. Meador and D. G. Blazer. 1999. "Does religious attendance prolong survival? A six-year follow-up study of 3,968 older adults." *Journals of Gerontology Series A: Biological Sciences and Medical Sciences* 54: M370-M376.
Krause, N., & T. Van Tran. 1989. "Stress and religious involvement among older blacks." *Journal of Gerontology* 44: S4-S13.
Kubler-Ross, E. 1969. *On Death and Dying.* New York: Macmillan.
Kubler-Ross, E. 1975. *Death: The Final Stage of Growth.* Englewood Cliffs, NJ: Prentice Hall.
Levin, J. S., and P. L. Schiller. 1987. "Is there a religious factor in health?" *Journal of Religion and Health* 26: 9-36.
Levin, J. S., and H. Y. Vanderpool. 1987. "Is frequent religious attendance really conducive to better health? Toward an epidemiology of religion." *Social Science and Medicine* 24: 589-600.
Ministry of Health. 1998. *Health Status in Israel.* Jerusalem: Israel Center for Disease Control.
Nisbet, R. A. 1975. *The Sociology of Emile Durkheim.* London: Heinemann.
Oman, D., and D. Reed. 1998. "Religion and mortality among the community-dwelling elderly." *American Journal of Public Health* 88: 1469-1475.
Peres, Y., and E. Yuchtman-Yaar. 1998. *Between Consent and Dissent.* Jerusalem: The Israel Democracy Institute.
Pescosolido, B. A., and S. Georgianna. 1989. "Durkheim, suicide, and religion: Toward a network theory of religion." *American Sociological Review* 54: 33-48.
Phillips, D. P., and K. A. Feldman. 1973. "A dip in death before ceremonial occasions: Some new relationships between social integration and mortality." *American Sociological Review* 38: 678-696.
Phillips, D. P., and E. W. King. 1988. "Death takes a holiday: Mortality surrounding major social occasion." *Lancet* 2 (8613): 728-732.
Phillips, D. P., and D. G. Smith. 1990. "Postponement of death until symbolically meaningful occasions." *Journal of the American Medical Association* 263: 1947-1951.
Roth, J. 1963. *Time Tables.* New York: Bobbs-Merrill.

Sherkat, D. E., and M. D. Reed. 1992. "The effect of religion and social support on self-esteem and depression among the suddenly bereaved." *Social Indicators Research* 26: 259-275.

Strawbridge, W. J., R. D. Cohen, S. J. Shema and G. A. Kaplan. 1997. "Frequent attendance at religious services and mortality over 28 years." *American Journal of Public Health* 87: 957-961.

Thoits, P. A. 1995. "Stress, coping and social support processes: Where are we? What next?" *Journal of Health and Social Behavior* (special number): 53-79.

Troyer, H. 1988. "Review of cancer among four religious sects: Evidence that life-styles are distinctive sets of risk factors." *Social Science and Medicine* 26: 1007-1017.

Witter, R. A., W. A. Stock, M. A. Okun and M. J. Haring. 1985. "Religion and subjective well-being: A quantitative synthesis." *Review of Religious Research* 26: 332-342.

Zuckerman, D. M., S. V. Kasl and A. M. Ostfeld. 1984. "Psychosocial predictors of mortality among the elderly poor." *American Journal of Epidemiology* 119: 410-423

14

Mortality Differentials among Women: The Israel Longitudinal Mortality Study

Orly Manor, Zvi Eisenbach , Avi Israeli, and Yechiel Friedlander

Introduction

In the industrialized world socio-economic status (SES) mortality differentials have been documented and analyzed extensively (Marmot, Shipley, and Rose 1984a; Sorlie, Backund, and Keller 1995; Kunst, Groenhof, and Mackenbach 1998). Frequently, such analyses have focused on male inequalities (Macintyre and Hunt 1997; Kunst et al. 1998). Studies, which address women, indicate that SES inequalities exist for women as well (Moser, Pugh, and Goldblatt 1988; Martelin 1994; Sorlie et al. 1995, Arber 1997). However, there is some evidence that the magnitude of SES inequalities differ, with women having smaller differentials than men (Valkonen 1989; Blane, Davey Smith, and Bartley 1990; Koskinen and Martelin 1994; Elo and Preston 1996).

One of the main indicators of social position used for investigating mortality differentials has been occupation. However, women's labor market experience, while varying among industrialized countries, is frequently characterized by a large percentage of women who are employed part-time or who are out of the paid labor market as full-time homemakers. Thus occupational class has been considered a less suitable measure of social circumstances (Arber 1989; Moser et al. 1988) and alternative indicators have been put forward and subsequently related to mortality and morbidity. Measures suggested include educational attainment (Lahelma, Manderbacka, Rahkonen, and Karisto 1994; Kunst and Mackenbach 1994; Manor, Matthews, and Power 1997) home ownership (Moser et al. 1988, Power, Manor, and Fox 1991), crowding (Martelin 1994) and access to cars (Fox and Goldblatt 1982). These socio-economic indicators are associated with health through complex mechanisms such as material deprivation, health related behaviors, and access to and utilization of health care (Townsend and Davidson 1982; Power et al. 1991).

Women's health also appears to be influenced by their marital and parental status (Weatherhall, Joshi, and Macran 1994); married women have lower mortality and better health than single or previously married women (Kotler and Wingard 1989; Elstad 1996; Hu and Goldman 1990) and mothers are healthier than childless women (Kotler and Wingard 1989; Green, Beral, and Moser 1988). Most studies assessing the effects of marital and parental status on women's health were carried out within the framework of social roles, although there has been a debate about whether women's involvement in multiple roles is associated with health benefits or role strain (Arber 1991; Macran, Clarke, and Joshi 1994; Verbrugge 1983; Bartley, Sacker, Firth, and Fitzpatrick 1999). However, an evaluation of these effects in conjunction with women's socio-economic circumstances is more sparse.

In Israel, for many years, studies of differential mortality have focused on country of origin (Peritz and Tamir 1979; Goldbourt and Kark 1982). Studies in other countries also showed mortality and morbidity differentials associated with country of origin or ethnicity (Kingston and Smith 1997; Marmot, Adelstein, and Balusu 1984b). However, some of these studies aimed at evaluating mortality differentials between migrants and indigenous populations (Senior and Bhopal 1994; Uniken-Venema, Garretsen, and van der Mass 1995), whereas in the Israeli population all the groups are immigrants who differ by their continent of origin. The ethnic composition of the adult Jewish population of Israel is unique, consisting mainly of immigrants from about 100 countries. A number of cross sectional studies carried out in Israel (Peritz 1986; Friedlander, Schellekens, and Sharashov-Cohen, see chapter 11) showed an excess mortality associated with North African origin. In a recent report based on the Israel Longitudinal Mortality Study, the excess mortality of men originating in North Africa appeared to be due to differences in SES (Manor, Eisenbach, Peritz, and Friedlander 1999). This report also showed substantial mortality inequalities among Israeli men according to a number of SES indicators including occupation, education, and income. But, as yet, there has been no systematic evaluation of mortality differentials among Israeli women.

The present study investigates differentials in mortality among Israeli adult women, with respect to socio-economic and demographic characteristics. Our objectives are: a) to estimate differences in mortality among women according to ethnic origin, marital status, living arrangements, and several variables measuring social status; b) to compare the above mortality differences with those reported for Israeli men; and c) to investigate explanations for socio-demographic mortality differences among women.

Methods

This chapter uses the Israel Longitudinal Mortality Study (Eisenbach, Manor, Peritz, and Hite 1997), which links census records from a 20 percent systematic sample of households in the 1983 census, with records of death occurring in the subsequent 9.5 years, until the end of 1992. Israel has a population register in which a unique ID number identifies every resident, newborn, or immigrant. The linkage was performed by means of the ID number, which appears in both the census records and on death notifications, and was carried out by the Israel Central Bureau of Statistics (ICBS), which omitted from the data set any personal identification information. The quality of the linked data set was enhanced by the high coverage in the census of 1983, where only 2.6 percent of the population escaped enumeration, and by the fact that practically all deaths in Israel are reported. In addition, the linkage was ascertained by comparing six demographic variables available in both data sources (Eisenbach et al. 1997).

The analyses presented here are based on Jewish women aged 45-89 excluding persons living in kibbutzim or institutions as well as those with undefined ethnic origin (see below). The study includes 79,623 women, with 14,332 reported deaths in the sample and 72,527 men with 17,378 reported deaths. The data file for the analysis includes demographic and socio-economic variables of the census and the date of death for women who died during the follow-up period.

The dependent variable is dichotomous with a value of one for death during the study period, and zero otherwise.

The independent variables used were:

Age at the time of the census: subdivided into five-year groups.

Marital status at the time of the census.

"Ethnic" origin: according to country of birth. Father's country of birth was used for individuals born in Israel (mother's country of birth is not available in the census; in most cases mother's and father's country of birth are identical). The variable was categorized as "North Africa," "Asia," and "Europe." The last category also includes a small proportion of women (2.8 percent) originating from North America, South America and Australia.

Education: number of years of school attended, grouped into 0-8, 9-12 and 13 years and over.

Employment status: whether or not the individual was employed during the year preceding the census.

Number of rooms (excluding kitchen): grouped into three categories, below, equal to or above three.

Possession of car by a household member, categorized as Yes or No.

Amenities: a derived variable, based on household possession of the following items: food processor, electric oven, telephone, color TV, vacuum cleaner, and bath (rather than only a shower). This variable is the first factor produced by a factor analysis model.

Living arrangements: categorized as living alone or not.
Number of children: categorized as 0, 1, 2, 3, 4-5, or 6 and above.

Statistical Analysis

Logistic regression models were used to assess differences in mortality according to demographic and socio-economic variables. The effect of each variable was estimated first separately and then in a multivariate analysis. All analyses controlled for age as a linear variable (a quadratic term of age was not significant). The multivariate analyses were carried out in stages, thus incorporating the temporal order of events. In the first stage (Model 1) only ethnic origin and age, both acquired at birth, were examined. Model 2, representing the second stage, included education, usually acquired in early adulthood. The third model also incorporated marital status and employment status, related to the time of the census. Number of rooms, possession of a car and an index of socio-economic status based on household amenities, were added in Model 4. The fit of sequential models was evaluated by log-likelihood, and significance of each independent variable was assessed by a Wald-type Chi-square test. Results also include a test for each category (relative to the reference category) of every variable. Such tests should be viewed with caution since they involve multiple comparisons.

Analysis was carried out in two groups according to the age at the census: 45-69 and 70-89. Two additional analyses, for restricted subgroups of women, were performed. The first, which aimed at assessing mortality differences associated with childbearing history, was restricted to married and widowed women. The second, which was restricted to married and widowed women aged 70-89, aimed at further assessment of mortality differentials associated with household composition at an older age. Due to the strong association between marital status and living arrangements, a combined variable, "household composition," was created using the following categories: married, widowed not living alone, and widowed living alone. The percentages of women in each category were 40, 19, and 41 respectively. These additional analyses followed the stages described above, that is, adjusting at first only for age, and then for additional variables.

The gender difference in the age-adjusted effect of each socio-demographic variable was tested by an interaction term in a logistic model for both sexes (Manor, Eisenbach, Peritz, and Friedlander 1999).

To further validate our results, analyses were repeated using Cox's proportional hazards model. The two models have been shown to give similar results when the event under consideration is rare and the follow-up period is relatively short (Green and Symons 1983). Results of Cox's proportional hazards model were similar to those of the logistic regression. Similarity was evident regarding both the significance and the size of the effects, where the differences in the size of effects between the two models ranged between 0 and 7 percent.

A potential problem in the analyses used is co-linearity arising from the correlation between the independent variables. We assessed the size of this problem and its impact on the estimated parameters and found that the results are not affected by co-linearity (Wax 1992).

Results

Eighteen percent of the women died during the 9.5 years of follow-up; 10 percent of those aged 45-69 and 45.9 percent of 70-89 year olds. The distribution of the study population according to the explanatory variables is given in table 14.1 (table 14.6 includes the distribution according to the number of children).

In the younger age group, mortality was higher among women originating from North Africa (table 14.2), while in both age groups, mortality was lower

Table 14.1
Socio-Demographic Distribution (%) of the Sample

Variable	All women	Age 45–69	Age 70–89
Sample size	79,623	61,807	17,816
Died during follow-up	18.0	10.0	45.9
Age			
45–54	33.2	42.8	
55–64	32.1	41.3	
65–69	12.3	15.8	
70–74	11.6		51.8
75–79	6.5		29.2
80–84	3.2		14.4
85–89	1.0		4.6
Origin			
Asia	20.7	22.2	15.4
Africa	16.3	18.2	9.7
Europe	63.0	59.5	74.9
Education			
0–8	55.7	53.9	61.9
9–12	31.2	31.9	28.6
13+	13.1	14.2	9.6
Marital status			
Married	68.6	77.2	38.7
Divorced	3.6	3.9	2.3
Widowed	26.0	17.2	57.0
Single	1.8	1.7	2.0
Living alone	20.0	13.3	42.5
Employed in 1983	28.9	35.5	5.8
Number of rooms			
< 3	39.5	34.1	58.1
3	35.5	37.5	28.5
> 3	25.0	28.4	13.4
Had a car	33.9	39.6	13.8

among those originating from Asia, relative to women of European origin. An increase in mortality rates with decline in the level of education was evident, with a stronger trend for the older age group. Table 14.2 also shows lower odds of death for married women for both age groups. Among non-married women, single women showed the highest mortality risk and the widowed showed the lowest. Women living alone had higher odds of dying among the younger age group and lower odds among the older age group, compared to women not living by themselves.

Women who were employed at the year of the census had half the odds of dying, of those not employed. All three asset-based measures of SES, namely, number of rooms, car possession, and amenities, showed strong and significant differences among younger women, with mortality declining with improved

Table 14.2
Age-Adjusted Odds Ratios of Death by Selected Variables

Variable	Age 45–69	Age 70–89
Origin	[b,c]	[b]
Europe	1.00	1.00
Asia	0.89[b]	0.90[a]
Africa	1.21[b]	1.10
Education	[b]	[b]
13+	1.00	1.00
9–12	1.10	1.18[b]
0–8	1.38[b]	1.45[b]
Marital status	[b]	[b]
Married	1.00	1.00
Divorced	1.34[b]	1.09
Widowed	1.20[b]	1.09[a]
Single	1.62[b]	1.46[b]
Living arrangements		
Alone	1.00	1.00
Not Alone	0.81[b]	1.10[b]
Employment in 1983		
Employed	1.00	1.00
Not employed	1.51[b]	1.48[b]
Number of rooms	[b]	
> 3	1.00	1.00
3	1.23[b]	0.98
< 3	1.44[b]	1.06
Car		
Yes	1.00	1.00
No	1.35[b]	0.98
Amenities	0.80[b]	0.85[b]

[a] $p < 0.05$.
[b] $p < 0.01$.
[c] An [a] or a [b] on the first line of a variable corresponds to the overall effect of that variable.

socio-economic position. Differences were smaller and non-significant for the older age group, with the exception of household amenities.

Socio-demographic indicators for which significant gender differences in mortality differentials were detected are presented in figures 14.1 and 14.2. Among the younger age group (figure 14.1), differences were found for ethnic origin, where the difference between European and Asian origin was larger for women than men; and for education and possession of car, where inequalities among women were smaller than those for men. Among the older age group (figure 14.2) gender differences were evident for education, with greater inequalities among women than among men; while for number of rooms (results not shown in the figure) and car possession differences were smaller for women than for men. The effect of living alone differed between men and women in both age groups. Younger men showed a larger effect than women, whereas older men showed a smaller effect than older women.

In the multivariate analysis for women aged 45-69, the elevated mortality risk among North Africans was no longer significant after controlling for years of education (table 14.3). In contrast, the lower mortality for women originating from Asia compared to European women increased when education was added to the model (table 14.3, Model 2) and also with the adjustment for additional variables (Models 3 and 4). The odds of death for women of Asian origin, relative to North African women, remained almost constant in Models 1, 2, 3 and 4. The effect of education, although reduced after adjustment, remained significant even when all other variables were included in the model (Model 4, table 14.3). Marital status also remained a significant factor after adjusting for all other variables, wherein single women had the highest odds of dying. Of the three SES measures only car ownership became non-significant with

Figure 14.1
OR of Death by Gender for Origin, Education, Living Arrangement and Car, 45-69

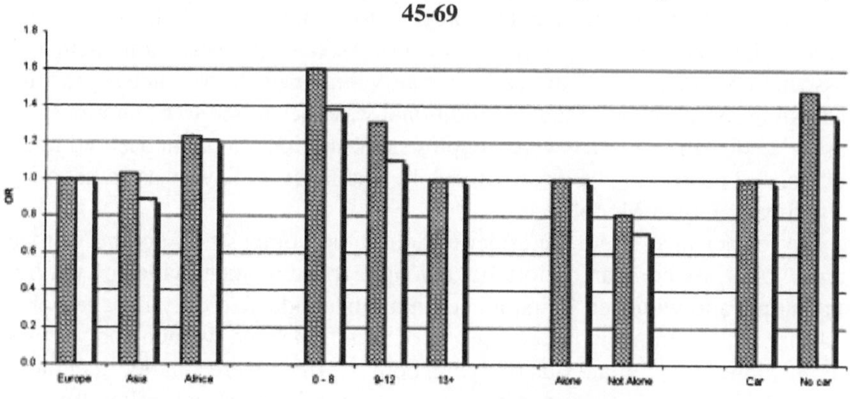

Figure 14.2
OR of Death by Gender for Origin, Education, Living Arrangement and Car, 70-89

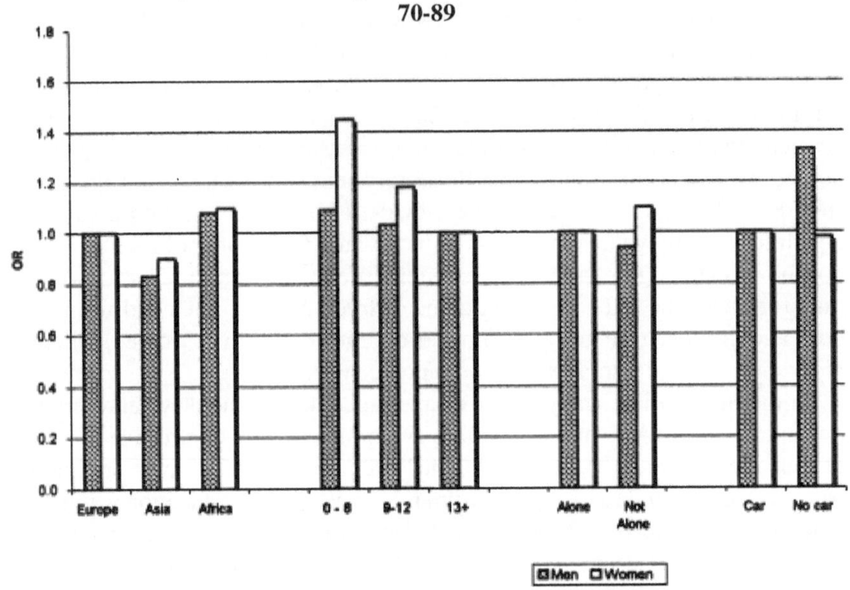

adjustment for other variables (table 14.3, Model 4), whilst the effect of number of rooms and amenities remained substantial and significant (Model 4). The marked effect of employment at the census on mortality remained substantial after adjusting for the other variables (Model 4, table 14.3).

Results of the multivariate analysis of women aged 70-89 are presented in table 14.4. The trends in the effect of origin, found for the younger age group, were also evident for the older age group. However, for the older age group a strong protective effect of North African and Asian origin relative to European origin emerged after adjustment for other factors (table 14.4, Model 4), whereas among the younger group only the effect of Asian origin was significant. The association between education and mortality remained almost unchanged after adjusting for all other variables. Additional variables found to be significantly associated with mortality were: employment, marital status, household amenities, and possession of a car (Model 4). The latter variable was statistically significant only in Model 4.

To further investigate the effect of household composition among women aged 70-89, we compared mortality among married women, widowed not living alone, and widowed living alone. In a model adjusted only for age (table 14.5), highly significant differences were found. Married women and widows living alone had similar odds of dying, both of which were smaller than those for widows not living alone. After all other variables were controlled for, this difference increased, such that the odds of dying among widows not living alone

Table 14.3
Adjusted Odds Ratios of Death, Women Aged 45-69

Variable	Model 1	Model 2	Model 3	Model 4
Origin	b,c	b	b	b
Europe	1.00	1.00	1.00	1.00
Asia	0.89[b]	0.78[b]	0.76[b]	0.71[b]
Africa	1.21[b]	1.08	1.03	0.94
Education		b	b	b
13 +		1.00	1.00	1.00
9–12		1.21[a]	1.06	0.99
0–8		1.44[b]	1.32[b]	1.11[a]
Employment in 1983				
Employed			1.00	1.00
Not employed			1.48[b]	1.39[b]
Marital status			b	b
Married			1.00	1.00
Divorced			1.46[b]	1.18[a]
Widowed			1.20[b]	1.05
Single			1.80[b]	1.39[b]
Number of rooms				b
> 3				1.00
3				1.15[b]
< 3				1.26[b]
Car				
Yes				1.00
No				1.07
Amenities				0.84[b]
−2 log likelihood	36,839	36,743	36,565	32,771
Model Chi-square	3378[b]	3472[b]	3651[b]	3419[b]

[a] $p < 0.05$.
[b] $p < 0.01$.
[c] An [a] or a [b] on the first line of a variable corresponds to the overall effect of that variable.

Table 14.4
Adjusted Odds Ratios of Death, Women Aged 70-89

Variable	Model 1	Model 2	Model 3	Model 4
Origin	b,c	b	b	b
Europe	1.00	1.00	1.00	1.00
Asia	0.90[a]	0.80[b]	0.79[b]	0.72[b]
Africa	1.10	0.99	0.97	0.85[b]
Education		b	b	b
13 +		1.00	1.00	1.00
9–12		1.19[b]	1.18[b]	1.22[b]
0–8		1.52[b]	1.50[b]	1.44[b]
Employment in 1983				
Employed			1.00	1.00
Not employed			1.43[b]	1.40[b]
Marital status			b	a
Married			1.00	1.00
Divorced			1.16	1.11
Widowed			1.10[a]	1.02
Single			1.58[b]	1.44[b]
Number of rooms				
> 3				1.00
3				0.93
< 3				0.92
Car				
Yes				1.00
No				0.84[b]
Amenities				0.83[b]
−2 log likelihood	23,327	23,245	23,199	20,431
Model Chi-square	1253[b]	1333[b]	1380[b]	1366[b]

[a] $p < 0.05$.
[b] $p < 0.01$.
[c] An [a] or a [b] on the first line of a variable corresponds to the overall effect of that variable.

were 1.5 those of married women. Inclusion of the household composition variable in the multivariate model did not alter the effect of other variables in Model 4 (table 14.4), except for car possession, which was no longer significant when household composition was included.

Number of children was found to be strongly related to mortality for both age groups (table 14.6). In the age-adjusted model (Model A, table 14.6) a "u" shape emerged for this association among the younger age group, with the lowest mortality among women with two children. The association remained highly significant after adjusting for ethnic origin and education. When the analysis was restricted to women with at least one child (results not shown), significant differences associated with number of children were evident. A comparison of the effect of number of children by ethnic origin indicated a similar non-significant effect among women of Asian and North-African origin, and a substantial effect among women of European origin (results not shown). The interaction term, however, was found to be only borderline significant.

Discussion

This study is the first systematic evaluation of demographic and socio-economic mortality differentials among Israeli Jewish women. Mortality differentials during the period 1983-1992 were examined by linking a sample of 20 percent of the 1983 census records with records of deaths occurring during that period. The large number of records, the high coverage of the population, the prospective design, and the variety of socio-economic indicators all make the ILMS a highly suitable source for investigating mortality differentials. Results reveal substantial mortality differentials among Israeli women in the 1980s according to ethnic origin, SES, living arrangements, marital status, and number of children. The study therefore extends previous work on mortality differentials among women. Until recently, most studies of health inequalities have focused on male populations (Macintyre and Hunt 1997) and a systematic evaluation of gender differences has been rare. However, there are now several exceptions in which both sexes were investigated (Koskinen and Martelin 1994; Arber 1997; Elo and Preston 1996), women were solely addressed (Macran et al. 1994; Elstad 1996; Bartley et al. 1999) as well as one study reporting a systematic gender comparison (Matthews, Manor, and Power 1999). By evaluating mortality differentials among women according to a broad spectrum of demographic and SES indicators and by systematically examining gender differences, our study contributes to the understanding of women's health and gender differences in health inequalities.

The approach adopted in this paper differs from that taken by a number of other studies evaluating the associations between women's health and their marital, parental, and employment status. Most previous studies were carried out within the framework of social roles, while others focused on differentials associated with occupational class (Arber 1991; Macran et al. 1994, Sorensen

Table 14.5
Adjusted Odds Ratios of Death by Household Composition, Women Aged 70-89

	Model A	Model B	Model C	Model D
Household composition	b,c	b	b	b
Widows living alone	1.00	1.00	1.00	1.00
Married	1.00	0.99	0.98	1.10[a]
Widows not alone	1.32[b]	1.26[b]	1.29[b]	1.53[b]

[a] $p < 0.05$.
[b] $p < 0.01$. Model A=age+household composition, Model B=Model A+origin, Model C=Model B+education, Model D=Model C+rooms+car+amenities.
[c] An [a] or a [b] on the first line of a variable corresponds to the overall effect of that variable.

and Verbrugge 1987; Verbrugge 1979; Weatherall et al. 1994). We aimed for an approach that would enable us to estimate mortality differentials among women as well as to carry out a methodical gender comparison. Thus, while we have assessed mortality differentials associated with employment status, we did not evaluate differentials by occupational class. Among women aged 45-69 only 43 percent were employed outside their home at the time of the census or five years prior to the census. Use of occupational class within a multivariate analysis would have yielded a major reduction in the sample size. This, in conjunction with other limitations associated with the usage of occupation as an SES indicator (Blaxter 1986; Whitehead 1988), have led us to employ several other SES indicators including education, housing, household amenities and the possession of a car.

Ethnic Origin

We found that women who originated from North Africa had higher mortality rates and women originating from Asia lower mortality rates, compared with women of European ancestry. However, after allowing for the cumulative effect of several socio-economic indicators, the differences in mortality associated with ethnic origin were altered. The excess of mortality of women originating from North Africa was transformed and the protective effect associated with Asian origin, relative to European, increased. However, the difference between Asian and North African women remained constant. Excess mortality of individuals of North African origin has been presented in previous studies of the Israeli population. These studies showed that the excess mortality, which has persisted over time and over all age groups, was evident for both sexes (Peritz 1986). Results presented here are similar to those found for men, using the ILMS (Manor et al. 1999). Studies in other countries also show mortality and morbidity differentials associated with country of origin or ethnicity (Kingston and Smith 1997; Marmot et al. 1984b, Senior and Bhopal 1994; Uniken-Venema et al. 1995). Possible explanations offered for the differentials in mortality associated with ethnic origin, include socio-economic factors, socio-cultural factors, and genetic factors (Friedlander et al., see chapter 11; Peritz 1986; Uniken-Venema et al. 1995). Indeed, differences were notable among Europeans, Asians, and North African Jews when they immigrated to Israel, with respect to socio-demographic background as well as to genetic markers (Cohen 1971). Evidence for genetic differences includes the recent findings on genetic factors associated with breast cancer among Jewish women of European origin (Roitberg-Tambur et al. 1995; Karlin, Kenett, and Bonne-Tamir 1979; Sterwing, Hartge, and Wacholder 1997; Abeliovich et al. 1997). Reports on socio-economic differences are related to the persistent association, in the Israeli population, between ethnic origin and socio-economic position, where individuals originating in North Africa and Asia are more likely to have a lower social class (Smooha 1993). This is evident in our data. For example, younger women who completed at least nine years of schooling account for 21 percent among both the Asian and North African groups and 72 percent among the European group. Our results suggest that differences in mortality associated with ethnic origin are strongly related to socio-economic factors, and that additional factors also play a role in this association.

Family Composition

We found that mortality was lowest among married women while among those not married, single women had the highest odds of dying and the widowed women the lowest odds. Differences in mortality according to marital status have been investigated and documented (Hu and Goldman 1990; Goldman, Koreman and Weinstein 1995; Waldron, Hughes, and Brooks 1996; Central Bureau of Statistics 1973). While our results accord with a number of studies addressing this issue (Hu and Goldman 1990; Goldman et al. 1995, Rogot, Sorlie, Johnson, Glover, and Treasure 1988), they contrast with recent studies suggesting that never-married women have better health than separated and divorced women, especially among older women (Waldron, Weiss, and Hughes 1997; Sorlie et al. 1995; Martikainen 1995; Elstad 1996). Interestingly, the proportion of single women in Israel is similar to that found in Japan and lower than that of Western societies. However, mortality differences reported here between single and married women are smaller than those of Japanese women and similar to those found in Western countries (Goldman and Hu 1993).

Potential causal pathways that have been suggested for the link between mortality and marital status include: 1) a protective effect of material resources and life-style of those currently married compared to those of non-married; 2) a selection effect of being married; and 3) the selection effect of re-marriage for the widowed and the divorced (Murphy 1996; Waldron et al. 1996). However, a recent longitudinal study of marital transition in Holland indicated that the effect of selection in marital transitions is limited (Joung, van de Mheen, Stronks, van Poppel, and Mackenbach 1998). Although our data set does not allow us to distinguish between the "protection" and the "selection" effects, both

Table 14.6
Adjusted Odds Ratios of Death by Number of Children Married and Widowed Women

	Model A	Model B	Model C	No. of children (%)
Women aged 45–69				
No. of children	[b,c]	[b]	[b]	100.0
0	1.00	1.00	1.00	5.6
1	0.86[a]	0.86[a]	0.88[b]	11.9
2	0.68[b]	0.69[b]	0.70[b]	30.8
3	0.72[b]	0.72[b]	0.73[b]	20.1
4–5	0.75[b]	0.75[b]	0.73[b]	15.4
6 +	0.83[b]	0.80[b]	0.76[b]	16.2
Women aged 70–89				
No. of children	[a]	[a]	[b]	100.0
0	1.00	1.00	1.00	12.6
1	0.91	0.91	0.92	20.4
2	0.84[b]	0.84[b]	0.83[b]	28.6
3	0.87[a]	0.87[a]	0.84[b]	13.8
4–5	0.92	0.92	0.86[a]	11.2
6 +	0.83[b]	0.83[a]	0.77[b]	13.4

[a] $p < 0.05$.
[b] $p < 0.01$. Model A = age + number of children, Model B = Model A + origin, Model C = Model B + education.
[c] An [a] or a [b] on the first line of a variable corresponds to the overall effect of that variable.

effects are likely to contribute to the better health of married persons compared to the non-married. Moreover, the results show that the never married have the highest mortality and the widowed have the lowest mortality among those not married, that is, there is an indication for the accumulation of the two effects over the life span. The marked difference in mortality found between married and widowed women, especially among the younger age group, may be related to what is referred to in the literature as "the broken heart syndrome." This effect increases mortality of widowed persons, especially among relatively young individuals (Parkes, Benjamin, and Fitzgerald 1969). Additional influences are the economic changes yielded by the changes in family income and expenditure associated with the death of a spouse. For both age groups, the effect of marital status remained significant after adjusting for all independent variables. This finding accords with that reported on Finnish (Martikainen 1995) and American women (Sorlie et al. 1995) but contrasts with a report focusing on American elderly women, for whom the effect of marital status on mortality diminished after adjustment for a wide range of confounders (Goldman et al. 1995).

Among widowed women aged 70-89, living alone was associated with lower mortality, an effect that increased after adjusting for other variables. Additional analyses (results not shown) indicated that widowed women living alone had higher education and were more likely to have a European origin, compared with those widows not living alone. Thus the more disadvantaged widows were more likely to reside with others (probably children). Furthermore, a larger percentage of these women reported possession of a car within their household, hence explaining the excess mortality associated with possession of a car among the elderly women.

Substantial mortality differentials were associated with the number of children ever born to a woman. Furthermore, similar effects prevailed for both younger and older women. Other studies have also suggested that mothers are generally healthier than childless women (Elstad 1996; Weatherall et al. 1994; Kotler and Wingard 1989). Health selection has been put forward as one possible explanation for the observed excess mortality among childless women (Weatherall et al. 1994). However, our results showed that an analysis restricted to women with children, which is less affected by selective factors, revealed significant differences associated with the number children. The lowest mortality was found for women with two children. Similar results have been reported for British and Norwegian women, where women with three children had the lowest mortality (Green et al. 1988; Lund, Arnesen, and Borgen 1990). Both social and biological explanations have been suggested for the association between the number of children and mortality. Social elements include social-familial networks, whose negative effect on mortality may be explained in terms of a reduction in stress related to social support (Fox 1988; Clausen 1987), reinforcement of preventive health behavior (Gottlieb and Green 1984) and access to instrumental aid (Berkman 1985). Biological effects include endogenous hormonal influences (Beral 1983, Lochen and Lund 1997). Reports on cause-specific mortality indicate divergent trends. For example, mortality from diabetes mellitus and cervical cancer increase with the number of children, whereas mortality from breast and ovarian cancer decrease with number of children (Green et al. 1988, Lund 1992). Our data indicated differences among ethnic groups in the association between number of children and mortality. This may be due to differences in mortality in causes of death that are related to both number of children and ethnicity, for example breast cancer (Sterwing et al. 1997; Abeliovich et al. 1997).

Socio-Economic Status

Substantial and consistent differences in mortality were found, among women aged 45-69, according to each of the socio-economic indicators considered. These results support studies showing social class gradients in mortality and morbidity (Marmot et al. 1984a; Sorlie et al. 1995; Kunst and Mackenbach 1994; Mustard, Derksen, Berthelot, Wolfson, and Roos 1997; Power 1994). Also welfare states that enable universal access to medical care, of which Israel is one, demonstrate substantial socio-economic differences in health (Townsend and Davidson 1982; Power 1994; Valkonen 1989). Various explanations have been put forward for the observed association between socioeconomic position and mortality including a selection effect (Illsley, 1991), the effect of material circumstances as well as behavioral patterns (Townsend and Davidson 1982). Health selection is likely to be relatively unimportant in a longitudinal study such as ours, particularly with measures such as years of education, which is usually completed by early adulthood.

Educational attainments play a major role in determining positions in the social hierarchy and are related to knowledge and attitudes that influence health behaviors and practices. Education has been suggested as preferable to other indicators of socio-economic position, such as occupation or income (Elo and Preston 1996; Valkonen 1993), and is strongly associated with mortality (Valkonen 1989; Sorlie et al. 1995, Mustard et al. 1997). Such an association is also evident from our study. We found that, irrespective of age, differences in mortality associated with education were significant even after adjusting for a series of other variables. It is perhaps surprising that the association between education and mortality among the elderly Israeli women is stronger than that for younger women. This result contrasts with the recent finding for Israeli men, for which no association between mortality and education was found among the elderly (Manor et al. 1999).

Socio-economic differentials in mortality were assessed here using a number of indicators of social position, including both education-based and asset-based indicators, such as housing and amenities. Our results suggest that most indicators also have an independent component in their relationship with mortality, especially among the younger age group. The differences associated with asset-based indicators may reflect differences associated with wealth, self-esteem or, alternatively, these indicators may be seen as 'health-promoting' and play the role of mediating between wealth and health. A recent study suggested that housing and car access have direct health promoting and health-damaging effects, beyond that associated with wealth (Macintyre, Ellaway, Der, Ford, and Hunt 1998). While our results for younger women indicate substantial socio-economic mortality differentials, the magnitude of these differentials among Israeli women tends to be somewhat smaller than those reported for other countries (Sorlie et al. 1995; Valkonen 1989). Methodological issues such as the type of model used for analysis, the composition of the population included (e.g., non-institutionalized), the meaning of the socio-economic indicators selected, the structure of health services and social characteristics, may all contribute to these dissimilarities.

Our study shows that participation in the labor force was strongly associated with lower mortality. This result accords with other studies showing that employed women are healthier than non-employed women (Elstad 1996; Weatherall et al. 1994; Kotler and Wingard 1989). Our measure of employment reflects the women's status during the year preceding the census. Non-employed women aged 45-69 are a heterogeneous group including women seeking work, housewives, permanently sick, and retired women. While the association between unemployment and health has been documented before (Moser, Goldblatt, Fox, and Jones 1987; Fox and Sherwy 1988), this is unlikely to be the main influence here. Although the data do not enable us to distinguish between subgroups, unemployment in Israel during the period under consideration was relatively low and most individuals seeking work were younger than the age groups examined here. Hence, other explanations need to be considered, such as selection, material circumstances, social support, empowerment, and self-confidence associated with women's work (Nathanson, 1980; Sorensen and Verbrugge 1987).

Mortality differentials among women aged 70-89 were generally smaller than those found for the younger age group. Several other studies also show a reduction in mortality differentials with increasing age (Fox, Goldblatt, and Jones 1985; Martelin 1994; Mustard et al. 1997). Selective mortality is one explanation for this finding, whereby only the fittest, and most healthy individuals from subgroups with high mortality at relatively early ages are still alive at a later age. Another plausible explanation is the differential recruitment of individuals into institutional settings such as nursing homes, with those from the less advantaged sections of society being more likely to be institutionalized. Such a process was indeed identified in the sample under consideration. Residents under institutional care were excluded from the data set under consideration (Eisenbach et al. 1997).

Gender Differences

Generally, results presented here for Israeli women are similar to those reported recently for Israeli men (Manor et al. 1999). Both women and men show substantial mortality differentials by socio-demographic indicators, with smaller inequalities among elderly individuals. Furthermore, similarities were found in trends detected after adjustment. For example, in both sexes adjustment for SES eliminated the excess mortality associated with North African origin and revealed a lower mortality among those originating from Asia. However, a systematic comparison of the magnitude of mortality differentials indicated a number of gender differences in relation to both demographic and socioeconomic characteristics. Our comparison is relevant to the understanding of gender differences in health in general as well as specifically to the Israeli population. Israeli longevity patterns by gender are somewhat unique: men's life expectancy is ranked third in a worldwide comparison whereas women are ranked only at the fourteenth place (Central Bureau of Statistics 1998).

With respect to SES we found inconsistent evidence regarding gender differences in the magnitude of mortality inequalities. For several indicators, specifically education and possession of a car among younger individuals, mortality differentials were smaller among women than men, while for other indicators (specifically, household amenities and employment status for both age groups) no gender differences were evident. In contrast, for education among the elderly our results showed that inequalities among women were larger than those found for men. A number of studies reported on larger SES inequalities in mortality and morbidity among men compared with those of women (Koskinen and Martelin 1994; Stronks, van de Mheen, van den Bos, and Mackenbach 1995). However, in some studies men and women have similar SES gradients, for example:

coronary heart disease (Diez-Roux, Javier-Nieto, Tyroler, Crum, and Szklo 1995), self-perceived health and psychological well being (Marmot, Ryff, Bumpass, Shipley, and Marks 1997). Moreover, there are other examples in which greater SES inequality has been found for women, specifically for asthma (Eachus et al. 1972) and for myocardial infarction (Morrison, Woodward, Leslie, and Tunstall-Pedoe 1997). Inconsistent evidence regarding gender comparisons has also been reported for young adults with a variety of health indicators (Matthews et al. 1999). Our results also suggest inconsistency by age: some SES indicators showed gender differences only for the younger age group, while for others differences were found solely among the elderly. This finding accords with previous observations that gender differences may vary by period, as well as by age (Blane, Bartley, Davey Smith, Filakti, and Bethume 1994; Elo and Preston 1996; Matthews et al. 1999). Furthermore, our study indicates divergent evidence on gender differences in relation to demographic variables. Whilst differences were apparent in relation to ethnic origin and living arrangements, no differences were detected for marital status. The latter finding contrasts with other studies reporting that the longevity advantage of marriage is greater for men than for women (Hu and Goldman 1990).

Gender differences in cause-specific mortality, or in the processes linking SES with health, and in other factors associated with SES such as employment status, may all contribute to the observed gender patterns (Macintyre and Hunt 1997; Macintyre, Hunt, and Sweeting 1996; Matthews et al. 1999). Regarding ethnic differences, while it has been suggested that the interaction between mortality, gender and ethnicity might be crucial for understanding mortality differentials (Krieger 1990), this interaction is not usually considered (Hunt and Annandale 1999). Such an interaction may be due to both biological and social factors. Gender similarities in mortality inequalities by ethnicity, found in our analyses after adjustment for social class, suggest similarities in the social processes involved. However, further research on this topic, including gender comparisons of cause-specific mortality differentials and a systematic comparison of factors explaining these differentials, is needed.

In conclusion, this study has shown substantial mortality differentials among Israeli women, where those who were poor, less educated, non-married, childless, out of the labor force, and of North African origin had a higher risk of death. The excess mortality of women originating in North Africa appeared to be due to differences in SES. Gender differences in mortality differentials varied by the socio-demographic indicator examined as well as by age.

Acknowledgements

This research was supported by grant no. 93-00015/2 from the United States-Israel Binational Science Foundation, Jerusalem.

References

Abeliovich, D., L. Kaduri, I. Lerer, N. Weinberg, G. Amir, M. Sagi, J. Zlotogora, N. Heching and T. Peretz. 1997. "The founder mutations 185delAG and 538insC in BRACI and 617delT in BRAC2 appear in 60% of ovarian cancer and 30% of early-onset breast cancer patients among Ashkenazi women." *American Journal of Human Genetics* 60: 505-514.

Arber, S. 1989. "Gender and class inequalities in health: understanding the differentials." In A. J. Fox (ed.), *Health Inequalities in European Countries*, 250-279). London: Gower.

Arber, S. 1991. "Class, paid employment, and family roles: Making sense of structural disadvantage, gender, and health status." *Social Science and Medicine* 32: 425-436.

Arber, S. 1997. "Comparing inequalities in women's and men's health: Britain in the 1990s." *Social Science and Medicine* 44: 773-787.

Bartley, M., A. Sacker, D. Firth and R. Fitzpatrick. 1999. "Social position, social roles, and women's health in England: Changing relationships 1984-1993." *Social Science and Medicine* 48: 99-115.

Beral, V. 1983. "Parity and susceptibility to cancer." *Ciba Foundation Symposium* 96:182-203.

Berkman, L. F. 1985. "The relationship of social networks and social support to morbidity and mortality." In S. Cohen and S. L. Syme (eds.), *Social Support and Health*, 241-262. Toronto: Academic Press.

Blane, D., G. Davey Smith and M. Bartley. 1990. "Social class differences in years of potential life lost: Size, trends, and principal causes." *British Medical Journal* 301: 429-432.

Blane, D., M. Bartley, G. Davey Smith, H. Filakti and A. Bethume. 1994. "Social patterning of medical mortality in youth and early childhood." *Social Science and Medicine* 39: 361-366.

Blaxter, M. 1986. "Longitudinal studies in Britain relevant to inequalities in health." In R. G. Wilkinson (ed.), *Health, in Class and Health: Research and Longitudinal Data*, 125-211. London: Tavistock.

Central Bureau of Statistics. 1973. *Mortality among Adult Jews in Israel: 1950-1967.* Special Series no. 409. Jerusalem: Central Bureau of Statistics.

Central Bureau of Statistics. 1998. *Vital Statistics* 1994-1995, *Part D: Mortality.* Publication no. 1083. Jerusalem: Central Bureau of Statistics.

Clausen, J. A. 1987. "Health and the life course: some personal observations." *Journal of Health and Social Behavior* 28: 337-344.

Cohen, T. 1971. "Genetic markers in migrants to Israel." *Israel Journal of Medical Sciences* 7: 1509-1514.

Diez-Roux, A. V., F. Javier-Nieto, H. E. Tyroler, L. D. Crum, and M. Szklo. 1995. "Social inequalities and atherosclerosis." *American Journal of Epidemiology* 141: 960-972.

Eachus, J., M. Williams, P. Chan, G. Davey Smith, M. Grainge, J. Donovan and S. Frankel. 1972. "Deprivation and cause specific morbidity: Evidence from the Somerset and Avon survey of health." *British Medical Journal* 312: 287-292.

Eisenbach, Z., O. Manor, E. Peritz and Y. Hite. 1997. "The Israel longitudinal mortality study - differential mortality in Israel 1983-92: Objective, materials, methods and preliminary results." *Israel Journal of Medical Sciences* 33: 794-807.

Elo, I. T., and S. H. Preston. 1996. "Educational differentials in mortality: United States, 1979-85." *Social Science and Medicine* 42: 47-57.

Elstad, J. I. 1996. "Inequalities in health related to women's marital, parental and employment status: A comparison between the early 70s and the late 80s, Norway." *Social Science and Medicine* 42: 75-89.

Fox, A. J. 1988. "Social network interaction: New jargon in health inequalities." *British Medical Journal* 297: 373-374.

Fox, A. J., and P. O. Goldblatt. 1982. *Socio-demographic Mortality Differentials from the OPCS Longitudinal Study 1971–75* (series LS no. 1). London: HMSO.

Fox, A. J., P. O. Goldblatt and D. R. Jones. 1985. "Social class mortality differentials: Artifact, selection, or life circumstances." *Journal of Epidemiology in Community Health* 39: 1-8.

Fox, A. J., and M. Sherwy. 1988. "New longitudinal insights into relationships between unemployment and mortality." *Stress Medicine* 4: 11-19.

Goldbourt, U., and J. D. Kark. 1982. "The epidemiology of coronary heart disease in the ethnically and culturally diverse population of Israel." *Israel Journal of Medical Sciences* 64: 570-581.

Goldman, N., and Y. Hu. 1993. "Excess mortality among the unmarried: A case study of Japan." *Social Science and Medicine* 36: 533-546.

Goldman, N., S. Korenman and R. Weinstein. 1995. "Marital status and health among the elderly." *Social Science and Medicine* 40: 1717-1730.

Gottlieb, N. H., and L. W. Green. 1984. "Life events, social networks, life-style and health: An analysis of the 1979 National Survey of Personal Health Practices and Consequences." *Health Education Quarterly* 11: 91-105.

Green, M. S., and M. J. Symons. 1983. "A comparison of the logistic risk function and the proportional hazards model in prospective epidemiologic studies." *Journal of Chronic Disease* 36: 715-721.

Green, A., V. Beral and K. Moser. 1988. "Mortality in women in relation to their child-bearing history." *British Medical Journal* 297: 391-395.

Hu, Y. R., and N. Goldman. 1990. "Mortality differentials by marital status: An international comparison." *Demography* 27: 233-250.

Hunt, K., and E. Annandale. 1999. "Relocating gender and morbidity: Examining men's and women's health in contemporary western societies." *Social Science and Medicine* 48: 1-5.

Illsley, R. 1991. "Occupational class, selection and inequalities in health." *Social Science and Medicine* 33: 545-557.

Joung, I. M. A., H. D. van de Mheen, K. Stronks, F. W. A. van Poppel and J. P. Mackenbach. 1998. "A longitudinal study of health selection in marital transitions." *Social Science and Medicine* 46: 425-435.

Karlin, S., R. Kenett, and B. Bonne-Tamir. 1979. "Analysis of biochemical genetic data of Jewish populations, II; Results and interpretations of heterogeneity indices and distance measures with respect to standards." *American Journal of Human Genetics* 31: 341-365.

Kingston, R. S., and J. P. Smith. 1997. "Socioeconomic status and racial and ethnic differences in functional status associated with chronic diseases." *American Journal of Public Health* 87: 805-810.

Koskinen, S., and T. Martelin. 1994. "Why are socioe-conomic mortality differences smaller among women than among men?" *Social Science and Medicine* 38: 1385-1396.

Kotler, P., and D. L. Wingard. 1989. "The effect of occupational, marital and parental roles on mortality: The Alameda County Study." *American Journal of Public Health* 79: 607-612.

Krieger, N. 1990. "Racial and gender discrimination: Risk factors for high blood pressure?" *Social Science and Medicine* 30: 1273-1281.

Kunst, A. E., F. Groenhof and J. P. Mackenbach. 1998. "Mortality by occupational class among men 30-64 years in 11 European countries, EU Working Group on Social Inequalities in Health." *Social Science and Medicine* 46: 1456-1476.

Kunst, A. E., and J. P. Mackenbach. 1994. "Size of mortality differences associated with educational level in nine industrialized countries." *American Journal of Public Health* 84: 932-937.

Lahelma, E., K. Manderbacka, O. Rahkonen and A. Karisto. 1994. "Comparisons of inequalities in health: Evidence from national surveys in Finland, Norway and Sweden." *Social Science and Medicine* 38: 517-524.

Lochen, M., and E. Lund. 1997. "Childbearing and mortality from cancer of the corpus uteri." *Acta Obstetricia et Gynecologica Scandinavica* 76: 373-377.

Lund, E., E. Arnesen and J. K. Borgen. 1990. "Pattern of childbearing and mortality in married women – a national prospective study from Norway." *Journal of Epidemiology and Community Health* 44: 237-240.

Lund, E. 1992. "Mortality from ovarian cancer among women with many children." *International Journal of Epidemiology* 21: 872-876.

Macintyre, S., and K. Hunt. 1997. "Socio-economic position, gender, and health: How do they interact?" *Journal of Health Psychology* 2: 315-334.

Macintyre, S., K. Hunt and H. Sweeting. 1996. "Gender differences in health: Are things really as simple as they seem?" *Social Science and Medicine* 42: 617-624.

Macintyre, S., A. Ellaway, G. Der, G. Ford and K. Hunt. 1998. "Do housing tenure and car access predict health because they are markers of income or self-esteem? A Scottish study." *Journal of Epidemiology and Community Health* 52: 657-664.

Macran, S., L. Clarke and H. Joshi. 1994. "Women's health: Dimensions and differentials." *Social Science and Medicine*. 42: 1203-1216.

Manor, O., S. Matthews and C. Power. 1997. "Comparing measures of health inequality." *Social Science and Medicine* 45: 761-771.

Manor, O., Z. Eisenbach, E. Peritz and Y. Friedlander. 1999. "Mortality differentials among Israeli men." *American Journal of Public Health* 89: 1807-1813.

Marmot, M. G., M. J. Shipley and G. Rose. 1984a. "Inequalities in death-specific explanations of a general pattern." *Lancet* i: 1003-1006.

Marmot, M. G., A. M. Adelstein and L. Bulusu. 1984b. *Immigrant Mortality in England and Wales 1970-78: Causes of Death by Country of Birth*. London: HMSO.

Marmot, M., C. D. Ryff, L. L. Bumpass, M. Shipley and N. F. Marks. 1997. "Social inequalities in health: Next questions and converging evidence." *Social Science and Medicine* 44: 901-910.

Martelin, J. 1994. "Mortality by indicators of socio-economic status among the Finnish elderly." *Social Science and Medicine* 38: 1257-1278.

Martikainen, P. 1995. "Women's employment, marriage, motherhood and mortality: A test of the multiple role and role accumulation hypotheses." *Social Science and Medicine* 40: 199-212.

Matthews, S., O. Manor and C. Power. 1999. "Social inequalities in health: Are there gender differences?" *Social Science and Medicine* 48: 49-60.

Morrison, C., M. Woodward, W. Leslie and H. Tunstall-Pedoe. 1997. "Effect of socioeconomic group on incidence of, management of, and survival after myocardial infarction and coronary death: Analysis of community coronary event register." *British Medical Journal* 314: 541-546.

Moser, K. A., P. Goldblatt, A. J. Fox and D. Jones. 1987. "Unemployment and mortality: Comparison of the 1971 and 1981 Longitudinal Study sample." *British Medical Journal* 294: 86-90.

Moser, K. A., H. S. Pugh and P. Goldblatt. 1988. "Inequalities in women's health: Looking at mortality differentials using an alternative approach." *British Medical Journal* 296: 1221-1224.

Murphy, M. 1996. "Marital status and mortality: An epidemiological viewpoint." *Zeitschrift für Bevölkerungswissenschaft* 21: 303-317.

Mustard, C. A., S. Derksen, J. M. Berthelot, M. Wolfson and L. L. Roos. 1997. "Age-specific education and income gradients in morbidity and mortality in a Canadian province." *Social Science and Medicine* 45: 383-397.

Nathanson, C. 1980. "Social roles and health status among women: The significance of employment." *Social Science and Medicine* 14: 463-471.

Parkes, C. M., B. Benjamin and R. G. Fitzgerald. 1969. "Broken heart: A statistical study of increased mortality among widowers." *British Medical Journal* 1: 740-743.

Peritz, E. 1986. "Mortality of African-born Jews in Israel." In U. O. Schmeltz and G. Nathan (eds.), *Studies on the Population of Israel, in Honor of Roberto Bachi.* Jerusalem: The Magnes Press.

Peritz, E., and A. Tamir. 1979. "Remarks on the mortality of Ashkenazim with data on European-born Jews in Israel." In R. M. Goodman and A. G. Motulsky (eds.), *Genetic Disease among Ashkenazi Jews.* New York: Raven Press.

Power, C. 1994. "Health and social inequality in Europe." *British Medical Journal* 308: 1153-1156.

Power, C., O. Manor and A. J. Fox. 1991. *Health and Class: The Early Years.* London: Chapman & Hall.

Rogot, E., P. D. Sorlie, N. J. Johnson, C. S. Glover and D. W. Treasure. 1988. *A Mortality Study of One Million Persons by Demographic, Social, and Economic Factors:* 1979-1981 *Follow-Up.* National Institute of Health Publication no. 88-2896.

Roitberg-Tambur, A., C. S. Witt, A. Friedman, C. Safirman, L. Sherman, S. Battat, D. Nelken and C. Brautbar. 1995. "Comparative analysis of HLA polymorphism at the serologic molecular level in Moroccan and Ashkenazi Jews." *Tissue Antigens* 46: 104-110.

Senior, P. A., and R. Bhopal. 1994. "Ethnicity as a variable in epidemiological research." *British Medical Journal.* 309: 327-330.

Smooha, S. 1993. "Class, ethnic and national cleavages and democracy in Israel." In E. Sprinzak, and L. Diamond (eds.), *Israel Democracy under Stress*, 309-342. Boulder, CO, and London: Lymme Rienner.

Sorensen, G., and L. M. Verbrugge. 1987. "Women, work, and health." *Review of Public Health* 8: 235-247.

Sorlie, P. D., E. Backlund and J. B. Keller. 1995. "U.S. Mortality by economic demographic and social characteristic: The National Longitudinal Mortality Study." *American Journal of Public Health* 85: 949-956.

Sterwing, J. P., P. Hartge and S. Wacholder. 1997. "The risk of cancer associated with specific mutation of BRCAI and BRCA2 among Ashkenazi Jews." *New England Journal of Medicine* 336: 1401-1408.

Stronks, K., H. van de Mheen, J. van den Bos and J. P. Mackenbach. 1995. "Smaller socio-economic inequalities in health among women: The role of employment status." *International Journal of Epidemiology* 24: 559-568.

Townsend, P., and N. Davidson. 1982. *Inequalities in Health: The Black Report.* Harmondsworth: Penguin.

Uniken-Venema, H. P., H. F. Garretsen and P. J. van der Maas. 1995. "Health of migrants and migrant health policy, The Netherlands as an example." *Social Science and Medicine,* 41: 809-818.

Valkonen, T. 1989. "Adult mortality and level of education: A comparison of six countries." In J. Fox (ed.), *Health Inequalities in European Countries*, 142-162. London: Gower.

Valkonen, T. 1993. "Problems in measurement and international comparisons of socioeconomic differences in mortality." *Social Science and Medicine* 36: 409-418.

Verbrugge, L. M. 1979. "Marital status and health." *Journal of Marriage and Family* 41: 267-285.

Verbrugge, L. M. 1983. "Multiple roles and physical health of women and men." *Journal of Health and Social Behavior* 24: 16-30.

Waldron, I., M. E. Hughes and T. L. Brooks. 1996. "Marriage protection and marriage selection: Prospective evidence for reciprocal effects of marital status and health." *Social Science and Medicine* 43: 113-123.

Waldron, I., C. C. Weiss and M. E. Hughes. 1997. "Marital status effects on health: Are there differences between never married women and divorced and separated women?" *Social Science and Medicine* 45: 1387-1397.

Wax, Y. 1992. "Collinearity diagnosis for a relative risk regression analysis: an application to assessment of diet-cancer relationship in epidemiological studies." *Statistics in Medicine* 11: 1273-1287.

Weatherall, R., H. Joshi and S. Macran. 1994. "Double burden or double blessing? Employment, motherhood and mortality in the longitudinal study of England and Wales." *Social Science and Medicine* 38: 285-297.

Whitehead, M. 1988. "The health divide." In P. Townsend, N. Davidson and M. Whitehead (eds.), *Inequalities in Health: The Black Report and the Health Divide.* Harmondsworth: Penguin.

15

Mortality after Spousal Loss: Are There Socio-Demographic Differences?

Orly Manor and Zvi Eisenbach

Introduction

Mortality differentials by marital status have been examined in numerous studies, and show that married individuals have lower mortality rates than those who are widowed, divorced, or single (Hu and Goldman 1990; Goldman, Korenman, and Weinstein 1995; Sorlie, Backlund, and Keller 1995; Waldron, Hughes, and Brooks 1996). Among married people, loss of a spouse has been associated with excess mortality, even after controlling for potential confounding factors (Bowling 1987; Schaefer, Quesenberry, and Wi 1995; Martikainen and Valkonen 1996a). Given the stress associated with spousal loss, it is not surprising that bereavement greatly increases the risk of poorer physical and mental health (Parkes and Weiss 1983; Osterweis, Solomon, and Green 1984; Lund, Diamond, and Caserta 1985; Mor, McHorney, and Sherwood 1986; Jacobs et al. 1990; Bruce, Kim, Leaf, and Jacobs 1990; Parkes 1996). Other pathways leading from bereavement to poor health and mortality include role change (Lund, Caserta, and Dimond 1986; Bowling 1987; Lindstrom 1999) and loss of social and material support (Helsing, Szklo, and Comstock 1981; Zick and Smith 1991; Stylianos and Vachon 1993). With time, however, individuals gradually adapt to widowhood, and the risk of mortality decreases. Some studies suggest that the effect of death of a spouse is especially marked during the first weeks (Kaprio, Koskenvuo, and Rita 1987; Martikainen and Valkonen 1996a), months or years (Bowling 1987; Schaefer et al. 1995) after bereavement. Others, however, report both short-term and long-term excess mortality among widowed individuals (Mellstrom, Nilsson, Oden, Rundgren, and Svanborg 1982).

While much research has accumulated on mortality and morbidity differences by socio-demographic characteristics such as sex (Annandale and Hunt 1990; Arber and Ginn 1993) social class (Macintyre 1997; Mackenbach, Kunst, Cavelaars, Groenhof, and Geurts 1997; Lynch and Kaplan 2000) and ethnicity (Lillie-Blanton and LaVeist 1996; Manor et al. 1999; Curtis and Lawson 2000), little information is available on whether the effect of bereavement on mortality varies between socio-demographic groups. With regard to gender, a number of studies focus only on males (Parkes, Benjamin, and Fitzgerald 1969; Niemi 1979); studies of both genders generally indicate smaller effects among women (Stroebe and Stroebe 1983; Bowling 1987; Martikainen and Valkonen 1996a). However, there are exceptions, including a study showing increased mortality after widowhood but not after widowerhood (Jones, Goldblatt, and Leon 1984). A limited number of studies investigated the effect of age on mortality after spousal loss; the general trend emerging from these studies is a reduction in the effect of bereavement with increasing age in both sexes (Schaefer et al. 1995, Martikainen and Valkonen 1996b), or only among men (Helsing et al. 1981). There are, however, studies in which differentials in the effect of bereavement by age were not detected (Mendes de Leon, Kasl, and Jacobs 1993); this discrepancy could be attributed to the limited power of the latter study. Almost no evidence has been presented with regard to differences by social class or ethnicity in the survival of bereaved persons. One early exception is a study suggesting that the excess mortality among widowers in higher social classes is greater than that of widowers in lower classes (Parkes et al. 1969). Two more recent exceptions report no race differences (Schaefer et al. 1995) and no educational differences (Martikainen and Valkonen 1998) in the relative risk of mortality among the bereaved. Similarly, while it has been shown that household size and number of children are strongly associated with mortality (Lund, Arnesen, and Borgen 1990; Manor, Eisenbach, Israeli, and Friedlander, see chapter 14), mainly due to selection and social support (Berkman 1995; Elstad 1996), the effects of household size or number of children on the risk of mortality following spousal bereavement have not been previously reported.

Recent studies based on the Israel Longitudinal Mortality Study reported substantial mortality inequalities among Israelis according to socio-economic position and marital status (Manor et al. 1999; Manor, Eisenbach, Peritz, and Friedlander 1999). However, up to now there has been no systematic evaluation of the effect of spousal bereavement on mortality in Israel, nor an investigation of socio-demographic differentials in this effect. Given the public health importance of the effect of bereavement on mortality, a deeper understanding is required of socio-demographic differentials associated with this effect. Such an understanding may contribute to an assessment of the causal mechanisms relating bereavement to mortality. The main purpose of this paper is, therefore, to investigate differentials in mortality after death of a spouse. Specifically, we evaluate the effect of spousal death on mortality and examine differences in this effect by duration of bereavement, age, sex, education, ethnic origin, household size, and number of children.

Methods

Sample and Data

Data were obtained from the Israel Longitudinal Mortality Study (Eisenbach, Manor, Peritz, and Hite 1997), which links census records from a systematic 20 percent sample of households in the 1983 census with death records occurring in the subsequent 9.5 years, until the end of 1992. Israel has a population register in which a unique ID number identifies every resident, newborn, or immigrant. The linkage of records was carried out by the Israel Central Bureau of Statistics, using the ID number from both the census and death notifications. ID numbers were omitted from the data set. The quality of the linked data set was enhanced by the high coverage in the census of 1983, where only 2.6 percent of the population escaped enumeration, and by the fact that practically all deaths in Israel are recorded. Furthermore, the linkage was ascertained by comparing six demographic variables available in both data sources (Eisenbach et al. 1997).

In addition, information on emigration was ascertained through record linkage with data from the Israel Border Control Gates of the year of departure for each person who had not returned to Israel by the end of 1994. Thus we were able to estimate the time interval between census and emigration.

Using the linked file, married individuals who were either heads of households or spouses of heads of households were selected for the present analysis. The data set allows identification of couples who stayed married until the end of the follow-up period or until death or emigration, as well as those widowed since the census, each with the corresponding date of bereavement. Cases of divorce or remarriage during the follow up period were ignored.

The analysis presented here is based on Jewish men and women aged 50-79, who were married at the time of the census. It excludes persons living in kibbutzim or in institutions, and individuals whose ethnic origin could not be determined (see below). Deaths occurring for both spouses on the same day were excluded. The study population comprised 49,566 men and 41,264 women, of whom 4,402 (9 percent) and 11,114 (27 percent), respectively, were bereaved during the follow-up period. The data include demographic and socio-economic variables from the census and the date of death for people who died during the follow-up period.

Variables

The dependent variable was the time (in months) from the date of the census until the date of death. This variable was censored by either a permanent departure from the country or at the end of the follow up. The independent variables used were:

- *Age at the time of the census* - subdivided into 5-year groups.
- *Duration of bereavement* - time since bereavement, grouped into 4 categories: <7 months, 7–12 months, 13–24 months, >24 months.
- *"Ethnic" origin* - according to country of birth. Father's country of birth was used for individuals born in Israel. The variable was categorized as "North Africa", "Asia", or "Europe." The last category includes a small proportion (2.7 percent) of individuals originating in North or South America or Australia.
- *Education* - number of years of school attended, grouped into 0–8, and ≥9.
- *Household size* - categorized as a couple living alone or a couple living with others.
- *Number of children* - categorized as 0, 1–3, and ≥3.

Statistical analysis

Cox proportional hazards model was used to estimate the effect of spousal loss on mortality. Duration of bereavement was considered as a time-dependent covariate. The reference category was the group who remained married until death or censoring. The effect of spousal loss was assessed first separately and then after controlling for education and ethnic origin. All analyses were controlled for age, which was recorded in five-year groups. Within each age group, a comparison showed that the mean age of widowed persons was similar to that of married persons (with a mean difference of less than two months). Analysis was carried out separately for men and women. Socio-demographic differences in the effect of spousal loss were tested by an interaction term in the Cox model.

Results

Of the 49,566 men studied, 12,083 died during the follow-up period (1983–1992) and 4,402 lost their spouse during that period. Among the 41,264 women 6,057 died and 11,114 lost their spouse during the follow-up period (table 15.1). Spousal loss varied with age: among men aged 50-54 only 3 percent lost their spouse during the study period, whereas among men aged 75-79 the loss reached 20 percent. The corresponding figures for women were 13 percent and 49 percent.

Age-adjusted relative risks of mortality by sex and duration of bereavement are presented in table 11.2. In the first six months after the loss of a wife, men had a risk of mortality about 40 percent higher than that of married men. This effect decreased with the time elapsed since spousal loss. Additional analysis (results not shown) indicated that the relative mortality risk during the second year after bereavement was similar to that from the third year onward, hence the two categories were collapsed. Women showed similar trends to those of men, although their excess mortality during the first six months of bereavement was higher (table 15.2). However, the gender difference was not statistically significant.

Among men, the risk of mortality during the first six months after spousal loss, relative to married men, decreased with age (figure 15.1). A linear trend among men was statistically significant ($\rho<0.05$). Among women, the relative risk was fairly constant over the age groups.

Adjustment for education and ethnic origin resulted in only small changes in the relative risks. The adjusted figures are presented in table 15.3. For each age group the overall effect of bereavement was statistically significant, and for most age groups, the effect of bereavement decreased with duration of bereavement. The latter examination considers each age and duration group separately, and was naturally based on a smaller number of cases. At younger ages the effect of spousal loss was somewhat larger among men than among women, but no effect of bereavement was found for seventy-five to seventy-nine-year-olds of either sex.

Table 15.4 presents the relative risk of mortality from a model that includes age, ethnic origin, and education, as well as an interaction term for assessing differentials in the effect of bereavement by education. The model for men also includes an interaction term for bereavement and age. Here we focused on the largest effect of bereavement, namely the effect occurring during the first six months, and therefore the categories of seven to twelve months and over thirteen months were collapsed. A significant interaction of bereavement and education was found for men, where among less educated men the effect of bereavement on mortality was smaller than that of more educated men (RR=0.72, 95 percent CI: 0.62–0.97). A comparable trend was observed for women, but the interaction was not statistically significant. Further analyses showed no significant interaction effect of bereavement with either ethnic origin or household size, for either sex. However, an interaction with number of children was of borderline significance among women: women with one to three children showed a weaker bereavement effect than childless women (RR of 0.79, p ¼ 0:07). The effect for women with four or more children was similar to that of childless women (RR=0.95).

Discussion

This study provides the first systematic evaluation of mortality after spousal loss in the Israeli Jewish population. A number of previous studies in Israel have assessed the effect on health of bereavement associated with a loss of a child (Levav, Friedlander, Kark, and Peritz 1988; Levav et al. 2000). We examined mortality after spousal bereavement during the period 1983–1992 and identified socio-demographic differentials in the effect of bereavement by linking a

Table 15.1
Distribution of Socio-Demographic Characteristics of the Sample[a]

	Men	Women
Sample size	49566	41264
Died (%)	24.4	14.7
Bereaved (%)	8.9	26.9
Age (%)		
50–54	20.9	26.4
55–59	20.4	25.5
60–64	20.3	19.7
65–69	15.0	13.7
70–74	14.8	10.5
75–79	8.6	4.2
Origin (%)		
Asia	20.3	19.2
North Africa	15.9	14.3
Europe	63.8	66.5
Education (year) (%)		
0–8	48.1	56.1
9+	51.9	43.9
Household size (%)		
A couple	51.8	63.0
A couple + others	48.2	37.0
# of children (%)		
0	—	7.0
1–3	—	65.6
4+	—	27.4

[a] At the time of the census.

Table 15.2
Age-Adjusted Risk[a] of Mortality by Duration of Bereavement

	Men		Women	
Duration (months)	Relative risk	95% CI	Relative risk	95% CI
0–6	1.38	1.18–1.58	1.48	1.28–1.70
7–12	1.25	1.04–1.50	1.20	1.01–1.43
13+	1.23	1.14–1.32	1.21	1.13–1.30
All bereaved	1.25	1.18–1.33	1.26	1.19–1.33

[a]Not bereaved—relative risk = 1.

sample of 20 percent of the 1983 census records with deaths occurring during that period. The large number of records, the high coverage of the population, and the prospective design all make the Israel Longitudinal Mortality Study a highly suitable source for investigating mortality after spousal loss (Susser 1981). The results revealed an excess mortality among both men and women after the death of a spouse. During the first six months, the age-adjusted excess mortality was about 50 percent among women and about 40 percent among men. The effect of bereavement on mortality varied by duration of bereavement, age,

Figure 15.1
Relative Risk (RR) of Mortality during the First 6 Months after Bereavement by Age

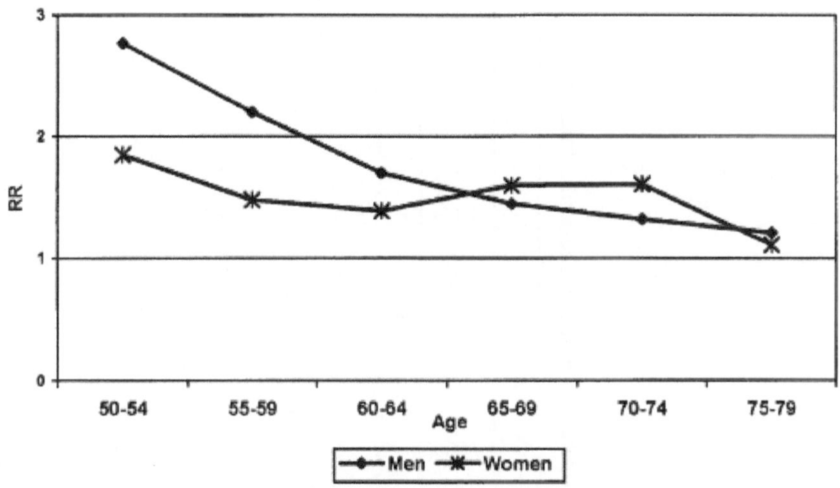

and education (the last one only among men); and the variation in the effect of bereavement by age differed between men and women. By evaluating mortality after death of a spouse in relation to a number of socio-demographic indicators, this study contributes to the understanding of the association between bereavement and health and extends previous work on bereavement. Furthermore, the gender comparison is relevant to the understanding of gender differences in health, in general, as well as to the Israeli population, specifically. For the latter, our comparison confirms the relative vulnerability of Israeli women regarding longevity. Israeli longevity patterns by gender are somewhat unique: men's life expectancy is ranked third in a worldwide comparison, whereas women are ranked only fourteenth (Central Bureau of Statistics 1998).

It has been suggested that mortality is lower among those who remarry, mainly due to selection effects (Helsing et al. 1981; Murphy 1996; Waldron et al. 1996), yet contradictory evidence emerges from a recent longitudinal study indicating that the effect of selection in marital transitions is limited (Joung, van de Mheen, Stronks, van Poppel, and Mackenbach 1998). However, since the aim of our study was to assess the effect of spousal loss on mortality, without taking into account moderating or fortifying events (such as remarriage) which might take place later on in life, our study did not incorporate remarriages among the widowed. Information on divorces taking place during the follow-up period, among those married at the time of the census was not available in our data. The bias associated with divorce, however, is likely to be small because of the low divorce rates during the 1980s among Israelis aged fifty and above (less than 1 percent per year; Central Bureau of Statistics 1999). Furthermore, since

Table 15.3

Risk of Mortality (95% CI) by Duration of Bereavement and Age, Adjusted for Education and Ethnic Origin

Duration (months)	Men						Women					
	Age						Age					
	50–54	55–59	60–64	65–69	70–74	75–79	50–54	55–59	60–64	65–69	70–74	75–79
0–6	3.06 (1.14–3.16)	2.24 (1.11–4.48)	1.70 (1.01–2.37)	1.45 (0.95–2.20)	1.32 (1.01–1.74)	1.21 (0.92–1.59)	1.85 (1.01–3.39)	1.58 (0.92–2.67)	1.54 (1.04–2.27)	1.72 (1.28–2.31)	1.61 (1.26–2.04)	1.11 (0.79–1.56)
7–12	—[b]	2.32 (1.16–4.65)	1.49 (0.84–2.61)	1.65 (1.11–2.48)	1.06 (0.75–1.49)	1.16 (0.85–1.58)	1.91 (0.91–4.03)	2.05 (1.30–3.33)	1.01 (0.62–1.63)	1.21 (0.71–2.05)	0.97 (0.67–1.35)	1.26 (0.88–1.80)
13+	1.73 (1.07–2.79)	1.50 (1.09–2.05)	1.30 (0.95–1.77)	1.25 (0.99–1.57)	1.18 (1.05–1.34)	1.20 (1.06–1.36)	1.21 (0.87–1.69)	1.28 (0.98–1.65)	1.25 (0.94–1.66)	1.19 (1.03–1.38)	1.18 (1.05–1.34)	1.15 (0.98–1.75)
All Bereaved	1.89 (1.11–3.21)	1.60 (1.21–2.11)	1.38 (1.12–1.58)	1.30 (1.10–1.51)	1.19 (1.06–1.33)	1.18 (1.04–1.34)	1.39 (1.03–1.88)	1.36 (1.11–1.66)	1.27 (1.08–1.36)	1.24 (1.09–1.41)	1.22 (1.08–1.36)	1.16 (1.00–1.35)

[a] Not bereaved—relative risk = 1.
[b] No cases of death among the bereaved.

divorce is likely to increase the risk of mortality (Murphy 1996), the true effect of spousal loss may be underestimated in our study.

The effect of bereavement on mortality remained almost unchanged after controlling for ethnic origin and education. This finding is in accordance with a number of other studies evaluating the effect of bereavement. Martikainen and Valkonen (1996a) found that adjustment for a number of factors, including socio-economic position and household characteristics, reduced only slightly the excess mortality among the bereaved. Similar results were reported by Schaefer et al. (1995), who adjusted for social class and health behaviors. These results, therefore, indicate that the excess mortality is indeed related to the death of a spouse, rather than a shared unfavorable environment.

We found that, in most age groups, the excess mortality among the bereaved men and women was highest in the first six months after spousal loss. Several authors have reported similar findings (Kaprio et al. 1987), including Martikainen and Valkonen (1996b), who reported such trends for death from all causes except cancer. A somewhat different tendency was noted by Schaefer et al. (1995), who observed the strongest effect during the second half-year following bereavement. Others have reported a delayed effect only for women, as

Table 15.4
Relative Risk[a] of Mortality by Duration of Bereavement, Age, Ethnic Origin and Education

Variable	Men	Women
Duration (months)		
0–6	4.00**	1.66 ***
7+	1.92***	1.26***
Age	1.60***	1.67***
Age × duration		
Age × 0–6	0.88*	—
Age × 7+	0.94*	—
Origin[b]		
Asia	0.92**	0.78**
North Africa	1.13***	1.00
Education[c]	1.16***	1.33***
Education × duration		
Education × 0–6	0.72*	0.82
Education × 7+	0.98	0.92

[a]Not bereaved—relative risk = 1.
[b]The reference group for origin is Europe.
[c]The reference group for education is 9+ years of schooling.
$^{*}p<0.05$, $^{**}p<0.01$, $^{***}p<0.001$.

described in an early review of mortality after bereavement (Jacobs and Ostfeld 1977). In contrast, some studies have failed to find any increase in mortality after spousal loss. Helsing et al. (1981), who used paired widowed and married controls, reported no effect among women, whereas Jones et al. (1984), using data from the British Longitudinal Study, reported only a slight early excess mortality among women, but not among men. Some of the inconsistencies between studies could be attributed to differences in sample sizes, where larger studies (Kaprio et al. 1987, Martikainen and Valkonen 1996b), including ours, tend to indicate higher risk of mortality shortly after bereavement. Further, the reduction in excess mortality over time corresponds with findings showing that the intensity of grief associated with spousal loss diminishes gradually over time (Hyrkas, Kaunonen, and Paunonen 1997). There is also evidence showing that the level of bereavement-associated depressive symptoms is attenuated over time, mainly among women (van Grootheest, Beekman, and Broese van Groenou 1999).

We did not find gender differences in the age-adjusted relative risk of mortality after spousal loss. This result contrasts with a number of studies suggesting that the effect of bereavement among men is greater than that among women (Stroebe and Stroebe 1983; Bowling 1987; Martikainen and Valkonen 1996b). Notably, systematic statistical testing of gender differences in the effect of spousal loss on mortality is rare. Further, there are some studies suggesting no gender differences in the effect of bereavement, and others reporting a larger effect for women (Lund et al. 1986; Jones et al. 1984). Notably, some of these studies focus on the elderly (Lund et al. 1986), yet others cover similar age groups to those addressed here (Jones et al. 1984). Inconsistencies have also been described in relation to gender differences in psychological distress associated with bereavement; some studies report larger effects among women and others show no gender differences (Hays, Kasl, and Jacobs 1994; Hyrkas et al. 1997; Chen et al. 1999; van Grootheest et al. 1999). Our results are consistent with findings of the Israel Longitudinal Mortality Study showing no gender differences in the protective effect of marriage on mortality (Manor et al., see chapter 14), as well as with the relatively disadvantaged position of Israeli women with respect to life expectancy (Central Bureau of Statistics 1998). Thus, it may be that our results reflect the specific Israeli situation, and that gender differences in the effect of bereavement, differ between countries. Furthermore, while the excess mortality associated with spousal loss found here for men was similar to that of women, it may well be that different factors operate for each sex. For example, it has been suggested that women's main source of vulnerability after spousal loss stems from an increase in financial strain. For men, however, a major source of concern is the reduction in social interaction and the need to fulfill tasks carried out in the past by their spouses (Wortman, Cohen-Silver, and Kessler 1993). In contrast, our data did indicate a gender difference in the effect of age at bereavement on mortality: among men the effect decreased linearly with age, whereas among women the effect varied little over the age range fifty to seventy-nine. A higher relative risk for young widowed than for older ones has also been suggested by others (Helsing et al. 1981; Martikainen and Valkonen 1996b). Nevertheless, analyses of mortality after bereavement rarely include an interaction term for the effect of age, which would permit adjustment for age differences. A different pattern was found in a recent study of emotional distress among bereaved men and women (Chen et al. 1999), where trends over time in emotional distress experienced by men were similar to those of women. Factors aside from emotional stress that were suggested for the association between bereavement and mortality included changes in risky health behaviors, such as alcohol consumption, smoking, and diet (Bowling 1987). It may well be that such changes are more prevalent among young widowers than among older widowers or widows. In addition, older men have generally experienced more life crises than younger men, hence the latter are less prepared for the adversities associated with spousal loss.

With regard to the moderating effect of education, bereavement had a greater impact on the more educated men than on the less educated. A similar, albeit non-significant trend was observed for women. Studies of the relationships between socio-economic factors, bereavement and mortality are limited and show inconsistent results. Our findings accord with those of a study reporting a larger effect among men of higher occupational class than among men of lower occupational class (Parkes et al. 1969), and contradict those of a study indicating no differential effect by education (Schaefer et al. 1995). Recently, Martikainen and Valkonen (1998), using a large sample of Finnish adults, reported no social-class differentials in the relative risk of mortality after spousal loss. However, when absolute differences in mortality rates were considered, they detected larger effects of bereavement among those in low social class, suggesting, therefore, mainly public health relevance rather than etiologic relevance. Role theory, which has been used to explain the pathways between bereavement and mortality (Gove 1973, 1984), may shed some light on the socio-economic differences in the effect of bereavement found in our study. After spousal loss, the survivor has to take over the household tasks formerly performed by the spouse. It may well be that coping with the new tasks of homemaking and housekeeping is harder for the more educated men. This hardship in coping was probably more prevalent among the cohort under study than it is today, when the division of roles by gender is more equal among highly educated people, at least in some Western countries. It has been argued that the role played by people in different marital setups may lead to differential exposure to risk (Stroebe, Stroebe, Gergen, and Gergen 1981). Thus, educated men who enjoy several roles, including head of household and chief breadwinner, may lose more in bereavement. Another explanation has been put forward by Wortman et al. (1993) who observed that individuals with the highest self-esteem and the greatest intellectual and financial resources were the hardest hit emotionally by the loss of their spouse. They suggest that individuals who have more control over their circumstances are more vulnerable on spousal loss. Clearly, more research is needed regarding the processes associated with the moderating effect of social class.

The support of social–familial networks is well recognized as having a beneficial effect on mental and physical well-being (House, Landis, and Umberson 1988; Berkman 1995; Berkman and Glass 2000). Death of a spouse has a direct influence on familial support. In addition, it has been postulated that social support will attenuate the effect of stressful life events such as bereavement (Berkman 1985). We found only limited support for this hypothesis. The effect of bereavement did not vary by household size; individuals living alone showed similar excess mortality to those living with other persons. However, household size reflects social support only partially, and this may account for our failure to establish an association (Antonucci 1990). Further, our analysis did not incorporate changes in the household size during the follow-up period, and thus could cause misclassifications, which might obscure the association between household size and mortality after bereavement. Nonetheless, our finding accords with that of another study reporting no effect of social support on the long-term survival of the bereaved (Bowling 1994).

In contrast, our study suggests that the number of children born to a woman moderates her risk of mortality associated with bereavement. The effect of bereavement on mortality was lowest for women with one to three children. Similar trends have been found for overall mortality by number of children: among Israeli women, those with two children experienced the lowest mortality (Manor et al., see chapter 14), while mortality among British and Norwegian women was lowest for those with three children (Green, Beral, and Moser 1988; Lund et al. 1990). Apart from social support, factors suggested as explanations for the association between the number of children and mortality include health selection, biological factors, and multiple roles (Beral 1983; Weatherall, Joshi, and Macran 1994; Lochen and Lund 1997); all four factors may be operating in our sample. For example, selection processes may explain the higher mortality among childless women than among women with one to three children. Among women with four or more children, the strain and risks associated with having a large number of children and with multiple roles may offset the possible benefits enjoyed by those with one to three children.

Interestingly, we found no association between the effect of bereavement and ethnic origin. This accords with a previous study of ethnicity and spousal loss (Schaefer et al. 1995). In contrast, there are substantial ethnic differences in this sample for overall mortality: individuals originating in North Africa showed higher risk of mortality than Europeans (Manor et al., see chapter 14). These differences, however, diminished after adjusting for socio-economic position.

In conclusion, for both men and women, loss of a spouse is associated with excess mortality, especially in the first six months following bereavement.

Among men, some groups are more vulnerable than others, including the young and the more educated. For women, having one to three children has a protective effect.

Acknowledgements

This research was supported by grant no. 93-00015/2 from the U.S.–Israel Binational Science Foundation, Jerusalem.

References

Annandale, E., and K. Hunt. 1990. "Masculinity, femininity and sex: An exploration of their relative contribution to explain gender differences in health." *Sociology of Health and Illness* 12: 24-46.

Antonucci, T. C. 1990. "Social supports and social relationships." In R. H. Binstock and L. K. Gorge (eds.), *Handbook of Aging and Social Sciences*, 3rd ed. New York: Academic Press.

Arber, S., and J. Ginn. 1993. "Gender inequalities in health in later life." *Social Science and Medicine* 36: 33-46.

Beral, V. 1983. "Parity and susceptibility to cancer." *Ciba Foundation Symposium* 96:182-203.

Berkman, L. F. 1985. "The relationship of social networks and social support to morbidity and mortality." In S. Cohen and S. L. Syme (eds.), *Social Support and Health*, 241-262. Toronto: Academic Press.

Berkman, L. F. 1995. "The role of social relations in health promotion." *Psychosomatic Medicine* 57: 245-254.

Berkman, L. F., and T. Glass. 2000. "Social integration, social networks, social support, and health." In I. Kawachi and L. F. Berkman (eds.), *Social Epidemiology*, 137-173. New York: Oxford University Press.

Bowling, A. 1987. "Mortality after bereavement: A review of literature on survival periods and factors affecting survival." *Social Science and Medicine* 24: 117-124.

Bowling, A. 1994. "Mortality after bereavement: An analysis of mortality rates and associations with mortality 13 years after bereavement." *International Journal of Geriatric Psychiatry* 9: 445-459.

Bruce, M. L., K. Kim, P. J. Leaf and S. Jacobs. 1990. "Depressive episodes and dysphoria resulting from conjugal bereavement in a prospective community sample." *American Journal of Psychiatry* 147: 608-611.

Central Bureau of Statistics. 1998. *Vital Statistics 1994-1995, Part D: Mortality*. Jerusalem: Central Bureau of Statistics.

Central Bureau of Statistics. 1999. *Vital Statistics, Parts A and B: Marriages & Divorces*. Jerusalem: Central Bureau of Statistics.

Chen, J. H., A. J. Bierhals, H. G. Prigerson, S. V. Kasl, C. M. Mazure and S. Jacobs. 1999. "Gender differences in the effects of bereavement-related psychological distress in health outcomes." *Psychological Medicine* 29: 367-380.

Curtis, S., and K. Lawson. 2000. "Gender, ethnicity and self reported health: The case of African–Caribbean populations in London." Social *Science and Medicine* 50: 365-385.

Eisenbach, Z., O. Manor, E. Peritz and Y. Hite. 1997. "The Israel longitudinal mortality study—differential mortality in Israel 1983-92: Objective, materials, methods and preliminary results." *Israel Journal of Medical Sciences* 33: 794-807.

Elstad, J. I. 1996. "Inequalities in health related to women's marital, parental and employment status: A comparison between the early 70s and the late 80s, Norway." *Social Science and Medicine* 42: 75-89.

Goldman, N., S. Korenman and R. Weinstein. 1995. "Marital status and health among the elderly." *Social Science and Medicine* 40: 1717-1730.
Gove, W. R. 1973. "The relationship between sex roles, marital roles, and mental illness." *Social Forces* 51: 34-44.
Gove, W. R. 1984. "Gender differences in mental and physical illness: The effects of fixed roles and nurturant roles." *Social Science and Medicine* 19: 77-91.
Green, A., V. Beral and K. Moser. 1988. "Mortality in women in relation to their childbearing history." *British Medical Journal* 297: 391-395.
Hays, J. C., S. V. Kasl and S. C. Jacobs. 1994. "The course of psychological distress following threatened and actual conjugal bereavement." *Psychological Medicine* 24: 917-927.
Helsing, K. M., M. Szklo and G. W. Comstock. 1981. "Factors associated with mortality after widowhood." *American Journal of Public Health* 71: 802-809.
House, J. S., K. R. Landis and D. Umberson. 1988. "Social relationships and health." *Science* 241: 540.
Hu, Y. R., and N. Goldman. 1990. "Mortality differentials by marital status: An international comparison." *Demography* 27: 233-250.
Hyrkas, K., M. Kaunonen and M. Paunonen. 1997. "Recovering from the death of a spouse." *Journal of Advanced Nursing* 25: 775-779.
Jacobs, S., F. Hansen, S. V. Kasl, A. Ostfeld, L. Berkman and K. Kim. 1990. "Anxiety disorders during acute bereavement: Risk and risk factors." *Journal of Clinical Psychiatry* 51: 269-274.
Jacobs, S., and A. Ostfeld. 1977. "An epidemiological review of the mortality after bereavement." *Psychosomatic Medicine* 39: 344-357.
Jones, D. A., P. O. Goldblatt and D. Leon. 1984. "Bereavement and cancer: Some data on deaths of spouses from the longitudinal study of office of population censuses and surveys." *British Medical Journal* 289: 461-464.
Joung, I. M. A., H. D. van de Mheen, K. Stronks, F. W. A. van Poppel and J. P. Mackenbach. 1998. "A longitudinal study of health selection in marital transitions." *Social Science and Medicine* 46: 425-435.
Kaprio, J., M. Koskenvuo and H. Rita. 1987. "Mortality after bereavement: A prospective study of 95,647 widowed persons." *American Journal of Public Health* 77: 283-287.
Levav, I., Y. Friedlander, J. Kark and E. Peritz. 1988. "An epidemiologic study of mortality among bereaved parents." *New England Journal of Medicine* 319: 457-461.
Levav, I., R. Kohn, J. Iscovisch, J. H. Abramson, W.Y. Tsai and D. Vigdorovich. 2000. "Cancer incidence and survival following bereavement." *American Journal of Public Health* 90: 1601-1607.
Lillie-Blanton, M., and T. LaVeist. 1996. "Race/ethnicity, social position and health." *Social Science and Medicine* 43: 83-92.
Lindstrom, T. C. 1999. "Coping with bereavement in relation to different feminine gender roles." *Scandinavian Journal of Psychology* 40: 33-41.
Lochen, M., and E. Lund. 1997. "Childbearing and mortality from cancer of the corpus uteri." *Acta Obstetricia et Gynecologica Scandinavica* 76: 373-377.
Lund, E., E. Arnesen and J. K. Borgen. 1990. "Pattern of childbearing and mortality in married women—a national prospective study from Norway." *Journal of Epidemiology and Community Health* 44: 237-240.
Lund, D. A., M. S. Caserta and M. F. Dimond. 1986. "Gender differences through two years of bereavement among the elderly." *The Gerontologist* 26: 314-320.
Lund, D. A., M. S. Dimond and M. S. Caserta. 1985. "Identifying elderly with coping difficulties two years after bereavement." *Omega: Journal of Death and Dying* 16: 213-224.

Lynch, J., and G. Kaplan. 2000. "Socioeconomic position." In I. Kawachi and L. F. Berkman (eds.), *Social Epidemiology*, 13-35. New York: Oxford University Press.

Mackenbach, J. P., A. E. Kunst, A. E. J. M. Cavelaars, F. Groenhof and J. J. Geurts. 1997. "Socioeconomic inequalities in morbidity and mortality in Western Europe." *Lancet* 349: 1655-1659.

Macintyre, S. 1997. "The Black Report and beyond: What are the issues?" *Social Science and Medicine* 44: 723-745.

Manor, O., Z. Eisenbach, E. Peritz and Y. Friedlander. 1999. "Mortality differentials among Israeli men." *American Journal of Public Health* 89: 807-813.

Martikainen, P., and T. Valkonen. 1996a. "Mortality after death of a spouse in relation to duration of bereavement in Finland." *Journal of Epidemiology and Community Health* 50: 264-268.

Martikainen, P., and T. Valkonen. 1996b. "Mortality after death of a spouse: Rates and causes of death in a large Finnish cohort." *American Journal of Public Health* 86: 1087-1093.

Martikainen, P., and T. Valkonen. 1998. "Do education and income buffer the effects of death of spouse on mortality?" *Epidemiology* 9: 530-534.

Mellstrom, D., A. Nilsson, A. Oden, A. Rundgren and A. Svanborg. 1982. "Mortality among widowed in Sweden." *Scandinavian Journal of Social Medicine* 10: 33-41.

Mendes de Leon, C. F., S. V. Kasl and S. Jacobs. 1993. "Widowhood and mortality risk in a community sample of the elderly: A prospective study." *Journal of Clinical Epidemiology* 46: 519-527.

Mor, V., C. McHorney and S. Sherwood. 1986. "Secondary morbidity among the recently bereaved." *American Journal of Psychiatry* 143: 158-163.

Murphy, M. 1996. "Marital status and mortality: An epidemiological viewpoint." *Zeitschrift für Bevölkerungswissenschaft* 21: 303-317.

Niemi, T. 1979. "The mortality of male old age pensioners following spouse's death." *Scandinavian Journal of Social Medicine* 7: 115-117.

Osterweis, M., F. Solomon, M. Green (eds.). 1984. *Bereavement: Reactions, Consequences and Care*. Washington, DC: National Academy Press.

Parkes, C. M. 1996. *Bereavement: Studies of Grief in Adult Life*, 3rd ed. London: Tavistock.

Parkes, C. M., B. Benjamin and R. G. Fitzgerald. 1969. "Broken heart: A statistical study of increased mortality among widowers." *British Medical Journal* 1: 740-743.

Parkes, C. M., and R. S. Weiss. 1983. *Recovery from Bereavement*. New York: Basic Books.

Schaefer, C., C. P. Quesenberry and S. Wi. 1995. "Mortality following conjugal bereavement and the effects of a shared environment." *American Journal of Epidemiology* 141: 1142- 1152.

Sorlie, P. D., E. Backlund and J. B. Keller. 1995. "U.S. mortality by economic demographic and social characteristic: The national longitudinal mortality study." *American Journal of Public Health* 85: 949-956.

Stroebe, M. S., and W. Stroebe. 1983. "Who suffers more? Sex differences in health risks of the widowed." *Psychological Bulletin* 93: 279-301.

Stroebe, M. S., W. Stroebe, K. J. Gergen and M. Gergen. 1981. "The broken heart: Reality or myth." *Omega: Journal of Death and Dying* 12: 87-105.

Stylianos, S. K., and M. L. S. Vachon. 1993. "The role of social support in bereavement." In M. S. Stroebe, W. Stroebe and R. O. Hansson (eds.), *Handbook of Bereavement*, 397-410. Cambridge: Cambridge University Press.

Susser, M. 1981. "Widowhood: A situational life stress or a stressful life event?" *American Journal of Public Health* 71: 793-795.

van Grootheest, D. S., A. T. F. Beekman, M. I. Broese van Groenou and D. J. H. Deeg. 1999. "Sex differences in depression after widowhood. Do men suffer more?" *Social Psychiatry and Psychiatric Epidemiology* 34: 391-398.

Waldron, I., M. E. Hughes and T. L. Brooks. 1996. "Marriage protection and marriage selection: Prospective evidence for reciprocal effects of marital status and health." *Social Science and Medicine* 43: 113-123.

Weatherall, R., H. Joshi and S. Macran. 1994. "Double burden or double blessing? Employment, motherhood and mortality in the longitudinal study of England and Wales." *Social Science and Medicine* 38: 285-297.

Wortman, C. B., R. Cohen-Silver and R. C. Kessler. 1993. "The meaning of loss and adjustment to bereavement." In M. S. Stroebe, W. Stroebe and R. O. Hansson (eds.), *Handbook of Bereavement*, 349-366. Cambridge: Cambridge University Press.

Zick, C. D., and K. R. Smith. 1991. "Patterns of economic changes surrounding the death of a spouse." *Journal of Gerontology* 46, S310-320.

16

Mortality in Two Jewish Populations-Montreal and Israel: Environmental Determinants of Differences

Bryna Shatenstein and Jeremy Kark

Reports on differences in disease occurrence and health-relevant characteristics between Jews and non-Jews (Mayberry and Rhodes 1984; Kune, Kune and Watson 1986), and among Jews of various ethnic origins (Kaufmann et al. 1982; Goldbourt and Kark 1982; Donchin et al. 1984; Gilat and Rozen 1979), suggest the existence of diversity in Jewish populations living in Israel and elsewhere, which may have a bearing on health-relevant behaviors and their outcome. Competing hypotheses have inferred that Israeli Jewish male: female mortality differences may relate to sociocultural factors concerning the role of women, or result from genetic characteristics particular to Jewish populations (Kark 1976; Beiran et al. 1991; Ore, et al. 1991; Neufeld and Goldbourt 1983). A lack of consistency across genetically-similar populations would support an environmental rather than genetic aetiology. While recent data on Jewish populations outside Israel are sparse, North American studies on Jewish mortality patterns have pointed to greater longevity in Jews (Spiegelman 1948), and cause-specific mortality rates, proportional mortality, and mortality patterns among men and women which differed from other ethnic and religious groups in North America (Newill 1961; King et al. 1965; Horowitz and Enterline 1970; Seidman 1871; Rosenwaike 1984; Goldstein 1986; Rosenwaike and Hempstead 1989; Rosenwaike and Hempstead 1990; Rosenwaike 1994).

However, some of these studies are limited by their use of proportional mortality instead of rates (Rosenwaike 1984; Goldstein 1986; Rosenwaike and Hempstead 1989; Rosenwaike and Hempstead 1990) or assumptions regarding rates, (Rosenwaike 1994) whereas others were done several decades ago (Newill

1961; King et al. 1965; Horowitz and Enterline 1970; Seidman 1871). In light of the unusual patterns of mortality which have been observed in the Israeli Jewish population (Central Bureau of Statistics 1992a), we sought to compare mortality rates between Canadian and Israeli Jews, and assess: a) whether the low Israeli Jewish male mortality and small excess longevity characteristic of Israeli women is evident in another Jewish community, as well as, b) whether Israeli death rates for selected conditions (Central Bureau of Statistics 1992a; World Health Organization 1992) are reflected elsewhere among Jews. Overall Canadian mortality data were included in the comparison (World Health Organization 1991). Unlike its U.S. counterpart, the Canadian census collects information on the religious affiliation of its citizens, providing denominators for the calculation of religion-specific rates. In this report, the data are presented for men and women aged ≥thirty-five years, for mortality due to all causes, and diseases of the circulatory system, the latter constituting the major cause of death in most western societies. Ill-defined causes have been included for methodological reasons, and suicide as a potential manifestation of community cohesiveness and religiosity. Comparisons of other causes of death, in particular neoplasms, will be addressed elsewhere.

Methods and Materials

Study Population and Sampling

Of the approximately 96,000 Jews resident in Montreal, a minority (around 5 percent) are adherents of various ultra-orthodox Hassidic sects. A recent survey of Montreal's Jewish community found that the majority classified themselves as "traditional" Jews belonging to one of several religious movements (orthodox [24 percent], conservative [31 percent], reform [3.6 percent], and reconstructionist [1.6 percent]), as secular Jews (9.1 percent), or "just Jewish" (24.6 percent). The remainder of those surveyed were married to Jews (0.6 percent) or refused to respond (5.4 percent). It is noteworthy that Montreal Jews are highly traditional, and their rate of intermarriage is very low compared to other Jewish communities in North America (Allied Jewish Community Services 1991). Some 66.2 percent of Jews living in Montreal in 1986 were born in North America (mainly Canada), 4.1 percent immigrated from Western Europe, 16.5 percent originated in Eastern Europe, 9.4 percent from North Africa, and 3.8 percent from Israel and the Near East (Shahar 1989). (By comparison, in Israel 60.4 percent of Jewish residents counted in 1985 were Israeli-born, 8.2 percent had immigrated from Asia, 9.4 percent from North Africa, and 22 percent from Europe and America combined (Central Bureau of Statistics 1992b)).

We reviewed death certificates (DC) of Jewish decedents in Montreal for the years 1986-1990. Studies elsewhere in North America have observed that virtually all Jewish dead are interred within the structure of Jewish law (Seidman 1871; Goldstein 1986). Due to the absence of accessible published information on the religious distribution of decedents in the general population (Smith, and Newcombe 1980), we approached Jewish burial institutions for data. There are only two funeral homes (FH) serving the Montreal Jewish population, where the "Attestation of Declaration of Death," transmitted to the burial institution by the hospital or coroner certifying death, is filed chronologically by date of burial. The FH records were abstracted for date of birth, age at death, marital status, place of birth, language spoken at home, local postal code, sex, date of death, cause(s) of death, and other morbid states.

Data Collection and Death Certificate Coding

As the annual number of decedents averages only seventy-five in the exclusively ultra-orthodox FH (FH1), all DC from 1986 to 1990 were abstracted by the first author and study coder (BS), for a total of 337. Approximately 900 deaths occur yearly in the majority Montreal Jewish community and are handled by the larger establishment (FH2). A systematic one-in-three selection of DC, carried out for the same five-year period by a trained FH2 staff member, provided data on 1594 Jewish decedents. The FH2 forms were then weighted by a factor of 3 to reflect the total population from which they were sampled, and subsequently combined with those from FH1.

The underlying cause of death was coded and selected using the International Classification of Diseases-9th Revision (ICD-9) coding manual (World Health Organization 1977) and the ICD-9-CM alphabetized index (World Health Organization 1978). A 10 percent blinded systematic random sample of DC (n = 196) was recoded and cause of death selected, by an Israeli and a Canadian nosologist, to assess inter-coder agreement. Perfect agreement among all three coders occurred in 156 (79.6 percent) DC; agreement was reached in 10 (5.1 percent) by the study coder and the Jerusalem nosologist only, and in 9 (4.6 percent) by the study coder and the Canadian nosologist only. There was no agreement between the study coder and one of the two nosologists in the remaining twenty-one DC; however, 11(5.6 percent) of the disagreements resulted in codes in the same disease category, thus having no effect on reliability or validity of the reported disease rates; the final ten (5.1 percent) involved discrepancies between coding of dementia, Alzheimer's disease and pneumonia. The Montreal decedents were also compared with a listing for 1986-1990 reported to Statistics Canada by the Bureau de la Statistique du Québec, for decedents from two Montreal municipalities with high proportions (76 percent) of Jewish residents. Remarkable similarity was observed in the proportional distribution of causes of death in this listing and the study sample, lending this comparison particular importance, as the latter subset was represented among individuals sampled in the FH.

Data Analysis

Frequency distributions were generated for selected underlying causes of death, by age, sex, funeral home, and country of birth. Individual diseases were grouped into categories according to World Health Organization (1991, 1992). Age- and sex-specific rates for selected causes of death were calculated using the 1986 Montreal Jewish population (Shahar 1989) in the denominators. After inspecting the data for each year to ascertain consistency of the estimates over the study period, the five-year mortality figures were averaged. Cumulative mortality (CM), a directly age-standardized measure which approximates cumulative risk of death, was calculated for ages 35-74 using the formula: $CM = 1 - e[-\Sigma ID\, \Delta t]$, where ID is the incidence density or rate of death for each age stratum, and Δt represents a ten-year age band. Ten-year age groups were used because the available published data are arrayed accordingly.

Causes of death among Montreal Jews were compared to those of the multi-ethnic Canadian and Israeli Jewish populations, using the World Health Statistics Annual (World Health Organization 1991), and the Israeli Central Bureau of Statistics (CBS) publication "Causes of Death 1987-1989" (CBS 1992a) respectively, for 1988, the midpoint of the present study period. The 1988 Israeli Jewish population figures were obtained from the CBS' Statistical Abstract of Israel (CBS 1989). Additional Israeli rates were taken for certain causes from the World Health Statistics Annual (World Health Organization 1992) to complement those not presented in the Israeli report. These latter figures pertain to the whole Israeli population, not only Jews (who constitute 81.9 percent of the total Israeli population). However, a comparison of the Israeli Jewish and overall Israeli mortality rates for causes of death published in the two sources revealed that they were extremely similar.

Data were compiled and analysed using SAS-PC statistical software (SAS Institute Inc. 1988) and programs from Gahlinger and Abramson (1993). Differences between rates were examined using Z-tests, equivalent in this context to the χ^2 test with correction for continuity. Due to the threefold weighting of results from FH2, variance estimates were adjusted, assuming a Poisson distribution of rates. Variances and standard errors were calculated using the method of Day (1987) and confidence intervals were then derived.

Results

The age structure of the Canadian, Montreal Jewish, and Israeli Jewish populations differed markedly (figure 16.1). The striking dip in the Montreal Jewish population at ages 45-54 corresponded to a birth cohort of the Second World War period (suggesting that fewer Canadian Jews were born during this period. or that fewer immigrated and/or survived). It also reflected the wave of out-migration some fifteen years ago among Jewish Montrealers then aged thirty to forty, contrasting sharply with the "baby boom" generation; however,

Figure 16.1
Comparative Population Structure

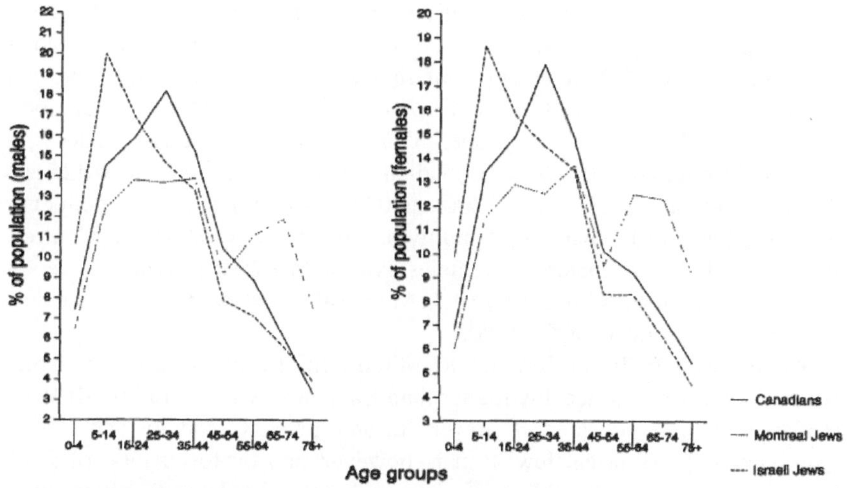

Sources Canadians (1988): WHO, 1991.
Montreal Jews (1986): Allied Jewish Community Services (AJCS), 1989.
Israeli Jews (1988): Central Bureau of Statistics (CBS), 1989.

for Montreal the latter cohort did not exhibit the peak one generally expects, due to the previously mentioned wave of out-migration. Overall, the Israeli population showed a relative excess at the youngest ages, and Canadians in young adulthood, whereas the distribution of Montreal Jews revealed a high proportion of those over sixty-five years—20.4 percent, versus 10.2 percent in Israeli Jews, and 11.1 percent in Canada. Canadians and Israeli Jews had similar proportions of elderly females (5.4 percent and 4.5 percent, respectively over age seventy-five), whereas elderly females made up 9.1 percent of the Montreal Jewish population.

All-cause age- and sex-specific mortality (figure 16.2) demonstrated favorable mortality rates for young Israeli Jews as compared to Montreal Jews and Canadians. Rate ratios (data not shown) were lower at ages thirty-five to forty-four in Israeli Jewish males (0.68, $P = 0.17$), and were similarly lower in young Israeli Jewish and Canadian females than their Montreal Jewish counterparts (0.63, $P = 0.19$ and 0.65, $P = 0.21$, respectively), although these differences were not statistically significant. However, at ages 45-54 Montreal Jewish males had the lowest mortality: the rate ratio for Israeli Jewish males was 1.52 ($P = 0.08$), and for Canadian males 1.62 ($P = 0.04$) compared to Montreal. Among women aged 45-54 differences were less pronounced and not significant, but Israeli Jews were lowest and Canadian women intermediate compared to Montreal Jewish females. Notably, at ages ≥fifty-five, Israeli Jews experienced significantly greater mortality compared to Montreal Jews (the rate ratios were 1.18, $P = 0.0003$ for males, and 1.2, $P = 0.0002$ for females), while Canadian men had intermediately higher rates (1.09, $P = 0.05$); mortality rates among Canadian and Montreal Jewish women were similar.

Comparative age- and sex-specific mortality rates are presented for the three populations for selected causes of death at ages ≥ thirty-five, in tables 16.1 (males) and 16.2 (females). Cumulative sex-specific mortality for ages thirty-five to seventy-four (CM) is given in table 16.3 for all three populations. Cumulative all-cause mortality, ages 35-74 for Montreal Jewish males was 0.312 and for females, 0.202; for Canadians, these proportions were 0.425 and 0.251. and among Israeli Jews, 0.406 and 0.299. As implied by the confidence intervals, these differences were highly significant (*P* < 0.001 for Montreal versus Israeli Jewish males and females and for Montreal Jewish men versus Canadian, men; the difference between, Montreal Jewish women and Canadian women was significant at $P = 0.003$).

Among women, Israeli Jewish rates of mortality from diseases of the circulatory system were noticeably higher than Canada's, whereas in Jewish Montrealers they were substantially lower. Among males, Canadians and Israelis fared similarly; Montreal Jewish men, however, had far lower rates of death from these diseases. The differences in rates between males and females were statistically highly significant (*P* < 0.001) in all three populations. A substantial proportion of the differences between Israeli and Montreal Jews, and between Canadians and Montrealers was explained by circulatory system disease mortality. Coronary heart disease (CHD) mortality was higher in Canadian than Israeli males; again, Montreal Jews had the lowest rates, with the gap closing

Figure 16.2
Comparative All-Cause Mortality by Age Group and Sex

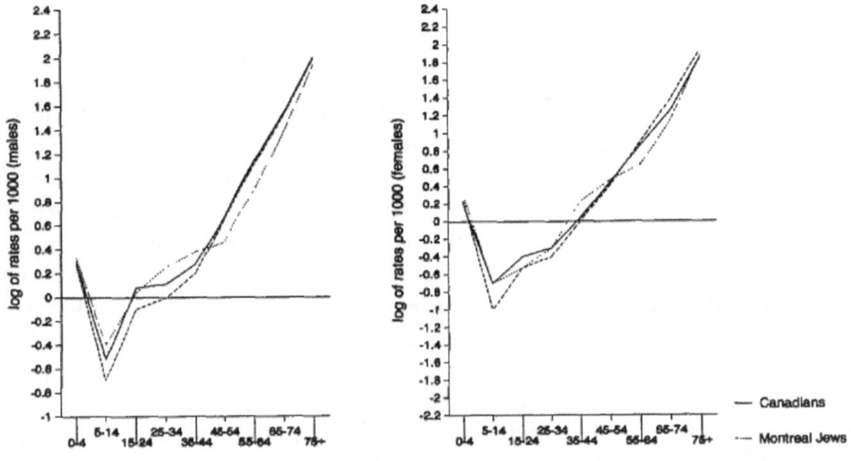

Sources Canadians (1988): WHO, 1991.
Israeli Jews (1988): Central Bureau of Statistics (CBS), 1989, 1992.
Montreal Jews: 1986 denominators, AJCS, 1989. Average mortality 1986–1990.

only in those over seventy-five. Females from Montreal's Jewish community showed strongly lower mortality rates due to coronary heart disease at all age groups examined, whereas Israeli women exhibited high rates relative to Canada. Cerebrovascular disease (CVD) mortality rates were highest in Israeli Jews, particularly so in Israeli females, while Montreal Jews exhibited substantially lower rates than either of the other two groups. The ratio of male: female all-cause cumulative mortality from ages 35-74 was intermediate in Montreal (1.54) between Israeli Jews (1.36) and Canadians (1.69).

Discussion

It has previously been observed that patterns of mortality among Jews differ from those of other population groups (Newill 1961; King et al. 1965; Goldstein 1986; Rosenwaike and Hempstead 1990; Rosenwaike 1994; Levin and Schiller 1987). Some Israeli investigators have examined the association of different Jewish ethnic origins (and to a lesser extent, religiosity) with health and health behaviors (Friedlander and Kark 1984; Friedlander et al. 1985; Friedlander et al. 1987). It was of interest to us therefore, to assess and compare the mortality experience of a well-defined and accessible Jewish population outside Israel, within the context of its home environment where the leading causes of mortality are diseases of the circulatory system and cancers (Gagnon and Comeau 1986). However, consideration of possible biases is in order before inference is made.

Possible Methodological Biases

A very small, albeit unknown proportion of Montreal Jewish decedents are buried outside Montreal. Since the funeral service is generally first held in one of the participating FH, with the body later shipped elsewhere for interment, these mortality data were indeed captured, and reported herein. Knowledge of the community (Allied Jewish Community Services 1991) and reports from the funeral homes thus lead to the reasonable assumption of almost total ascertainment of Jewish deaths. As the 1986 Census underestimated the total Montreal Jewish population (Shahar C, Allied Jewish Community Services of Montreal, personal communication, 1993), it is probable that rates for Montreal were in fact over-estimated, and the results of this study are even more striking than this report indicates.

Death certificates provide a valuable means for comparing mortality experience between populations. The literature on DC, and the quality and accuracy of information they furnish, generally agrees that there are numerous areas of doubt. Training the medical certifier in the completion of these forms, provision of clear guidelines for the nosologist, and consistency in the application of the ICD rules (World Health Organization 1977), are areas of paramount importance and potential causes for concern as to the reliability and validity of the data (Ore et al. 1991; Editorial 1987; Editorial 1989; Percy and Muir 1989; Balkau and Papoz 1992; Balkau et al. 1993). As such, variation in selection of the un-

Table 16.1

Mortality Rates for Selected Causes among Males—Canadians (1988)[a], Montreal Jews (1986-1990)[b,c], and Isreali Jews (1988)[d]

Cause of death	Population	Age groups and rates per 10 000 population				
		35–44	45–54	55–64	65–74	75+
all causes	Canada	18.9	47.5	139.0	347.5	1014.8
	Montreal	23.6	29.3	79.9	241.4	865.6
	Israel	16.0	44.5	130.3	330.4	975.9
diseases of circulatory system	Canada	4.0	16.2	53.9	148.4	474.4
	Montreal	2.1	9.0	22.8	115.8	400.6
	Israel	3.3	15.5	51.9	156.2	435.9
coronary heart disease	Canada	2.8	12.3	39.8	101.8	278.8
	Montreal	1.2	6.3	11.9	77.5	216.1
	Israel	2.1	9.2	33.0	90.8	206.0
cerebrovascular disease	Canada	0.5	1.4	4.9	17.6	84.5
	Montreal	–	–	2.2	8.8	53.3
	Israel	0.2	1.9	6.5	29.3	92.7
ill-defined	Canada	0.5	0.9	1.9	3.3	10.6
	Montreal	8.4	3.7	5.6	16.5	35.0
	Israel	1.7	4.5	9.9	18.9	51.0
suicide	Canada	2.6	2.4	2.8	2.6	3.1
	Montreal	–	1.4	–	1.4	–
	Israel	1.2	2.1	2.0	2.5	3.3

[a] WHO, 1991.

[b] Events collected from funeral homes.

[c] 1986 Montreal Jewish population age distribution (Allied Jewish Community Services [AJCS], 1989) used in denominators.

[d] Israeli Central Bureau of Statistics (CBS), 1989, 1992.

derlying cause of death (Balkau and Papoz 1992; Gitelsohn 1982; Thouez and Ghadirian 1988; Jougla et al. 1992; Jacobs et al. 1992) could have led to some of the marked differences in coronary heart disease and stroke between Montreal and Israeli Jews. "Ill-defined" causes of death, previously observed to be high in Jewish females (King et al. 1965), could actually have been attributable to circulatory system diseases, leading to underestimation of the rates of these diseases. However, the Montreal rates for ill-defined causes, as ascertained by our study, were in fact similar to those of Israel for both sexes. Thus, from the extent of the differences, the reliability and validity assessment we undertook, and the fact that these differences were evident prior to age seventy-five (when co-morbidity less often complicates coding of DC), we conclude that no notable bias in coding or selection of cause of death has occurred.

Overall Mortality

We have observed that Montreal Jews over age forty-five (but not at younger ages) generally experienced a large protective effect compared to Canadians and Israeli Jews, expressed as lower mortality rates overall. While low Jewish mortality relative to non-Jews has previously been reported (Seidman et al. 1962), it was surprising to find the cumulative mortality (35-74) rates to be 30 percent higher for Israeli Jewish men than for Montreal Jews, and 48 percent higher for Israeli women. In fact, the rates for Canadian men compared with Montreal Jewish men were higher by 36 percent, whereas for women they were higher by 24 percent, which is smaller than the difference between the two Jewish populations for women. These findings may be related to social class differences between the three populations, affecting health relevant behaviors and social relationships (Marmot et al. 1987), as well as differences in the ethnic structure of Montreal versus Israeli Jews. Montreal's Jewish population is an older immigrant community, established in the early part of the twentieth century, whereas in Israel, the majority are more recent immigrants. Divergent immigration patterns and selective migratory forces may contribute to difficulties in interpretation of mortality trends due to variation in exposure to risk factors (Modan 1991). While North African born Israeli Jews have higher mortality rates than Asian, European, or Israeli born, a similar proportion (around 9 percent) of Jews living in both Montreal and Israel were born in North Africa (Shahar 1989; CBS 1992b). It is thus unlikely that ethnic origin was a source of confounding; however, differences may manifest social class disparities in the populations that immigrated to the two countries (Kark 1976).

Sex (m:f) differences in all-cause cumulative mortality were consistently highest in Canadians, and lowest in Israeli Jews. Montreal's mortality sex ratios were intermediate, indicating that the relatively small excess female longevity characteristic of Israeli Jews (Kark 1976; CBS 1992a) may be modifiable. This finding emphasizes that determinants of women's health (Carmel et al.

Table 16.2

Mortality Rates for Selected Causes among Females—Candians (1988)[a], Montreal Jews (1986-1990)[b,c], and Isreali Jews (1988)[d]

Cause of death	Population	Age groups and rates per 10 000 population				
		35–44	45–54	55–64	65–74	75+
all causes	Canada	10.5	28.0	72.9	177.7	713.4
	Montreal	16.3	29.6	43.9	135.8	742.9
	Israel	10.3	26.0	80.1	238.7	864.1
diseases of circulatory system	Canada	1.5	5.3	19.1	68.2	384.4
	Montreal	0.3	3.0	4.6	36.1	311.8
	Israel	1.3	5.1	24.8	102.1	439.1
coronary heart disease	Canada	0.5	2.6	11.2	41.9	198.9
	Montreal	–	1.3	3.3	24.1	147.5
	Israel	0.3	1.9	13.3	52.1	187.3
cerebrovascular disease	Canada	0.6	1.4	3.6	11.9	88.6
	Montreal	0.3	–	0.3	2.0	42.1
	Israel	0.1	1.8	4.2	22.8	106.0
ill-defined	Canada	0.3	0.4	0.8	1.5	8.6
	Montreal	1.8	–	5.9	13.7	48.4
	Israel	0.6	1.5	3.6	13.2	45.2
suicide	Canada	0.9	0.9	0.7	0.6	0.6
	Montreal	1.8	1.3	–	–	–
	Israel	0.7	0.7	1.1	1.1	1.7

[a] WHO, 1991.

[b] Events collected from funeral homes.

[c] 1986 Montreal Jewish population age distribution (Allied Jewish Community Services [AJCS], 1989) used in denominators.

[d] Israeli Central Bureau of Statistics (CBS), 1989, 1992.

1991) may differ in Israel and other Jewish populations and deserve special investigation (Kark 1976), and provides less support for the contention that these differences are largely genetically determined. Sex-gene-environment interactions could play a role (Neufeld and Goldbourt 1983).

Mortality Due to Circulatory System Diseases

Israeli Jews experienced higher mortality rates from circulatory system diseases as compared to Montreal Jews, with a remarkable excess of cerebrovascular disease deaths. In the absence of incidence data it is unclear whether the differences in cardiovascular mortality reflect divergent incidence rates or case-fatality or both. The steep decline in circulatory system diseases mortality over the past two decades has been similar in both Israel and Canada (Thorn 1989). Unlike a study of proportional mortality comparing Jews to the total white population of Rhode Island (Goldstein 1986), and observations on heart disease in elderly New York Jews around 1980 (Rosenwaike 1994), we have found very large differences in circulatory diseases mortality rates (favoring the Jewish group) between Montreal Jews and Canadians, particularly for CHD and CVD. Rosenwaike and Hempstead (1989, 1990) likewise found lower CVD proportional mortality in New York foreign- and native-born Jews in relation to Irish New Yorkers, as did Rosenwaike (1994) in elderly Jewish men and women compared to their non-Jewish New York counterparts.

Risk Factors for Preventable Diseases

Differences in risk factors such as smoking, hypertension and its control, diet, blood lipids, obesity, and physical activity between Montreal and Israeli Jews could play a role. For example, the prevalence of cigarette smoking among Israelis is relatively high (Rennert et al. 1991) compared to Canadians (Statistics Canada 1994), and Israelis have an unusually high dietary intake of polyunsaturated fat (largely linoleic acid) (Kaufmann et al. 1982; Blondheim et al. 1976). Little is known about the health-relevant behaviors of Montreal Jews, with the possible exception of food habits and nutrient intakes in the small ultra-orthodox sector of the community (Shatenstein et al. 1993a; 1993b) or the patterns of observance of the Jewish dietary laws in the majority sector of Montreal's Jewish community (Shatenstein et al. 1992). While ritual dietary practices would seem an unlikely explanation for the relatively low rates of mortality from circulatory system diseases in Montreal Jews, it is plausible that differences in environmental determinants of disease susceptibility, including social structure and potentially-modifiable health behaviors (such as diet, exercise, and smoking), are responsible for differing rates of circulatory diseases. In this context, it is worth mentioning that considerable regional differences in standardized mortality ratios are observed in Israel (CBS 1992a; Ginsburg 1992), and may signal

Table 16.3

Cumulative Mortality (CM)[a] for Selected Causes: Ages 35-74—Canadians (1988)[b], Montreal Jews (1986-1990)[c,d], and Israeli Jews (1988)[d]

Cause of death	Sex	Cumulative mortality					
		Canadians	95% CI	Montreal Jews	95% CI	Israeli Jews	95% CI
all causes	Male	0.425[∫]	(0.414–0.435)	0.312	(0.273–0.351)	0.406[‡]	(0.379–0.434)
	Female	0.251**	(0.244–0.253)	0.202	(0.172–0.232)	0.299[∫]	(0.276–0.322)
diseases of circulatory system	Male	0.199[∫]	(0.192–0.207)	0.139	(0.114–0.164)	0.203[∫]	(0.185–0.221)
	Female	0.081[‡]	(0.076–0.086)	0.043	(0.029–0.056)	0.125[∫]	(0.109–0.141)
coronary heart disease	Male	0.145[∫]	(0.139–0.151)	0.092	(0.072–0.112)	0.126[∫]	(0.116–0.137)
	Female	0.055[‡]	(0.051–0.058)	0.028	(0.018–0.039)	0.065[∫]	(0.056–0.075)
cerebrovascular disease	Male	0.024**	(0.021–0.027)	0.011	(0.004–0.018)	0.037[∫]	(0.029–0.045)
	Female	0.017[∫]	(0.015–0.019)	0.003	(0.000–0.005)	0.028[∫]	(0.021–0.036)
ill-defined	Male	0.007[∫]	(0.006–0.008)	0.034	(0.022–0.045)	0.034	(0.028–0.041)
	Female	0.003[∫]	(0.002–0.004)	0.021	(0.012–0.030)	0.019	(0.014–0.024)
suicide	Male	0.010*	(0.009–0.011)	0.003	(0.000–0.006)	0.008	(0.006–0.009)
	Female	0.003	(0.003–0.004)	0.003	(0.000–0.007)	0.004	(0.002–0.005)

[a] Probability of death calculated from 10-year age bands, where CM = 1 − $e[-\Sigma \text{ ID} . \Delta t]$.

[b] WHO, 1991.

[c] Events collected from funeral homes.

[d] 1986 Montreal Jewish population age distribution (Allied Jewish Community Services [AJCS], 1989) used in denominators.

[e] Israeli Central Bureau of Statistics (CBS), 1989, 1992.

* $P \leq 0.05$, ** $P \leq 0.005$, ‡ $P \leq 0.0005$, ∫ $P \leq 0.0001$.

Note: Where significant CM differences are shown, they indicate (i) Canadians versus Montreal Jews, or (ii) Israeli Jews versus Montreal Jews, respectively.

social and behavioral-lifestyle variations between communities. The notable differences between the two Jewish populations described in this paper suggest, in our opinion, that causes of death may be due more to community-specific, lifestyle factors than to genetic differences, possibly reflecting observations on how certain types of community affiliation and cohesiveness can mediate life stressors and promote health (Carmel et al. 1991; Anson et al. 1990).

Religiosity and Health

With the exception of a few Israeli studies addressing diet and health by degree of religiosity (Friedlander and Kark 1984; Friedlander et al. 1985; Friedlander et al. 1987), there is little published empirical information on the influence of Jewish religious observance or cultural attributes on health-related behaviors. While the difference between active versus passive religious adherence might provide some insight into this issue (Hannay 1980), we are currently unable to present mortality rates by degree of religiosity among Jews in both Montreal and Israel.

The primary importance of family, sense of community and solidarity, may exert a salutary role in a cohesive Jewish context (Anson et al. 1990). Belonging to a religious community may enhance the ability to cope with stressful life events (Carmel et al. 1991; Anson et al. 1990). Significantly lower mortality due to suicide was observed among Jewish males aged 35-74 compared with Canadians, particularly in Montreal Jews ($P = 0.03$ for the difference between each group of Jewish males and Canadian males); these marked differences may be related to protective factors in Jewish communities, in line with Durkheim's thesis alluding to the protective quality of certain religions (Pescosolido and Georgianna 1989). To explain the difference between Montreal and Israel's Jewish communities in this light, we would have to assume considerable differences in community cohesiveness. Montreal's Jewish community has traditionally provided a supportive environment for its members, appearing to adhere to the Jewish cultural practice of viewing community as an extension of the family (Allied Jewish Community Services 1991). However, the absence of differences in suicide rates between women in the three populations complicates inference. This may be rationalized by suggesting that community cohesiveness could be more important to men, possibly implying that women have better social networks.

Conclusions

Our observations on mortality patterns in older Montreal Jews represent a snapshot of inhabitants from a time and place that no longer exists, a phenomenon true of resettled Jewish communities everywhere. The waves of emigration from Eastern Europe around the turn of the century, the demographic ravages of World War II, the emergence of the State of Israel, and the concurrent disappearance of the remnants of longstanding "traditional" Diaspora life in

Europe, the Near East and North Africa, have brought about gradual change in Jewish sense of community, lifestyle and behaviors. Indeed, many years ago it was suggested that low Jewish Canadian mortality rates were the result of adherence to "a traditional way of life, customs and rules of living," and that Jews would continue to exhibit favorable disease rates only if they maintained Jewish religious principles, and participated in the community's cultural life (Rosenberg 1939). The contemporary process of polarization (a modest increase in Jewish fundamentalism, alongside assimilation in some Jewish quarters) may contribute further to changes in frequency of intermarriage, dietary practices, and ultimately the degree of social integration and stability.

Despite their favorable mortality rates overall, particularly in circulatory system diseases, higher rates of death in Jewish Montrealers below age forty-five might signal incipient changes in mortality patterns. These may be a function of differences in sense of community and social integration, and increased exposure to stresses faced by the younger generations. Conversely, the lower rates at the younger age groups in Israel (particularly among women) may reflect altered exposures and reduced risk in these cohorts, implying some form of adaptation subsequently leading to lower relative rates of mortality among these younger cohorts as they age.

We suggest conducting similar studies in other Jewish communities to extend the present findings, which point to modifiable cultural or other environmental determinants of the mortality patterns seen in Israeli Jewish women. A clearer awareness of comparative population mortality patterns might provide aetiological leads. Investigations in different Jewish populations that compare incidence and case fatality for key causes of death, and examine genetic, psychosocial, behavioral and environmental attributes and their interactions might explain our striking findings.

Acknowledgements

Bryna Shatenstein is supported by a Hebrew University Postdoctoral Fellowship. We wish to express our gratitude to the administrators of the two Montreal funeral homes for permitting access to their records. We are also grateful to Charles Shahar of the Research Department, Federation CJA (formerly the Allied Jewish Community Services of Montreal), for providing valuable ancillary demographic data on the Montreal Jewish community. Susan St Laurent (Montreal) performed an excellent job of abstracting and transcribing the mortality data in FH2; finally the technical expertise of Barbro Lundberg (Jerusalem) and Sylvie Laperière (Montreal) was essential to this work.

References

Allied Jewish Community Services. 1991. *Montreal Jewish Community: Attitudes, Beliefs and Behaviours.* Montreal: Allied Jewish Community Services, Department of Community Planning.

Anson, O., S. Carmel, D. Y. Bonneh, A. Levenson and B. Maoz. 1990. "Recent life events, religiosity, and health: An individual or collective effect." *Human Relations* 43: 1051-66.

Balkau, B., and L. Papoz. 1992. "Certification of cause of death in French diabetic patients." *Journal of Epidemiology and Community Health* 46: 63-65.

Balkau, B., E. Jougla, L. Papaz and the Eurodiab Subarea C Study Group. 1993. "European study of the certification and coding of causes of death of six clinical case histories of diabetic patients." *International Journal of Epidemiology* 22: 11-26.

Beiran, I., L. Ore and L. Epstein. 1991. "Mortality trends among Jewish and non-Jewish men in Israel." *Israel Journal of Medical Sciences* 27: 36-42.

Blondheim, S. H., T. Horne, R. Davidovich, J. Kapitulnik, S. Segal and N. A. Kaufmann. 1976. "Unsaturated fatty acids in adipose tissue of Israeli Jews." *Israel Journal of Medical Sciences* 12: 658-661.

Carmel, S., O. Anson, A. Levenson, D. Y. Bonneh and B. Maoz. 1991. "Life events, sense of coherence and health: Gender differences on the Kibbutz." *Social Science and Medicine* 32: 1089-1096.

Central Bureau of Statistics. 1989. *Statistical Abstract of Israel.* Jerusalem: Central Bureau of Statistics.

Central Bureau of Statistics. 1992a. *Causes of Death, 1987- 1989.* Special Publication Series, No. 923. Jerusalem: Central Bureau of Statistics.

Central Bureau of Statistics. 1992b. *Statistical Abstract of Israel.* Jerusalem: Central Bureau of Statistics.

Day, N. 1987. "Cumulative rate and cumulative risk." In C. Muir, J. Waterhouse, T. Mack, J. Powell and S. Whelan (eds.), *Cancer Incidence in Five Continents,* vol. V, 787-789. Lyon: International Agency for Research on Cancer.

Donchin, M., J. D. Kark, J. H. Abramson, L. Epstein and C. Hopp. 1984. "Prevalence of diabetes among ethnic groups in Jerusalem: The Kiryat Hayovel Community Health Study." *Israel Journal of Medical Sciences* 20: 578-583.

Editorial. 1987. "Physicians, vital statistics, and disease reporting." *Journal of the American Medical Association* 258: 379-381.

Editorial. 1989. "Problems in measurement of accuracy of cause-of death statistics." *American Journal of Public Health* 79: 1349-1351.

Friedlander, Y., and J. D. Kark. 1984. "Familial aggregation of blood pressure in a Jewish population sample in Jerusalem among ethnic and religious groupings." *Social Biology* 31: 75-90.

Friedlander, Y., J. D. Kark, N. A. Kaufmann and Y. Stein. 1985. "Coronary heart disease risk factors among religious groupings In a Jewish population sample in Jerusalem." *American Journal of Clinical Nutrition* 42: 511-521.

Fricdlander, Y., J. D. Kark and Y. Stein. 1987. "Religious observance and plasma lipids and lipoproteins among 17-year-old residents of Jerusalem." *Preventive Medicine* 16: 70-79.

Gagnon, G., and M. Comeau. 1986. *Sociodemographic and Health Report: CLSC Métro-Westmount Sector.* Montreal: Montreal General Hospital, Department of Community Health.

Gahlinger, P. M., and J. H. Abramson. 1993. *Computer Programs for Epidemiologic Analysis.* Honolulu, Hawaii: Makapuu Medical Press.

Gilat, T., and P. Rozen. 1979. Epidemiology of Crohn's Disease and ulcerative colitis: Etiologic implications *Israel Journal of Medical Sciences* 15: 483-493.

Ginsburg, G. 1992. "Standardised mortality ratios for Israel, 1983-86." *Israel Journal of Medical Sciences* 28: 868-877.

Gitelsohn, A M. 1982. "On the distribution of underlying causes of death." *American Journal of Public Health* 72: 133-140.

Goldbourt, U., and J. D. Kark. 1982. "The epidemiology of coronary heart disease in the ethnically and culturally diverse population of Israel." *Israel Journal of Medical Sciences* 18: 1077-1097.

Goldstein, A. 1986. "Patterns of mortality and causes of death among Rhode Island Jews, 1979-1981." *Social Biology* 33: 87-101.

Hannay, D. R. 1980. "Religion and health." *Social Science and Medicine* 14A: 683-685.

Horowitz, I., and P. E. Enterline. 1970. "Lung cancer among the Jews." *American Journal of Public Health* 60: 275-282.

Jacobs, D. R., P. G. McGovern and H. Blackburn. 1992. "The US decline in stroke mortality: what does ecological analysis tell us?" *American Journal of Public Health* 82: 1596-1599.

Jougla, E., L. Papaz, B. Balkau, P. Maguin, F. Hatton and the Eorodiab Subarea C Study Group. 1992. "Death certificate coding practices related to diabetes in European Countries—The 'EURODIAB Subarea C' Study." *International Journal of Epidemiology* 21: 343-351.

Kark, S. L. 1976. "Variation in the sex ratio in cardiovascular mortality: A comparative analysis of mortality in adults of different populations." *Israel Journal of Medical Sciences* 1: 1194-1206.

Kaufmann, N. A., J. D. Kart, Y. Friedlander, B. H. Dennis, D. McClish and Y. Stein. 1982. "Nutrient intake in Jerusalem: Effects of origin, social class and education." *Israel Journal of Medical Sciences* 18: 1198-1209.

King, H., E. Diamond and J. C. Bailar, III. 1965. "Cancer mortality and religious preference: A suggested method in research." *The Milbank Memorial Fund Quarterly* 43: 349-358.

Kune, S., G. A. Kune and L. Watson. 1986. "The Melbourne Colorectal Cancer Study: Incidence findings by age, sex, site, migrants and religion." *International Journal of Epidemiology* 15: 483-493.

Levin, J. S., and P. L. Schiller. 1987. "Is there a religious factor in health?" *Journal of Religion and Health* 26: 9-36.

Marmot, M. G., M. Kogevinas and M. A. Elston. 1987. "Social/economic status and disease." *Annual Review of Public Health* 8: 111-135.

Mayberry, J. F., and J. Rhodes. 1984. "Epidemiological aspects of Crohn's disease: A review of the literature." *Gut* 25: 886-899.

Modan, B. 1991. "The fragility of mortality data in epidemiological research." *Israel Journal of Medical Sciences* 27: 51.

Neufeld, H. N., and M. A. Goldbourt. 1983. "Coronary heart disease: genetic aspects." *Circulation* 67: 943-954.

Newill, V. A. 1961. "Distribution of cancer mortality among ethnic sub-groups of the White population of New York City, 1953-1958." *Journal of the National Cancer Institute* 26: 405-417.

Ore, L., A. Tamir, I. Beiran and L. Epstein. 1991. "Mortality trends among Jewish and non-Jewish women in Israel, 1960-82." *Israel Journal of Medical Sciences* 27: 30-36.

Percy, C., and C. Muir. 1989. "The international comparability of cancer mortality data: Results of an international death certificate study." *American Journal of Epidemiology* 129: 934-946.

Pescosolido, B. A., and S. Georgianna. 1989. "Durkheim, suicide and religion: Toward a network theory of suicide." *American Sociological Review* 54: 33-48.

Rennert, G., H. S. Rennert and L. Epstein. 1991. "Lung cancer histology in Jews and Arabs in Israel, 1962-1982." *The American Review of Respiratory Disease* 143: 721-726.

Rosenberg, L. 1939. *Canada's Jews: A Social and Economic Study of the Jews in Canada.* Montreal: Canadian Jewish Congress, Bureau of Social and Economic Research.

Rosenwaike, I. 1984. "Changing patterns of lung cancer among socio-cultural groups in New York City." *American Journal of Public Health* 74: 839-840.

Rosenwaike, I. 1994. "Causes of death among elderly Jews in New York City." *International Journal of Epidemiology* 23: 327-332.

Rosenwaike, I., and K. Hempstead. 1989. "Differential mortality by ethnicity: Foreign-born Irish, Italians and Jews in New York City, 1979-81." *Social Science and Medicine* 29: 885-889.

Rosenwaike, I., and K. Hempstead. 1990. "Differential mortality by ethnicity and nativity: Foreign- and native-born Irish, Italians and Jews in New York City, 1979-81." *Social Biology* 37: 11-25.

SAS Institute Inc. 1988. *SAS/STAT User's Guide, Release 6.03 Edition.* Cary, NC: SAS Institute Inc.

Seidman, H. 1971. "Cancer mortality in New York City for country-of birth, religious and socioeconomic groups." *Environmental Research* 4: 390-429.

Seidman, H., L. Garfinkel and L. Craig. 1962. "Death rates in New York City by socioeconomic class and religious groups and by country of birth, 1949-51." *Jewish Journal of Sociology* 4: 254-273.

Shahar, C. 1989. *Montreal Jewish Community: 1986 Census Summary.* Montreal: Allied Jewish Community Services.

Shatenstein, B., P. Ghadirian and J. Lambert. 1992. "Patterns of observance of the Jewish dietary laws (kashruth) among secular Jews in Montreal." *Journal of the Canadian Dietetic Association* 53: 198-204.

Shatenstein, B., P. Ghadirian and J. Lambert. 1993a. "Nutritional intakes and some health-relevant behaviours in ultra-orthodox (Hassidic) Jewish sects in Montreal." *International Journal of Food Sciences and Nutrition* 44: 105-121.

Shatenstein, B., P. Ghadirian and J. Lambert. 1993b. "Influence of the Jewish religion and Jewish dietary laws (kashruth) on family food habits in an ultra-orthodox population in Montreal." *Ecology of Food and Nutrition* 31: 27-44.

Smith, M. E., and H. B. Newcombe. 1980. "Automated follow-up facilities in Canada for monitoring delayed health effects." *American Journal of Public Health* 70: 1261-1268.

Spiegelman, M. 1948. "The longevity of Jews in Canada, 1940-42." *Population Studies* 11: 292-304.

Statistics Canada. 1994. "Health status of Canadians, 1991." *General Social Survey Analysis Series.* Catalogue 11-612-E8. Ottawa: Ministry of Industry, Science and Technology.

Thorn, T. J. 1989. "International mortality from heart disease: Rates and trends." *International Journal of Epidemiology* 18 (suppl. 1): S20-S28.

Thouez, J. P., and P. Ghadirian. 1988. "Cancer mortality risk among the major immigrant and ethnic groups in Canada: from 1969 to 1973." *Geographia Medica* 18: 27-46.

World Health Organization. 1977. *International Classification of Diseases, 1975 Revision.* Geneva: World Health Organization.

World Health Organization. 1978. *The International Classification of Diseases, Ninth Revision, Clinical Modification (ICD-9-CM), vol. 2: Diseases Alphabetical Index.* Michigan: World Health Organization Center for Classification of Diseases for North America.

World Health Organization. 1991. *World Health Statistics Annual 1990.* Geneva: World Health Organization.

World Health Organization. 1992. *World Health Statistics Annual 1991.* Geneva: World Health Organization.

Part 4

Related Issues

17

The Extra Burden of Muslim Wives: Clues from Israeli Women's Labor Supply

Shoshana Grossbard-Shechtman and Shoshana Neuman

Introduction

This chapter offers an empirical study of labor supply among married women belonging to the three major religions in Israel: Judaism, Islam, and Christianity. In addition, this chapter offers clues on how religion affects women's value of time in marriage by examining religious differentials in the effect of husband's income, number of children, education, and age on women's labor supply. There are no direct means by which the value of time in marriage can be accurately estimated. To compare women's value of time in marriage cross-culturally, one can examine ethnographic evidence, which is a very subjective methodology. Alternatively, one can study laws and customs, but this approach does not tell us much about how different laws and customs actually affect people's lives.

The idea that labor supply and wages can provide clues on the value of time in the home is central to the modern study of labor supply. Labor economics recognizes the importance of family and home. Any estimate of participation in the labor force by married women takes account of the presence of children and estimates the effect of a husband's income on a wife's labor supply. The most popular economic theory that places labor supply in the context of the family is the Becker-Mincer theory of household production, which views women and men as producers of valuable "commodities" in the home (Becker 1965; Mincer 1962; and Gronau 1973). Accordingly, the value of time in the home is modeled as a function of productivity in the home, which is in turn a function of education and age and of the household's demand for an individual's time in home production (e.g., a function of income). Traditionally, this theory takes household composition as given and ignores marriage-market forces and bargaining inside the household.

The importance of ethnicity and religion as influences on labor supply has been recognized in empirical models. For instance, most U.S. studies of women's participation in the labor force distinguish between black and white women's behavior. Religion is included less often in empirical studies of labor supply in the United States, in part because of lack of data. Recent empirical studies using U.S. data indicate that religion is an important variable (Chiswick 1988; and Lehrer 1995). Some empirical models indicate that ethnicity and religion, as well as socioeconomic variables, interact in affecting labor supply, but these interaction terms have not been elaborated on in terms of an economic theory of marriage (Chiswick 1988; Lehrer 1992 and Grossbard-Shechtman 1995a).

This study offers a new way of interpreting religious differentials in the impact of women's education, age, number of children, husband's income and husband's schooling on women's labor supply. Religious groups differ in the institutions they create to regulate marriage and divorce. In Section II, we derive rules of inference that enable us to learn more about how such institutions influence women's (and men's) value of time in marriage, on the basis of patterns of labor supply.

Section III applies our insights to a sample of Israeli women who belong to the three major religious groups in Israel: Jews, Muslims, and Christians. That section outlines the descriptive and statistical analysis and presents our findings. Our major finding is that the labor supply patterns of Christian Arab Israeli women resemble more closely those of Jewish women than those of Muslim Arab Israeli women. Given that such resemblance does not follow from institutional differences in labor markets, we conclude that institutional differences in marriage do play a role in explaining variations in labor supply across the religious groups. Our findings suggest that Muslim Israeli women living in a traditional setting find it relatively harder to translate their personal resources into a higher value of time in marriage than do Jewish or Christian women in Israel that there are only minor differences in the value of time in marriage between Jewish and Christian women, and that the contrast between Muslim Israeli women and other Israeli women seems to dwindle at higher educational levels.

Labor Supply and Marriage Institutions

In this section, we explain why laws, customs, and other institutions that influence marriage and divorce may influence labor supply. We will discuss some marriage institutions that may possibly distinguish the major religions represented in Israel. On the basis of these observations, we derive five rules of inference that help us use the findings of the determinants of labor supply to obtain clues regarding cultural variations in the relative status of women in marriage.

A New Institutional Perspective on Labor Supply

Economic models of labor supply are based on the assumption of rational choice and view the decision to enter the labor force as a comparison between the attractiveness of work, measured by the wage or potential wage *(w),* and the attractiveness of staying home, which is typically called the "reservation wage" (w^*), Labor force participation (LFP) tends to occur if the wage for outside labor exceeds the reservation wage, that is, $w > w^*$,

Rational choice theories such as the Becker-Mincer theory focus on individual differences in resources, on the assumption that the institutional framework remains constant for all individuals who are being compared cross-sectionally or over time. The bulk of the economic literature on this subject makes this assumption and focuses the analysis on individual characteristics that affect either the wage rate, w, the reservation wage, w^*, or both.

Marriage and family have been incorporated into labor economics in the context of rational choice models, with the institutional background taken as given. Economic models of women's labor supply have included variables that are expected to influence LFP via their effect on reservation wages, such as the husband's income, the number of children, and the ages of children. In households with either more income or more children, there is a higher demand for a married woman's time in household production, and therefore her reservation wage is higher.

Other factors included in such models, such as education and age, are expected to influence both the wage and the reservation wage. Younger and more educated women are expected to be in higher demand in labor markets, leading to higher wages. These women could also be more productive in household production, leading to higher reservation wages. The net predicted effect of education and younger age on LFP (controlling for other factors) is therefore ambiguous. It will depend on whether the effect on wage exceeds the effect on reservation wage, or vice versa.

Household production models that lead to the above insights take many factors for granted. Households are assumed to exist and marital status is assumed to remain unchanged. Even though G. Becker is a major architect of the household production theory of labor supply and authored a pioneering economic analysis of marriage, he never tied the home production-based theory of labor supply to his theory of marriage (Becker 1973, 1974, 1981). As a result, economic analyses of marriage based on the Becker framework have led to few new insights regarding the effects of marriage and marriage markets on the reservation wage.[1] This may explain why most recent empirical research on labor supply, which has been heavily influenced by Becker-Mincer theories, is typically unaware of the potential impact of marriage institutions on the labor supply behavior of members of different cultures.

In the past, labor economists haw recognized the role played by institutions, but they have mostly focused their attention on labor institutions, such as labor unions. National policies affecting labor supply, such as child-care policies, or labor demand, have also received a great deal of attention from researchers. It is this line of thought that has led cross-country and time-series empirical studies of women's labor supply to take account of differences in laws and policies such as family leave and child-care subsidies. However, in the past, labor economists were mostly unaware of the possible labor market effects of institutions that regulate the marriages of people living in a given culture. Each culture, which varies not only with nationality but also with ethnicity, language, and religion, tends to have its own marriage institutions.

Marriage Institutions

The reservation wage is a function of marriage market and bargaining-in-marriage conditions.[2] On the assumption that men earn more than women, a woman's access to her husband's income can be viewed as a material compensation for the value of her time in their marriage. The higher the value of time, the higher this compensation and the higher the reservation wage. The higher the reservation wage, the less likely married women are to participate in the labor force. Reservation wage and labor supply vary with conditions in marriage markets and rules for bargaining in marriage, which in turn depend on institutional constraints imposed by culture.

Religion and Marriage

Religions such as Islam, Christianity, and Judaism contribute to the establishment of institutions that influence the marriages of people living in a given culture. These institutions include laws and customs as well as the means by which they can be enforced. It is noteworthy that these world religions do not have exactly the same institutions in every country where they arc represented. For instance, the institutions of Muslim Arabs are different from those of Muslim non-Arabs, and there are significant differences in the institutions found among Muslim Arabs living in different countries (Hale 1995). It is preferable to restrict comparisons of religious groups to a given country, at a given time.

The following marriage institutions related to religion are expected to affect value of time in marriage. Each of these institutions is predicted to have its own singular effect on the marriage market value of women and on the bargaining power in marriage. Women's actual value of time in marriage depends on the total effect of all institutions found in a given culture and is also a function of the prevalence of a market mechanism in the allocation of brides and grooms into marriages. The first five institutions discussed below will principally affect demand and supply of brides and grooms and thereby the market value of time in marriage.

1. Religious groups may differ in the value they place on having children and especially on the value of having a large number of offspring. To the extent that in one particular religion men value children more than they would in another, men's aggregate demand for women as procreators would be larger, and therefore, for any given supply, the market value of time of women in marriage is expected to be higher. In Israel, fertility norms seem to be much higher for Muslims than for Jews or Christians. According to the *Statistical Abstract of Israel,* in the period 1980-1984 the fertility rate among all Muslim women stood at an average of 5.54 children per woman, whereas it was 2.80 for Jewish women and 2.41 for Christian women. In the past ten years, fertility has declined among all groups, with the fastest decreases observed among Muslims and Christians. By 1994, the fertility rate stood at 4.60 for Muslim women, 2.60 for Jewish women, and 2.04 for Christian women.

2. Religious groups may differ in their rules about the age at which men and women may marry.[3] In all societies, on average, husbands are older than wives. Where the average age difference at marriage between husbands and wives tends to be greater, one expects that the value of young women in the marriage market will be higher because men over a wider continuum of ages are competing for young women than is the case among groups in which young men and younger women typically marry each other. Groups with significant age differences at marriage also often have strong male preferences for virginity in women, which can add to the value of time of young women in the marriage market. (However, women may never see this value. as discussed in points 6 and 7.) In groups that encourage marriages between young women and older men, the market value of time in marriage of older women will be lower than it is in groups that do not encourage such unions, as older women are particularly vulnerable to competition from younger women. From this point of view, the differences between the various religious groups in Israel are not dramatic. According to the *Statistical Abstract of Israel,* in 1983, on average, at first marriage Jewish husbands were 2.9 years older than their wives, Muslim husbands were 3.3 years older than their wives, and Christian husbands were 4.3 years older than their wives. The average age at first marriage of women was 23.1 years among Jews and Christians, whereas it was 20.8 years among Muslims. The *Statistical Abstract* also reports that in the period 1980-1984, 24 percent of all Jewish women had entered their first marriage by nineteen years of age, whereas 56 percent of all Muslim women had entered their first marriage by age nineteen. (No comparable statistic was available for Christian women.) Also, 3.9 percent of Jewish men and 7.7 percent of Muslim men were older than thirty-five years at first marriage. This indicates a higher proportion of Muslim marriages involving teenage wives and possibly a higher proportion of Muslim marriages involving large age differences at marriage.

3. Religious groups (and other groups such as Indian castes) often have gender-asymmetric rules regarding exogamy (marriage outside one's group).

For instance, there is no religious restriction on Muslim men's marriages to non-Muslim women. In fact, it is even considered commendable when a Muslim man marries a non-Muslim woman. In contrast, Muslim women are not expected to marry outside their religion. Such asymmetry will hurt women's market value of time in marriage. This institutional aspect is related to the next institution, discussed below.

4. Religions often determine the rules for divorce: whether divorce is permitted, under what circumstances, who gets custody rights over children, and so on. Many countries recognize such religious laws, as was the case in Italy until recently. In Israel, everyone has to follow the marriage and divorce laws of his or her particular religion. The divorce laws in some of the religions appear to be relatively more favorable to husbands than to wives. For instance, according to the Koran, custody over children is clearly allocated to the husband at divorce, whereas the opposite is generally the case among Christians and Jews. Divorce laws that favor men imply a lower value of time for women; this is not the case for women who live in cultures where rules are more gender-symmetric.[4] This institutional feature interacts with the laws of exogamy discussed above. The possible costs of an interfaith marriage—being alienated from one's children's religion—are lower for men (who expect to obtain child-custody rights) and higher for women (whose husbands are expected to get child-custody rights).[5]

5. Some religious groups permit polygamy, whereas others do not. The availability of multiple marriage partners for men but not for women translates into a higher demand among men for women's time in marriage and at home, leading us to expect that under a polygamous regime women's market value in marriage and married women's reservation wages will exceed those of women in a monogamous regime (Becker 1973, Grossbard 1978, Grossbard-Shechtman 1993).[6] That women in polygamous societies actually have a value of time in marriage exceeding that of women in monogamous societies does not necessarily follow, because there may be other institutional differences pointing in the opposite direction.[7]

The next two kinds of institutions we discuss principally determine whether a market mechanism or a command mechanism regulates the allocation of eligible men and women into marriages. In cases in which the command mechanism prevails, one expects more divergence from the (free) market value of time in marriage.

6. Religious groups also differ in their endorsements and punishments of physical domestic violence. In some cultures men may even kill their female relatives over issues of sexual behavior and expect to receive light or no punishment at all. The more lenient the punishment for such acts of violence, the more women's freedom to make their own marriage choices will be limited. This results in women's inability to capture the market value of their time as wives. Forced elopement is another institutional feature that involves violence against women and leads to the same result.

The more prevalent violence against women is in a culture, the lower women's actual value of time is in marriage. Violence against women may be endogenous. For instance, endorsement of male domestic violence may be more prevalent in situations in which the market value of women's time would otherwise be very high, such as in polygamous societies and in marriages between young virgins and rich old men in a culture that promotes the ideal of virginity.

7. Religious groups differ in their endorsement of marriages forced by parents. Forced marriages are often related to parental violence. To the extent that parents, usually fathers, can force their children to marry a particular mate, the bride or groom is less likely to receive his or her market value of time in marriage and more likely to receive a mix of monetary and non-monetary compensation for value of time in marriage, which satisfies the parents more than it does the children. Freedom of mating choice is also likely to be endogenous. For instance, men have a greater interest in restricting freedom of mating choice where the market value of young brides is especially high and where men stand to gain more from interfering with market mechanisms.

8. Further features of marriage often associated with religion, which are related to whether women are compensated at their market value in marriage are the institutions of bridewealth and dowry. In cultures in which marriages entail bride wealth payments (i.e., transfer payments prior to marriage from the groom and his family to the bride's family) women's compensations in marriage are likely to be below the market value of their time in marriage. In contrast, dowry payments at marriage by the bride and her relatives may compensate for above-market level compensations for women's time in marriage.[8]

We have focused on institutions that could possibly help us interpret our findings. Depending on the context, one can modify this list of marriage institutions that may be related to an individual's value of time in marriage.

Inferring Value of Time in Marriage from Labor Supply

We will now reason backward.[9] There is no direct way of estimating reservation wage, and certainly no way to estimate value of time in marriage. We do observe labor supply, however, which is a function of reservation wage. Therefore, by comparing labor supply patterns across various individuals or groups, we can infer comparisons of the reservation wage and the value of time in marriage. In the following discussion, cultures *A* and *B* represent a religious group, nationality, or ethnic group.

Rule of inference 1: If married women of culture *A* are found to participate in the labor force at a lower level than do married women of culture *B* we infer that: 1) the reservation wages of married women are higher in culture *A* than in culture *B and* 2) marriage institutions of culture *A* may have caused a higher value of women's time in marriage.

These two inferences do not necessarily follow. We recognize that instead of step 1 we could infer that wages available to women in culture *A* are lower. Instead of step 2 we could infer that in culture *A* fewer women are available for marriage. Even if the link connecting married women's LFP to value of time in marriage is not very strong, it exists and deserves to be analyzed.

Rule of inference 1 considers that all women in a given culture are part of a homogeneous marriage market. In every culture, marriage market values vary with individual characteristics, such as education, age, and income. The value of time in marriage of people with valuable characteristics is expected to be higher, because of both market forces and bargaining in marriage. In a culture in which marriage markets function freely with little regulation through coercive marriage institutions, one expects wide variations in the value of time in marriage of women of varying characteristics. In contrast, where coercive marriage institutions exist, one expects women to receive less than their market value of time in marriage. Such coercion hurts primarily the women who would otherwise receive higher compensations for the value of their time in marriage.

Husband's Income

Valuable characteristics make women more desirable as marriage partners. Women with such characteristics are more likely to marry rich men. We expect that there exists less of a gap between the value of time of women married to rich husbands and the value of time of women married to poor husbands in a culture in which marriage institutions are coercive to women than is the case in a culture with relatively free marriage markets.[10] Less variation in the value of time by husband's income implies less variation in the reservation wage by husband's income and therefore less variation in married women's LFP by husband's income. The next rule reverses the order of reasoning.

Rule of inference 2: If the LFP of married women is found to be less sensitive to husband's income in culture *A* than it is in culture *B* we may infer that: 1) the reservation wages of married women in culture *A* vary less by husband's income than they do in culture *B* and that 2) marriage institutions of culture *A* may prevent the value of women's time in marriage from reaching high levels, even when husbands earn a high income.

Another factor one expects to be positively associated with the value of a woman's time in marriage is the number of children.[11] One expects a positive association between number of children and reservation wage of women and a negative association with LFP.[12] The effect of the number of children on women's value of time in marriage and LFP is expected to be lower in a culture with institutional mechanisms that favor men, such as pro-husband custody laws. Again, we can infer clues about the effect of children on women's value of time in marriage by examining children's effect on labor supply.

Rule of inference 3: If the LFP of married women in culture *A* is found to be less sensitive to the number of children than is the case in culture *B* we infer that the marriage institutions of culture *A* may prevent women with more children from obtaining a value of time in marriage as high as the value they might have obtained had they lived in culture *B*.

Next, we consider two characteristics that are expected to affect both a woman's reservation wage and her wage in the labor market.

Age

Women older and younger than a particular age are typically considered less attractive for marriage (this optimal age varies across cultures). The more desirable a particular age is considered for marriage, the higher is the market-determined value of a woman's time in marriage if market forces operate. Young age is more likely to be an asset to a woman's value of time in Western society, in which brides and grooms allocate themselves more according to the market mechanism than in other societies in which the allocation of individuals into marriages operates principally on the base of command mechanisms.

The effect of age on a woman's wage in the labor market may differ from that effect on her reservation wage in the workplace. The wage rate is expected to increase with age, because of more experience in the labor market up to an age of optimal earnings. The reservation wage based on the value of time in marriage is also expected to increase up to an optimal age, assuming that free market forces prevail. However, the age for marriage is likely to be much earlier than the optimal age for earnings in the labor market. Past the optimal age for marriage, we expect age to be associated with an intensified tendency to participate in the labor force, because the effect of age on wage and reservation wage reinforce each other.[13] Again, we can use findings about LFP to derive (cautiously) the next rule of inference.

Rule of inference 4: If the LFP of married women in culture *A* is found to increase less with age than is the case in culture *B* we infer that in culture *A* marriage institutions may prevent women at a prime age for marriage from capturing their higher value of time in marriage more so than such institutions do in culture *B*.

Education

Education is a positive determinant of wages and is associated with higher satisfaction from work. This explains the generally greater participation of educated women in the labor force. The value of time in marriage and the reservation wage can also be positively affected by education, to the extent that a substantial number of men in the marriage market perceive that education raises the productivity of women's time in marriage, This implies that more educated women will have a higher market value of time in marriage and a higher reservation wage and will be less likely to supply labor in the labor force. An additional reason that educated women may have a higher reservation rate is related to bargaining in marriage, To the extent that more educated women may translate this resource into a higher degree of bargaining power in marriage and then apply it to the attainment of better material living conditions, they will also have a higher reservation wage and be less likely to supply labor in the labor force.

Incorporating the effect of education on women's value in marriage therefore significantly weakens the commonly accepted hypothesis that more educated women are more likely to work in the labor force. Education may encourage women's labor supply at the highest levels of schooling which are most likely to affect wage levels and satisfaction from work, and are not likely to have a positive impact on women's value of time in marriage and thus their reservation wages. However, at low levels of schooling, it is very possible that a year of schooling might add to a woman's value of time in marriage more than it does to her wages, which would imply that education would have a discouraging effect on labor supply.[14] Where marriage markets are relatively free to establish a woman's value of time in marriage, the value of education as a resource in marriage will be reflected in higher compensations received by women in marriage and therefore higher reservation wages. Education is not as likely to translate into a higher reservation wage where value or women's time in marriage is restricted by the equivalent of price controls or other coercive rules (unless coercion is less likely to occur in educated marriages). This leads to the next inference.

Rule of inference 5: If the LFP of married women in culture *A* is found to increase more with education than is the case in culture *B,* we infer that education contributes less to women's value of time in marriage in culture *A* than in culture *B* possibly because marriage institutions of culture *A* may prevent women with optimal educational levels from capturing the full value of their time in marriage.

Our goal in this chapter is to apply these rules of inference in order to derive some conclusions as to the effect of religion on married women's value of time in Israel. In Israel, all three major monotheistic religions are represented and have relatively autonomous marriage institutions.

By considering the differences in Israel's religious institutions, we cannot reach an unambiguous prediction as to how women belonging to the various religious groups are treated in marriage. Points 1, 2, and 5 above lead us to predict that Muslim married women have a higher value of time than do their Christian or Jewish counterparts. In terms of point 1, Muslims seem to encourage fertility the most and actually have the highest fertility of the three religious groups (see table 17.1): in terms of point 2, the average age difference between husband and wife is higher among Muslims (expected to increase the value of time of young women) than among Christians and Jews: and in terms of point 5, Muslims have some degree of polygamy, whereas the other religious groups have none in the age groups we are covering.

However, points 3, 4, and 6-8 lead us to predict that Muslim married women have a lower value of time than their Christian or Jewish counterparts have. Exogamy laws favor men more among Muslims (point 3); rules of divorce favor men more among Muslims (point 4); domestic violence against women and restriction on freedom of mating choice are more common among Muslims (points 6 and 7); and bridewealth payments are found among Muslims but not among Christians or Jews (point 8). In view of these contradictory influences, we do not have a clear prediction about the total effect of religion on the value of time in marriage.

As mentioned above, when applying rules of inference 4 and 5, which deal with women's age and education, one has to be aware of alternative links between women's LFP, age, and education. There could be religious differences in the effects of age and education on wages. However, when interpreting religious differences in the effects of age and education on women's LFP, it is difficult to disentangle religious differences in the effects of age and education on wages from religious differences in the effects of age and education on value of time in marriage. Neuman's study indicates no differences in the effect of education on women's wages across the three religious groups in Israel, which increases our confidence in rule of inference 5 (Neuman 1996).

Empirical Study

Data

In order to examine the labor force pattern of Israeli married women, we used the 20 percent sample of the Israeli 1983 Census of Population and Housing conducted by the Bureau of Statistics. This was the most recent census available at the time of our study. Our sample covers some 147,173 married Israeli women—89 percent Jewish, 9 percent Muslim, and 2 percent Christian (Druze and others excluded; see table 17.1). Each household member (fifteen years of age or older) was interviewed separately and personally and answered a battery of forty questions relating to his or her socioeconomic background (age, sex. marital status, religion, place of birth and of residence, children, education, and work history). Our sample covers 146,173 first-time married couples: 130,082 Jewish couples, 13,103 Muslim couples, and 2,988 Christian couples. This composition is quite similar to the religious composition of the Israeli population.

The population of Israel is composed of two major ethnic groups: Jews, who are the majority (3,412.5 thousand, or 82.86 percent of the population in 1983), and Arabs. The latter are subdivided into Muslims (542.2 thousand, or 13.6 percent of the population), Christians (95.9 thousand, or 2.33 percent of the population), and Druze and others (68.0 thousand, or 1.65 percent of the population) (Central Bureau of Statistics 1985).[15] Because of the small number of employed Druze women, this group is excluded from the following discussion.

Table 17.1 offers some additional information about our sample. It shows that the occupational distribution is different for the three groups of working women. The great majority of Muslim women (62.5 percent) is employed in technical jobs, mainly as primary school teachers (53.3 percent; not shown).[16] About half of the female Christian employees are also in technical occupations (34.3 percent are primary school teachers). Israeli Arabs have a separate educational system in which most Arab female employees are employed. The largest percentage of Jewish women is employed in clerical jobs (32.5 percent), and 27.9 percent of employed Jewish women are working in technical jobs. The second largest occupation for Muslim women is in services—16.1 percent of working Muslim women are employed in service jobs, mainly as nurses (13.1 percent). The percentages are a bit lower for Christians (12.1 percent) and

Table 17.1
Mean Values and Standard Deviations (in Parentheses) of Married Israeli Women by Religion

	All Women			Working Women		
Variable	Jewish	Christian	Moslem	Jewish	Christian	Moslem
Years of schooling	10.33	8.72	4.64	12.18	11.96	11.52
	(4.35)	(4.25)	(4.48)	(3.82)	(3.48)	(4.40)
Age (years)	42.93	39.67	35.18	37.40	36.05	30.81
	(14.62)	(12.81)	(12.30)	(10.60)	(9.90)	(7.35)
No. of children	2.81	3.64	5.32	2.39	2.27	2.94
	(2.01)	(2.61)	(3.62)	(1.58)	(1.68)	(2.47)
Employed (%)	46.9	22.7	4.5	. . .	. . .	. . .
Worked full time (%)	23.9	11.2	1.6	49.7	47.1	36.2
Years of schooling of husband	10.85	9.36	6.67	12.29	12.07	11.57
	(4.41)	(4.49)	(4.52)	(4.06)	(4.40)	(4.68)
Husband's monthly income (shekels)	29,752	20,304	15,729	35,210	26,026	24,586
	(38,400)	(22,382)	(15,826)	(40,808)	(20,959)	(27,906)
Immigrated before 1947 (%)	9.2	. . .	. . .	4.5	. . .	. . .
Immigrated 1948–64 (%)	41.8	. . .	. . .	34.4	. . .	. . .
Immigrated 1965–71 (%)	5.8	. . .	. . .	5.0	. . .	. . .
Immigrated after 1971 (%)	9.2	. . .	. . .	11.1	. . .	. . .
Of Western origin (%)	55.6	. . .	. . .	59.6	. . .	. . .
Of Eastern origin (%)	44.4	. . .	. . .	40.4	. . .	. . .
Economic sector (%):						
Agriculture and fishing	. . .	. . .	. . .	1.0	.5	1.9
Industry	. . .	. . .	. . .	13.8	14.5	7.4
Electricity and water	. . .	. . .	. . .	.5	.6	. . .
Construction	. . .	. . .	. . .	1.1	.8	.7
Commerce, restaurants, and hotels	. . .	. . .	. . .	9.2	9.8	3.0
Transport, storage, and communication	. . .	. . .	. . .	2.8	1.8	1.2
Finance and business services	. . .	. . .	. . .	12.9	5.3	2.6
Public and community services	. . .	. . .	. . .	54.4	63.5	80.9
Personal and other services	. . .	. . .	. . .	4.3	3.1	2.3
Occupation (%):						
Scientific and academic workers	. . .	. . .	. . .	9.2	5.8	3.2
Other professional, technical, and related workers	. . .	. . .	. . .	27.9	48.7	62.5
Administrators and managers	. . .	. . .	. . .	2.4	.2	.5
Clerical and related workers	. . .	. . .	. . .	32.5	16.5	7.7
Sales workers	. . .	. . .	. . .	4.5	3.2	1.2
Service workers	. . .	. . .	. . .	14.9	12.1	16.1
Agricultural workers	. . .	. . .	. . .	.5	.2	.9
Skilled workers	. . .	. . .	. . .	6.5	10.4	6.0
Unskilled workers	. . .	. . .	. . .	1.6	3.1	1.9
Sample size	130,082	2,988	13,103	52,264	620	571
Relative frequency of religious group (%)	89.0	2.0	9.0	97.7	1.2	1.1

Source.—Israeli Census, 1983.
Note.—Ellipses points (. . .) indicate that the data are not relevant or that there were no observations.

Jews (14.9 percent). In all other occupations, the numbers of women from all religious groups are quite negligible.

Inspection of the distributions by economic sector reveals that the vast majority of all women is employed in the public sector: 54.4 percent of Jewish women, 63.5 percent of Christian women, and 80.9 percent of Muslim women. The very high share for Muslims and Christians in the public sector results from the fact that the education and health systems in Israel are public. The fact that the public sector is the major employer of all Israeli women, regardless of their religion, implies that insignificant differences in wages with respect to the different religious groups are expected. All the government workers have similar work contracts, implying similar wages for similar levels of human capital.

Jewish women appear to have considerably more schooling and fewer children than do Christian women, who in turn have more schooling and fewer children than do Muslim women. Muslim women had an average of 4.6 years of schooling and 5.3 children, in contrast to 10.3 years of schooling and 2.8 children for Jewish women and 8.7 years of schooling and 3.6 children for Christian women.[17] An estimation of wage equations reveals that the three religious groups of women had similar rates of return to education.

The very significant gaps in educational attainments and in fertility patterns of the three groups almost close when we focus on working women. The average number of years of schooling for Jewish, Christian, and Muslim women are 12.18, 11.96, and 11.52 years, respectively, as compared to 10.22, 8.72, and 4.64 years, respectively, for the entire female sample. The average number of children is also very similar for the three groups: 2.39, 2.27, and 2.94 children, respectively, compared to 2.81, 3.64, and 5.32 children, respectively, for the larger sample of all women. Years of schooling for husbands are also very similar when we look at the households with a wife in the labor force, compared to all households in the sample. The similarity in educational attainments leads to more similarity in monthly income of husbands of working women, as contrasted with husbands of all women.

For the Jewish women studied, we have a subdivision by ethnic origin: 59.6 percent of working women are of Western origin (from Europe or America) and 40.4 percent are of Eastern origin (from Asia or Africa). Eastern women have a lower tendency to join the labor force, and their share in the labor force is therefore smaller than their proportion of the population. About 50 percent of these women are Israeli born or immigrated before statehood in 1948, about 35 percent immigrated after statehood and up to 1965, and the rest did so after 1965.

Methodology

To test whether the effects of husband's income, children, age, and schooling on LFP rates of women differ for the various religious groups, we estimate regressions of employment with a pooled sample of women of all religious origins. The method of estimation is logit, an appropriate method in view of the dichotomous nature of the dependent variable.

A regression of participation in the labor force was estimated to include the following explanatory variables: age, age squared, schooling, number of children, husband's schooling, husband's income, and dummy variables for Christian and Jewish (Muslim being the reference group).[18] Husband's schooling was included either as an alternative measure of income—it has been used as a measure of permanent income in the past—or because of differences in the value of time in marriage of women married to husbands with higher education. Their value of time in marriage may differ for a number of reasons: educated men may be more supportive of their wife's career, women may appreciate educated husbands for other reasons, or educated men may have a different demand for women's work in marriage.

Each explanatory variable other than the religion dummies was entered three times and interacted each time with one of the three religions. We opted for this version of a full-interaction model so that when we translated the logit coefficients into partial derivatives we could obtain effects of each continuous explanatory variable for each group on the basis of the average probability of participation for each religious group. To transform the logit coefficients into partial derivatives, we multiplied each coefficient with $p_i\,(1 - p_i)$, where p_i is the average probability that a woman of religious group i participates in the labor force. The reported partial effects in tables 17.2 and 17.3 refer to a woman with an average probability to participate. In table 17.4 we report estimated probabilities of LFP for selected values of the explanatory variables.

Findings

As mentioned in the introduction. Muslim women are significantly less likely to participate in the labor force than are Jewish or Christian women (see table 17.1). While 46.9 percent of Jewish married women are employed, the rate drops to 22.7 percent for Christian women and to 4.5 percent for Muslim women. The differences in full-time employment are even larger: 23.9 percent, 11.2 percent, and 1.6 percent for Jewish, Christian, and Muslim women, respectively.[19]

Table 17.4 presents the estimated probabilities of LFP for women with average characteristics based on the logit participation equations estimated in table 17.2. As shown in table 17.4, on average, Israeli Jewish women had an estimated probability of LFP of 43.6 percent. The corresponding LFP rates are 15.3 percent for Christian women and 1.1 percent for Muslim women. When one controls for the various explanatory variables, the participation rate of Jewish women in the labor force was 3.15 times that of Muslim women, and Christian women's participation was 167 percent that of Muslim women.

Table 17.2
Logit Regression of a Labor-Force Participation Equation Married Israeli Women

Dependent Variable	Parameter Estimate	Standard Error	Partial Effect
Intercept	−18.6766	1.2199	. . .
Jewish	12.6201	1.2278	. . .
Jewish × schooling	.1670	.0031	.0416
Jewish × age	.2714	.0055	.0677
Jewish × age squared	−.00335	.00007	−.0008
Jewish × number of children	−.2258	.0067	−.0563
Jewish × husband's schooling	.0204	.0027	.0057
Jewish × husband's income (ln)	−.0315	.0124	−.0078
Moslem × schooling	.4324	.0203	.0237
Moslem × age	.4165	.0495	.0229
Moslem × age squared	−.0041	.0007	−.0002
Moslem × number of children	−.3348	.0367	−.0184
Moslem × husband's schooling	.0051	.0157	.0003
Moslem × husband's income (ln)	.4774	.1001	.0263
Christian	8.6454	1.7005	. . .
Christian × schooling	.2519	.0256	.0485
Christian × age	.3023	.0438	.0583
Christian × age squared	−.0036	.0006	−.0007
Christian × number of children	−.3718	.0435	−.0716
Christian × husband's schooling	.0199	.0187	.0038
Christian × husband's income (ln)	.1375	.0988	.0265

SOURCE.—Israeli Census, 1983.

NOTE.—Sample used for the regression is composed of 80,045 Jewish women, 8,873 Moslem women, and 1,931 Christian women. The reference group is "Moslem." The partial effects have been calculated, using the approximation rule $b_iP(1-p)$, where b_i is the regression coefficient, and p is the average probability to participate in the labor force. p is calculated for each group separately by use of a labor-force-participation equation for that group. An individual p has been estimated for each woman in the group, and then the average for the whole group has been calculated. This resulted in the following average probabilities: p_{Jews} = .5259; p_{Moslems} = .0582; and $p_{\text{Christians}}$ = .2605. To calculate the partial effects of variables that refer to Jewish workers, p_{Jews} was used and the other two values of p were used for Moslem and Christian, respectively. The choice of independent variables in the above logit equation has been made in order to facilitate such an estimation procedure.

Rule of inference 1 stated that Muslim women may have a higher reservation wage and value of time in marriage than non-Muslim women. If that is the case, the marriage institutions found among Israeli Muslims would have caused a higher value of time for Muslim married women than for their non-Muslim counterparts. Alternatively, there are additional restrictions on the participation of Muslim married women in the labor force, such as greater distance to jobs (many Muslims live in villages that offer limited employment opportunities) or restrictions on interactions with men other than family members.

Tables 17.2-17.4 present the empirical findings on which we can apply rules of inference 2-5. Table 17.3 reports partial effects in percentage points for a

Table 17.3
Partial Effects on Labor-Force Participation (%). By Religion, of Married Israeli Women

Variable	Jewish Women	Christian Women	Moslem Women
Schooling	4.16*	4.85*	2.37
Age	6.77*	5.83	2.29
Age squared	−.08	−.07	−.02
No. of children	−5.63*†	−7.16	−1.84
Husband's schooling	.57	. . .	. . .
Husband's income (ln)‡	−.0078*	. . .	.026‡

SOURCE.—Israeli Census, 1983.

NOTE.—Data are used on partial effects reported in table 2 and are estimated at the points of average probabilities. All reported partial effects are significant at $\alpha = .05$. Ellipses points (. . .) indicate an insignificant effect.

* Effect on labor force participation significantly different than corresponding effect for Moslem women.

† Effect on labor-force participation significantly different than corresponding effect for Christian women.

‡ Husband's income is transformed into ln, and therefore the respective partial effects measure income elasticities.

woman with an average probability to participate (see table 17.2 note), and table 17.4 presents estimated probabilities to participate for women with selected characteristics. Husband's income had been used in logarithmic form in the logit regression, so the partial effects in table 17.2 can be interpreted as the husband's income elasticities of the wife's participation in the labor force.

Discussion

A positive elasticity of .026 of wife's LFP to husband's income was found in the case of Israeli Muslim women, and a negative elasticity of -.008 in the case of Jewish Israeli women (the husband's income was not significant in the case of Israeli Christian women).[20] Following rule of inference 2, it appears that the husband's income is associated with a higher reservation wage for Jewish Israeli women and that it is associated with a lower reservation wage for Muslim women. The case of Christian Israeli women is in-between. This suggests that marriage institutions in the Muslim Israeli culture prevent the value of women's time in marriage from reaching higher levels when the husband's income is higher more so than is the case with Jewish marriage institutions. Alternatively, the positive effect of husband's income on wife's LFP among Muslims could simply be due to lack of control for other variables correlated with husband's income. For instance, Muslim women whose husbands earn more could also live closer to a major city than Muslim women whose husbands earn less. Unfortunately, we do not have information on local labor markets in our data set, so we cannot separate these alternative explanations.

Table 17.4
Estimated Probablitites of Labor-Force Participation (%) for Selected Values of the Exploratory Variables

	Jewish Women	Christian Women	Moslem Women
Reference case:			
Women with average characteristics	43.56	15.27	1.13
Selected cases:			
Women's schooling:			
4 years	20.95	5.18	.84
8 years	34.08	13.01	4.58
12 years	50.21	29.06	21.31
16 years	66.29	52.97	60.43
Women's age:			
Average age −2 SD	18.32	3.66	.015
Average age −1 SD	63.79	18.52	.65
Average age +1 SD	41.66	16.05	2.37
Average age +2 SD	21.57	18.65	5.41
No. of children:			
0	58.41	38.15	4.34
Average no. −1 SD	52.84	29.84	2.27
Average no. +1 SD	31.23	6.22	.22
Average no. −2 SD	22.42	2.13	.058
Husbands' schooling:			
Average −2 SD	39.65	13.01	1.09
Average −1 SD	41.62	14.06	1.11
Average +1 SD	45.03	16.36	1.16
Average +2 SD	47.66	17.63	1.18
Husbands' income (ln):			
Average −2 SD	44.64	13.61	.63
Average −1 SD	44.25	14.43	.80
Average +1 SD	43.09	16.22	1.29
Average +2 SD	42.71	17.17	1.63

NOTE.—The estimated probabilities are calculated using the regression of table 2. The reference case is a woman with average characteristics, reported in table 1. The partial effects reported in tables 2 and 3 are at the points of average probabilities (see note in table 2). Here we refer to the probabilities of women with average characteristics. Because our model is not linear, the two sets of probabilities obviously are different. The various selected cases differ from the reference woman in only one characteristic, as indicated in the table.

The effect of husband's income on wife's LFP could be related to the effect of husband's schooling on wife's LFP. The reported regressions included both husband's income and husband's schooling. We found that the husband's variable schooling had a significant and positive sign only in the case of Jewish couples, with no parallel findings for Muslim or Christian couples. Because both the husband's income and his schooling are used, the coefficient of schooling represents a net effect of education beyond its effect via income. The positive effect of the husband's schooling that we report can be interpreted in at least two ways. First, husbands with more education may encourage their wives to enter the labor force. Second, Jewish Israeli men with more schooling may use this asset as a bargaining tool to allow them to lower their wife's value of time in marriage. Jewish women may pay more for the benefit of having an educated husband than do non-Jewish women.[21]

When income is excluded, the husband's schooling has a significant positive effect on the LFP of Jewish women, whereas it has no effect on the LFP of Christian and Muslim women. When the husband's schooling is excluded from the regressions, the husband's income has an insignificant effect on Jewish women's LFP, probably as a result of the opposite effects of schooling and income canceling each other. The husband's income continues to have an insignificant effect on Christian wives' LFP and continues to have a significant positive effect on Muslim women's LFP.

Our finding of a positive effect of husband's income for Muslim women thus does not depend on the inclusion of husband's schooling in the regression. This does not imply that the classical theory of a leisure-income trade-off needs to be discarded. It implies that Muslim marital institutions may prevent married women from benefiting much from their husband's higher income, whereas this is apparently not the case with Christian or Jewish marital institutions. It also implies that women's labor supply analysis should integrate classical labor supply theory with a theory of marriage.

We find that the number of children has a negative effect on the participation of Muslim, Jewish, and Christian Israeli women in the labor force. Table 17.4 shows that differences in the estimated LFP probabilities of Israeli women of different religions continue to be large at every level of fertility. However, we find that the discouraging effect of children on married women's LFP is stronger for non-Muslims than for Muslims. Each additional child discourages mothers from participating in the labor force: by 1.84 percent for Muslims, 7.16 percent for Christians, and 5.63 percent for Jews. On the basis of rule of inference 3, this suggests that Muslim Israeli marriage institutions may prevent the value of time of mothers of more children from reaching higher levels to a greater degree than do non-Muslim marriage institutions.

The different effect of the presence of children on LFP of Muslim and non-Muslim women could also be due to differences in opportunities to combine income-generating work and child care, a function of the type of work and type of mother substitutes available. This does not seem to be the case here. There are, in fact, few child-care services in the Arab villages (mainly day-care centers), but Arabs tend to live in close proximity to their parents, siblings, and other members of the family, and they help each other with household work and childcare. The Arab women in our sample also participate in types of work that facilitate combining work with motherhood—most of them work part time (this is particularly true for Muslim women of childbearing ages; see table 17.1), and many of them are primary school teachers.

A nonlinear relationship with age was found for all three groups. We find that, beyond a certain point, age is positively related to labor supply of women for all religious groups, which possibly indicates that there is a positive effect of age on wage and a negative effect of age on reservation wage or both. Age has a stronger effect on the labor supply of Jewish women than on that of Muslim women. Each year added to a woman's age increased her chances of participating in the labor force, less so for Muslim women than for Jewish women (2.29 percent vs. 6.77 percent). The effect of age is nonlinear. At higher ages, an additional year has a smaller positive effect on participation, a mitigating effect that is also stronger for Jewish women than for Muslim women. The effect of age on Christian women's LFP was not significantly different from that effect for women of other religions.

On the basis of rule 4, we infer that Israeli Muslim women may be less likely to benefit from the value of youth in marriage than is the case with their Jewish counterparts. Alternatively, there could be more generational differences in desire to work among Muslim women than among Jewish women. Younger Muslim women may have lost more of the traditional attitudes that kept their older counterparts from entering the labor force than is the case among Jewish women.

Finally, we found that education had a very strong and positive effect on the LFP of Israeli married women of all religions. This is especially obvious from table 17.4, which shows that differences across the religious groups disappear at the level of a college education. For all education levels, however, our tests indicate that the effect of education on married women's LFP is less positive for Muslim women than for Jewish or Christian Israeli women. According to table 17.3, a year of schooling adds 2.37 percent to the probability that a Muslim woman participates in the labor force, whereas it more than doubles the likelihood that a Christian or Jewish woman participates in the labor force (4.85 percent and 4.16 percent, respectively). On the basis of rule of inference 5, we infer that Israeli Muslim women benefit more from the contribution of education to value of time in marriage than is the case for Christian or Jewish women. This, in turn, may indicate diminishing productivity of schooling in marriage or a weaker impact of traditional religious institutions when the level of education increases (Grossbard-Shechtman 1993).[22] Alternatively, the finding of a weaker effect of education on Muslim women's LFP could be due to more opportunities for the educated Israeli non-Muslim women in the labor market or more labor market discrimination against educated Israeli Muslim women than against less educated Israeli Muslim women.

Each of the findings we have reported has alternative ad hoc explanations. What appears, however, is that all of the findings reinforce each other, Muslim Israeli culture seems to be more like culture *A* in our rules of inference, and non-Muslim Israeli cultures more like culture *B*. The finding about religious differences in the effect of education on labor supply does not contradict our other findings. It could be that the institutions that make the Muslim culture an A-type culture do not apply as much to more highly educated people.

Clues on Traditional Muslim Culture

One of our most striking findings is that the LFP of Christian Israeli Arab women resembles that of Jewish Israeli women more so than that of Muslim Arab Israeli women. Initially, we found this surprising, given that the Christian women's participation in the labor force appears to be closer to that of the Muslim women than to the Jewish women's participation rate. Our findings help us interpret the statistics reported in table 17.1 for working women only, where Christian women appear more similar to Jewish women than to Muslim women. The contrast between Muslim women, on the one hand, and both Christian and Jewish women, on the other, makes sense in terms of our analysis of marriage institutions and labor supply.

Our findings suggest that Muslim Israeli women are less able to translate resources in marriage into a higher value of time than is the case with Israeli Jewish and, at times, Christian women. This applied to resources such as husband's income, youth, and children. Education, however, is a resource that appears to be associated with greater variation in reservation wage among Muslim Israeli women than among their non-Muslim counterparts.

Our findings are consistent with the substantial differences that exist between the marital institutions of Muslim Israeli culture, on the one hand, and Christian and Jewish Israeli culture, on the other. If Islamic laws and customs regarding marriage and divorce are significantly different from Christian and Jewish laws and customs, and the latter two religions are similar to each other, it is only natural that we find the labor supply of Christian and Jewish women responding similarly to differences in socioeconomic variables.

Our inferences indicate that Muslim marital institutions may interfere more with women's opportunities to benefit from their market value in marriage than do parallel Jewish and Christian marital institutions. These Muslim institutions include divorce laws that give automatic custody to fathers, exogamy rules favoring men, and relatively light punishment for men who use severe physical violence on female relatives for what are considered sexual transgressions.

This explanation also makes sense of the apparent contradiction between religious differences in the LFP effects of age, husband's income, and children, on the one hand, and of education, on the other. For the most part, education means Western education, and educated Muslim women may be a self-selected group marrying compatible men. These couples may not accept Muslim traditions as fully as do their less educated counterparts, enabling educated Muslim women to receive closer to their market value of time in marriage. If higher education discourages religious adherence, it is understandable why Muslim traditionalists argue that female education weakens the Islamic family unit (El-Mahairy 1985). [23]

Another implication of our analysis is that labor-market factors, such as discrimination against the Arab minority, explain few of the differences in women's labor supply. If discrimination by Jews against Arabs played an important role, we would expect to find similar results for all Arab women, Muslim or Christian. Discriminatory Jewish Israeli policies—such as prohibition of army service—tend to discriminate against all Arabs and do not make distinctions between Muslim and Christian Arabs. However, if marriage factors explain the religious differences in determinants of women's labor supply, it makes sense that more similarities were found between Jewish and Christian women than between Christian and Muslim women.

Conclusions

In this article, we compared patterns of married women's labor supply across religious groups in Israel. We used findings on differential impacts of the husband's income, the number of children, level of education, and age of women on LFP in order to infer how marriage institutions affect women's value of time in marriage. In view of the limited methods available to assess the value of time outside the labor market, this study is a valuable contribution.

Women belonging to different religious groups with different marriage institutions behave differently in the same national labor force. More specifically, the effects of the husband's income, the number of children, and the wife's age were weaker on Muslim women's labor supply than they were for Jewish women. The effects of the wife's schooling and the husband's income on Muslim women's labor supply were also significantly different from those for Christian women. Only the effect of children on Christian married women's labor supply differed significantly from that for Jewish women. We relate these findings to contrast between laws and customs regulating marriage and divorce among Muslim Israelis and the equivalent laws and customs among Christians and Jews in Israel. Christian Arab Israeli institutions regulating marriage and divorce resemble more closely the institutions regulating marriage and divorce among Israeli Jews than those among Muslim Arab Israelis. Muslim women seem to be less likely to translate their resources into a higher value of time in marriage than are either Christian or Jewish women. However, this conclusion does not appear to hold for educated women. Also, our findings indicate that it is not simply the husband's income that influences the wife's labor supply but, rather, it is the amount of the husband's income that reaches the wife. Marriage institutions apparently govern the degree to which husbands and wives share their income. This is one of the many ways by which marriage influences labor supply.

Our economic analysis of religious institutions, marriage, and labor supply strengthens interpretations of religious institutions as products of political and historical factors. In both the Christian West and the Muslim East, there is a tendency to think about religion in black and white and to categorize Muslim religious institutions as rigid obstacles to modernity (Arkoun 1995). We found that educated Muslim Arab Israeli women have achieved some success in using their education toward the achievement of higher values of time in marriage relative to their uneducated counterparts. This possibly indicates that religious institutions related to marriage are not rigid but instead respond to changes in what people expect from marriage as they become more educated.

The command mechanisms of marriage in traditional societies are being challenged universally, including within Muslim societies. Educated women in other economically developed Muslim societies have started to challenge Islamic rulings that influence marriage and are seen to be detrimental to women. For instance, Malaysia, one of the most developed Muslim economies, in 1995 passed a national law against domestic violence. Malaysian Islamic feminists are now putting pressure on Muslim clerics to induce them to follow this law (Mydans 1996).

Our study opens new avenues for related empirical research. It would be appropriate to apply the theoretical inferences and empirical methodology presented here to comparisons between other groups, whether they are classified by religion, ethnicity, or class and whether they are located in Israel or in any other country, such as the United States. It is possible that our results showed significant religious differences because of the clearly different ways of life among the various religious groups in Israel, who live in separate institutional settings. Israel has few national laws governing marriage and divorce for all citizens. Other comparisons will indicate whether the results we show are valid elsewhere. For instance, it would be interesting to compare Jews from the West and Jews from Arab countries in Israel or blacks and whites in the United States.

Finally, this analysis makes a case for integration between marriage theory and labor-supply theory. We can learn more about labor supply by analyzing marriage and marriage institutions and more about marriage by analyzing labor supply.

Acknowledgements

An earlier version of this article was presented at the annual meetings of the Population Association of America, San Francisco. April 1995. We gratefully acknowledge helpful comments of the editor, an anonymous referee, and Robert Taylor, as well as the econometric advice of Danny Steinberg and the financial help of the Schnitzer Foundation for Research on the Israeli Economy and Society.

Notes

1. Exceptions include Grossbard-Shechtman (1984), Peters (1986), Grossbard-Shechtman (1993) and Gray (1998).
2. See Grossbard-Shechtman (1993), especially chapter 2, for a more detailed analysis of how marriage markets influence reservation wage and how marital institutions influence marriage markets. According to Grossbard-Shechtman, marriage markets are defined as markets for spousal labor. For an empirical study of how characteristics valued in the marriage market are related to the wife's labor supply, see Grossbard-Shechtman and Neuman (1988).
3. A large age difference could also be endogenous in the sense that it is another result of relatively high demand for wives by husbands.
4. The impact of costs of divorce and remarriage faced by the spouses on value of time in marriage has been analyzed by Grossbard-Shechtman (1993) and Grossbard-Shechtman (1995b). See also Peters (1986). It can also be analyzed in light of the economic literature on bargaining in marriage. See Manser, and Brown (1980), and McElroy and Homey (1981). All these economic theories of marriage were influenced by Becker's theory of marriage (Becker 1973, 1974, 1981).
5. Also in Judaism, divorce costs are higher for women than for men, because men find it easier to circumvent their, wives' unwillingness to consent to a divorce than is the case for women facing husbands who will not grant consent. However, in contrast to Islamic courts, Jewish religious courts tend to allocate custody to mothers more often than they do to fathers. Therefore, the prospective costs of divorce to Muslim mothers is higher than it is to Jewish mothers.
6. Our Muslim sample consists of families with one wife only, but the fact that, according to Islam, it is possible for a man to marry more than one woman is expected to lead to a higher reservation wage for Muslim women.
7. If it is indeed the case that women in polygamous cultures are worse off than they are in monogamous cultures, it could be because of these other differences. The low status of women in polygamous societies does not prove that the demand-supply analysis of polygamy is wrong, as claimed in Bergmann (1995). Other institutions may be designed to specifically prevent women from enjoying a higher market value, as suggested by Guttentag and Secord (1983).
8. This follows reasoning first developed by Becker (1973, 1974, 1981). See also Grosshard-Shechtman (1993), chapter 4.
9. Similarly, Gronau (1973) provided estimates of value of time at home based on labor behavior. However, marriage markets and institutions did not appear in his analysis.
10. One expects married women's value of time to vary with husband's income for at least two reasons: 1) positive sorting between desirable qualities of men and women in the marriage markets and 2) men with more income wanting more to be produced in marriage. an argument also found in most recent analyses of labor supply.
11. More children may indicate more resources on the part of either the husband or the wife and therefore be associated with a higher value of the wife's time. However, the divorce costs of a woman with more children are higher than the divorce costs of a woman with fewer children, especially if divorce laws are adverse to women's interests. The presence of children may create more of an asymmetry in the costs of divorce, as argued by Becker (1981) and by Carmel, Chiswick and Lehrer, (1990).
12. One also expects that mothers of young children will have a higher value of time than mothers of older children. In the United States, the depressing effect of children on women's labor supply was found to be stronger for Jewish mothers of children in

preschool and in school, compared with women from other religions. See Chiswick (1988).

13. One has to be careful not to mix age effects with cohort effects. Some cohorts face dimmer prospects in either the labor market or the marriage market or both. See Grossbard-Shechtman (1993). In turn, low values of time in marriage faced by a cohort such as the first baby-boomers imply low reservation wages and high rates of female LFP. See Grossbard-Shechtman and Granger (1996).
14. Evidence for positive effects of low levels of schooling on women's value of time in marriage has been provided using the likelihood of marriage versus cohabitation and the presence of other wives as indicators. See Grossbard-Shechtman (1993) chapters 3, 6, 9, and 11.
15. Valid for the end of 1983, when the Census of Population and Housing, on which our empirical analysis is based, was conducted The sample distribution by religion is quite similar to that of the population. We refer only to Israeli Arabs and not to those living in the occupied territories (Central Bureau of Statistics 1985).
16. For the historical reasons for the entry of women into the teaching profession, see Mar'i and Mar'i (1985: 251-59).
17. These numbers are inferred from our sample. Number of children born includes those that died. The sample employed does not include data on age of children. Comparing the average number of years of schooling, based on the 1961 and 1983 censuses, reveals a dramatic rise for Muslim women—4.64 years of schooling in 1983 (table 17.1) as compared to 0.5 years in 1961 (more than ten times as large!). For Christian and Jewish women the changes are smaller in percentage terms. For Christians 8.72 in 1983 compared to 4.6 in 1961, and for Jews 10.33 and 7.3, respectively. Checking fertility rates for the three religions, in 1960 and 1983, we have rates of 9.31 dropping to 5.32 for Muslims, 4.61 and 3.64 for Christians, and 3.49 in 1960 and 2.81 in 1983 for Jews.
18. The square of age is included to test for a possible nonlinear effect of age on LFP. We did not include an estimated wage in our regressions. Wages are usually estimated as a function of age and schooling. This would have complicated our interpretations of religious differences in the effect of education and age on LFP.
19. These are, in fact, employment rates rather than LFP rates, since they do not include unemployed women. We use the two terms "labor force participation rates" and "employment rates" interchangeably. However, we always mean" employment rates."
20. The difference between the effect of income on Muslim women's LFP and that effect for either Jewish or Christian women is statistically significant.
21. The average years of schooling is much lower for Muslim women. The average for Christian women is almost double that for Muslim women, and approximately two years less than the average for Jewish women (see table 17.1). The point about selection of combinations of educational and religious levels was contributed by Robert Taylor.
22. See discussion on compensating differentials in marriage in Grossbard-Shechtman (1993), chapter 4 and 7-9.
23. Even social planners with a modern perspective concerning women's education are wary of copying the Western experience (El-Mahairy 1985). Hassouna (1977), a physician and development planner in the Ministry of Health in Egypt, states that the more educated women who tend to join the labor market are double losers: they suffer a reduction in their status in domestic roles and are assigned menial, cryptoservant jobs in the labor force. He relates this to Egyptian women, but such views may be prevalent among traditional Israeli Arabs as well. Such views are also

shared by some observant orthodox Jews, but, since they compose a relatively small fraction of our sample (there is no possibility of identifying them in the sample as there is no question relating to religiosity), the average results for Jewish women are only marginally affected by this group.

References

Arkoun, M. 1995. *Rethinking Islam*. Boulder, CO: Westview.

Becker, G. S. 1965. "A theory of allocation of time." *Economic Journal* 75: 493-515.

Becker, G. S. 1973. "A theory of marriage: Part I." *Journal of Political Economy* 81: 813-846.

Becker, G. S. 1974. "A theory of marriage: Part II." *Journal of Political Economy* 82: 511-526.

Becker, G. S. 1981. *A Treatise on the Family.* Cambridge, MA: Harvard University Press.

Bergman, B. 1995. "Becker's theory of the family: Preposterous conclusions." *Feminist Economics* 1: 141-150.

Carmel, U., B. Chiswick and E. L. Lehrer. 1990. "On marriage specific human capital: Its role as a determinant of remarriage." *Journal of Population Economics* 3: 193-213.

Central Bureau of Statistics. 1985. *Populations and Localities: Census of Population and Housing, 1983*. Publication no. 12. Jerusalem: Central Bureau of Statistics.

Chiswick, B. 1988. "Labor supply and investment in child quality: A study of Jewish and non-Jewish Women." *Contemporary Jewry* 9: 35-61.

El-Mahairy, T. 1985. "Status and education of women: A perspective on Egypt." In M. Safir, M. T. Mednick, D. Israeli and J. Bernard (eds.), *Women's Worlds*, 239-245. New York: Praeger.

Gray, J. S. 1998. "Divorce law changes, household bargaining, and married women's labor supply." *American Economic Review* 88: 628-642.

Gronau, R. 1973. "The interfamily allocation of time: The value of housewives' time." *American Economic Review* 63: 643-651.

Grossbard, S. A. 1978. "Towards a marriage between economics and anthropology and a general theory of marriage." *American Economic Review* 68: 33-37.

Grossbard-Shechtman, S. A. 1984, "A theory of allocation of time in markets for labour and marriage." *Economic Journal* 94: 863-882.

Grossbard-Shechtman, S. A. 1993. *On the Economics of Marriage.* Boulder. CO: Westview.

Grossbard-Shechtman, S. A. 1995a. "An integrated analysis of labor and marriage and explanation of black/white differences in marriage, labor, and welfare participation." Paper presented at the Conference on Economics and Sociology in Honor of Gary Becker and James Coleman, San Diego, CA.

Grossbard-Shechtman, S. A. 1995b. "Marriage market models". In M. Tommasi and K. Ierulli. (eds.), *The New Economics of Human Behavior*, 92-112. Cambridge: Cambridge University Press.

Grossbard-Shechtman, S. A., and C. Granger. 1996. "Women's jobs and marriage: Baby-boom versus baby-bust." Working paper. San Diego, CA: University of California, Department of Economics.

Grossbard-Shechtman, S. A., and S. Neuman. 1988. "Women's labor supply and marital choice." *Journal of Political Economy* 96: 1294-1302.

Guttentag, M., and P. F. Secord. 1983. *Too Many Women: The Sex Ratio Question.* Beverly Hills, CA: Sage.

Hale, S. 1995. "Gender and economics: Islam and polygamy—a question of causality." *Feminist Economics* 1: 67-80.

Hassouna, W. 1977. "Education of women: For what?" In *Women's Health and Development*. Cairo Papers in Social Science 1 (1). Cairo: American University in Cairo Press.

Lehrer, E. L. 1992. "The impact of children on married women's labor supply: Black-white differentials revisited." *Journal of Human Resources* 27: 422-444.

Lehrer, E. L. 1995. "The effects of religion on the labor supply of married women." *Social Science Research* 24: 281-301.

Manser, M., and Brown, M. (1980). "Marriage and Household Decision Making: A Bargaining Analysis." *International Economic Review* 21: 31-44.

Mar'i, M. M., and Mar'i, S. Kh. (1985). "The Role of Women as Change Agents in Arab Society in Israel." In, Safir, M., Mednick, M. T., Israeli, D. and Bernard, J. (Eds.). *Women's Worlds*. New York: Praeger.

McElroy, M. B., and Homey, M. J. (1981). "Nash-Borg Bargained Household Decisions: Toward a Generalization of the Theory of Demand." *International Economic* Review 22: 333-349.

Mincer, J. (1962). " Labor Force Participation of Married Women: A Study of Labor Supply." In Lewis, H. G. (Ed.). *Aspects of Labor Economics*, pp. 63-97. Princeton, NJ: Princeton University Press.

Mydans, S. (1996, October). "Blame Men, Not Allah. Islamic Feminists Say," *New York Times*, p. A4.

Neuman, S. (1996). *"Gender versus Ethnic Wage Differentials and Discrimination: Methodological Considerations and Evidence from Israel."* Ramat- Gan: Department of Economics, Bar-Ilan University, mimeographed.

Peters, E. H. (1986). "Marriage and Divorce: Informational Constraints and Private Contracting." *American Economic Review* 76: 437-454.

18

From Pronatalism to Social Welfare? Extending Family Allowances to Minority Populations in France and Israel

Leslie King

Introduction

With the exception of the United States, most wealthy nations provide family benefits to citizens, and often to non-citizen residents, with children. These benefits usually include family allowances, housing subsidies, tax breaks for dependent children, and paid family leave, to name some of the most important. Those excluded from eligibility are most often non-citizen immigrants; thus, research on exclusion from social programs often tends to focus on immigrant groups (e.g., Castles and Miller 1998). In some instances, however, citizens have been excluded from family-related social programs. Focusing on the cases of France and Israel, this paper explores how certain groups of citizens came to be excluded from family benefits and only recently, in the 1990s, gained access to these benefits. I argue that the citizens of France's Overseas Departments and the Arab citizens of Israel were originally denied access to certain family benefits because of the pronatalist agenda behind these programs. I then examine how and why these groups eventually gained access to pronatalist-inspired family benefits. Exploring the development of family benefits in these two countries illuminates questions of nation and citizenship, specifically the often hazy distinction between citizenship in the state (based on participation in a political community) and membership in "the nation" (which often entails belonging to a specific ethno-national group). It also draws attention to the uneasy relationship between pronatalism as an ideology and the actual policies that have been enacted to address pronatalist goals.

Family Policies and Pronatalism

Numerous forms of assistance to families were instituted in some European countries before the twentieth century (see various articles in Bock and Thane 1991) but comprehensive and universal benefits were introduced only in the first half of the twentieth century. Family policies were originally instituted in response to a number of political and societal concerns. These concerns included ideas about appropriate roles for women in society, concern over child poverty and, possibly most importantly, concern about low fertility. The earliest comprehensive family policies owe their existence, in large part, to the desire of some national leaders to increase national fertility rates (Pedersen 1993; Ohlander 1992). As fertility declined in Western Europe, many leaders worried that their nation's economy and military strength would eventually suffer because of slow growth rates. Others felt that low birth rates reflected declining morals. Thus, many Western European countries—including Germany, France, Sweden, Italy, and Spain—had some type of pronatalist-inspired family policy in place by the end of the 1930s. Family benefits, especially family allowances, which were designed to ease the financial burden of raising children, were the cornerstone of these pronatalist policies.

Without support from pronatalists, other groups seeking benefits for families had met with little success. Early in the twentieth century, non-pronatalist groups, such as feminists and/or socialists, had sought unsuccessfully to convince lawmakers to provide benefits to families with children. In Sweden, some Social Democrats had supported the idea of family programs to mitigate social inequality, but they had never gained enough support to make significant legislative changes. However, when family policy became associated with the population question, specifically with the notion of encouraging births, it gained widespread support (Ohlander 1992). In the 1930s, Swedish lawmakers developed a family policy designed to increase the national birth rate, which had fallen from about four children per woman at the turn of the century to two children per woman at the time the policy was instituted (Ginsburg 1992; Ohlander 1992).

In other countries, ideology was likewise important. Comparing family programs in Britain and France in the early twentieth century, Susan Pedersen (1993), illustrates the importance of ideology in the institution of family policies. In Britain, where family benefits became associated with feminism and socialism, lawmakers had little interest in programs to help families. In France, by contrast, family benefits were seen as pronatalist tools; they were associated with nationalism and conservatism and they eventually found support among business leaders and policymakers.

In France, pronatalism remained strong after World War II; but in most European countries, pronatalist ideology lost much of its appeal in the post-war years. The term "population policy" had become associated with Nazi atrocities (Ohlander 1992: 215). By this time, however, family benefits had become an integral part of the social welfare systems of countries like Sweden and France, with as much a social as a demographic imperative (Jonsson 1974; Ohlander 1992). Pronatalism did not disappear after the war but it ceased to be the dominant ideology driving family policy; politicians eventually tended to downplay any pronatalist intent. In Western Europe and elsewhere, pronatalist ideology experienced a resurgence in the 1970s and 1980s, as politicians and other national leaders became concerned once more with falling birth rates.

Pronatalist ideology has historically been closely linked to nationalist ideology. In seeking to encourage demographic growth, pronatalist policies imply competition among nations for power. Thus, national leaders, when discussing pronatalist programs often make comments about "the greatness of our nation" and speak about low birth rates in terms of a national crisis (see Yuval-Davis 1989; Heng and Devan 1992; Kligman 1992). To illustrate the idea that pronatalist efforts are, ultimately, expressions of nationalism it is instructive to look at immigration policies. If they wanted to ensure population growth, lawmakers might opt to encourage immigration. However, according to the United Nations *Global Population Policy Database* (1996), of the forty-seven countries that have policies designed to maintain or increase fertility only three claim to be intervening to raise immigration as well. Twenty-three have policies to lower immigration. And Israel, one of the few pronatalist countries seeking to raise immigration, encourages the immigration only of one specific racial/ethnic group (Goldscheider 1996). Immigration is clearly a sensitive issue for governments because social services for immigrants, such as housing or special school programs to help immigrant children gain language skills, are expensive and because native residents may resent immigrants, especially in times of economic recession. Pronatalist policies, however, are controversial and expensive as well. Teitelbaum and Winter (1985: 150) suggest that the most important reason governments may be loath to increase immigration is because "it unavoidably leads to rapid changes in the cultural, racial, linguistic, or ethnic composition of the national population."

In fact, pronatalist policies have historically been most concerned, implicitly or explicitly, with raising the fertility of a specific ethnic, racial, or national group[1] (Glass 1940; Gauthier 1996; Myrdal 1940; Yuval-Davis 1989). While the bifurcated fertility policies of Nazi Germany may be the first to come to mind (Aryans were encouraged to have more children, Jews and Gypsies were discouraged and/or forced not to have them—see Bock 1984), this undercurrent can be witnessed in contemporary policies. The most telling examples are those that are explicitly bifurcated. For example, in Singapore during the 1980s, the government sought to increase births to educated people, overwhelmingly ethnic Chinese, through pronatalist incentives, and to decrease births to less educated and less affluent people, mostly Malays and Indians, with anti-natalist programs (Heng and Devan 1992; Lee et al. 1991). South African population policy during the apartheid era was similarly bifurcated along racial lines as the government tried to reduce births to the black population through family planning programs and increase the fertility of the white population through pronatalist incentives (Chimere-Dan 1993).

Because family benefits comprise a large part of most modem welfare states (the United States, of course, is a notable exception) they must be understood not only as "population policy" but also as "social policy." The fact that family benefits are simultaneously part of a nationalist agenda, and also part of a social welfare agenda, may cause conflict. This conflict derives in part from a fundamental contradiction between "citizen" and "nation" (see Castles and Miller 1998). Citizens, according to liberal political theory, must all be free and equal within the political sphere, regardless of their membership in specific groups—race, ethnicity, religion, etc. In addition, ideally all citizens should all have equal access not only to the political sphere, but also to state-funded social programs (Marshall 1950). According to Castles and Miller (1998: 41) however, the idea of the citizen "conflicts with the reality of nation-state formation . . . in which being a citizen depends on membership in a certain national community, usually based on the dominant ethnic group of the territory concerned." Changes in access to family benefits in France and Israel illustrate the tensions between the nationalist agenda that would seek to raise fertility of specific groups only and that of a social agenda which has as its goal the distribution of benefits to increase the welfare of the nation's citizens and residents.

Family Policies in France and Israel

Governments of France and Israel have sought to raise birth rates through family-related incentives—France since the 1930s, Israel since the 1960s. The social welfare systems of France and Israel are based on ideals of national solidarity and equality for all citizens; but in each country, lawmakers instituted pronatalist policies that excluded certain citizens: in Israel, the Veteran's Child Allowance Scheme, instituted in 1970, excluded Palestinian citizens of Israel by distributing allowances only to veterans of the Israeli Defense Force; in France, citizens residing in the Overseas Departments[2] of Martinique, Guadeloupe, French Guyane, and Réunion received, from the time they joined the French nation shortly after World War II, only a fraction of the family benefits enjoyed by those living in metropolitan France. After decades of exclusion, in the mid-1990s these groups in Israel and France gained access to the full range of family benefits offered in each country.

In the following sections, I examine how and why these minority populations in France and Israel were first excluded from, and later became eligible for, pronatalist-oriented family benefits. In both countries, pronatalist and social welfare imperatives co-existed from the start. Pronatalist-inspired family benefits were originally instituted through the efforts of conservative, nationalist-pronatalists[3] who were joined by more left-leaning lawmakers seeking to broaden social welfare regimes (King, 1998). Members of the latter group may have opposed the idea of trying to encourage births through government policies; however, they were willing to support the initial programs because they provided increased social support for the much of the citizenry.

Family Policy in the French Overseas Departments

France has used family policy as a vehicle for encouraging births since the 1930s, especially since 1939, when the comprehensive Family Code was instituted.[4] The Family Code consolidated already-existing family programs and increased family-oriented benefits, including birth premiums, loans to young married couples, and housing subsidies. The code sought to create an environment in which parents would want to raise children. This legislation was the culmination of decades of concern about slow population growth on the part of national leaders. Joseph Spengler (1979: 134) wrote, in the late 1930s, "it may be said that the current alarm at depopulation, while not the first in the historical experience of France, is the most intensive and protracted in the history of France . . . " There is little doubt that the main goal of the Family Code was clearly to increase the birth rate (also see Lenoir 1991: 149).

By the late 1980s and early 1990s, government leaders emphasized that family policy had not only a demographic objective but also a social one—national solidarity. Thus, Family Secretary Laurent Cathala stated in a 1991 interview that the basic principles of family policy should include: 1) individual freedoms; 2) aid to those in greatest need and; 3) encouragement of solidarity between generations (Cathala 1991). Yet, by the late 1980s, residents of France's Overseas Departments (Départements d'Outre-Mer or DOM), though officially incorporated into the French nation-state since 1946, still did not benefit equally from the generous set of family benefits enjoyed by residents of the metropole ("mainland" France). The exclusion of DOM residents from family benefits was long-standing.

According to Helen Hintjens (1992: 70), "During the first two decades of departmentalization, there were long delays in the application of social and labor legislation to the new French departments." Thus, it has not only been in the area of family policy that social benefits are unequal in the metropole and the DOM. However, certain family benefits have lagged even further behind than other social provisions over the past several decades, probably in part because French policy makers did not want to encourage more births in the DOM, where fertility rates have been higher than in the metropole (see table 18.1). For example, in his book about Reunion, even staunch pronatalist politician Michel Debré (1974), suggested that this overseas department needed a different population plan than the metropole. He argued that while mainland France needed more children, Réunion needed fewer and he called upon doctors, social workers, and educators to help make people in Réunion aware of birth control.

Table 18.1
Total Fertility Rates in the French Overseas Departments and the Metropole, 1967-1994

	1967	1974	1982	1989	1991	1994
Guadeloupe	5.33	4.37	2.62	2.25	2.18	2.05
Martinique	5.12	3.85	2.11	2.09	1.96	1.17
Guyane	NA	4.10	3.90	3.35	3.73	3.69
Réunion	6.07	3.88	2.86	2.60	2.60	2.39
Metropole	2.67	2.10	1.91	1.79	1.77	1.65

[a]The Total Fertility Rate (TFR) is a measure of fertility calculated from period-specific data. It is an estimate of the average number of children that would be born to each woman if the age-specific birth rates at a given time were to remain constant.
Adapted from Rallu, 1997a and 1997b.

Extending family benefits to the DOM has been a gradual process. French family policy was strengthened in 1945 and 1946; family allowances were raised, tax breaks for families were increased, and pre-natal allowances were instituted, but none of these family benefits were extended to residents of the Overseas Departments. Some DOM leaders and activists complained, and slowly the French state began the partial extension of specific family benefits to the Overseas Departments. Civil servants in the DOM gained access to family benefits in 1953, after a lengthy strike (Gautier 1986). Over the next decade, certain other categories of workers in the DOM began receiving benefits, although at lower rates of payment than in the metropole. Disparities between mainland France and the Overseas Departments remained great. In 1960, an employed father of three in Guadeloupe or Martinique received about 4,000 francs in contrast to 20,000 francs in the metropole (Gautier 1986).

Gautier (1986) lists three main reasons typically offered for why DOM residents were denied access to the full range of family benefits. First, the socio-economic situations in the DOM have been very different from those of the metropole. On average, DOM residents are much poorer than residents of metropolitan France, and thus pay fewer taxes. Second, demographic trends in the DOM are different from those of the metropole. Specifically, fertility has been higher in the DOM. Third, family structure in the DOM tends to be different from the metropole. There is a higher percentage of cohabiting couples, nonmarital births, and lone-parent households. Gautier (1986) argues that one of the main reasons for the DOM's exclusion from France's family benefits is that the system is geared towards a male breadwinner, male head-of-household model. According to Gautier, since DOM families fit this model much more rarely than do metropole residents, lawmakers have been hesitant to extend family benefits to the DOM.

Despite resistance to distributing family benefits to residents of the DOM, however, there have also existed strong ideological and economic incentives in favor of extending benefits to the DOM. One of these has been the practical need to discourage residents of the DOM from seeking independence from France. Why do French leaders want to retain control of these departments? First, some French leaders want to maintain a French cultural presence around the world. Perhaps even more importantly, the DOM provide strategic outposts (for example, French Guyane on the east coast of South America is the site for French space launches) and provide France with the world's third largest exclusive maritime area (Aldrich 1996). During the anti-colonial movements of the early 1960s, the French government began providing more family-oriented benefits to the DOM residents in hopes of weakening any separatist movement (Hintjens 1991). Prior to Mitterrand's election as president of France in 1981, an uprising had occurred in Guadeloupe and a separatist movement in Martinique was gaining popularity (Murray 1997). Mitterrand came to the presidency committed to equalizing social benefits between the DOM and the metropole. At least, in part, because of Mitterrand's inclusive agenda, the separatist parties in the DOM lost some of their momentum (Hintjens 1991).

Although some family benefits continued to have a pronatalist orientation during his presidency, Mitterrand was concerned with national solidarity (King 1998).[5] In fact, when some French leaders (e.g., Jacques Chirac and Jean Marie Le Pen) argued for cutting off pronatalist benefits to non-citizens, Mitterrand's government continued to provide pronatalist benefits to all citizens and legal residents of France, including legal immigrants as well as residents of the DOM (this will be discussed in more detail below). One interpretation of this is that Mitterrand's vision of the French national community was inclusive, consisting of all citizens and potentially even all residents of France, whereas some other French leaders viewed "France" in a more limited way, mainly as "white" and "European" (e.g., Le Pen 1984).

Within a few years after he took office, Mitterrand's government announced a new family allowance system, spearheaded by Minister of Social Affairs and National Solidarity Georgina Dufoix. The new program was basically pronatalist; but Dufoix's family program extended more family benefits to the DOM. However, DOM residents continued to receive most benefits at lower rates than in the metropole and continued to be denied some benefits altogether.

During Parliamentary debates over Dufoix's plan, some Socialist deputies, representing the DOM, called for a greater equalization of benefits than was proposed in the new plan. Addressing the National Assembly, Representative Wilfrid Bertile clarified the status of DOM residents vis-à-vis family policy (*Journal Officiel* 1984: 6641). First, a few benefits were extended at the same rates to DOM and metropole residents. Second, DOM residents received other benefits, such as a parenting allowance, a single parent's allowance, and a housing allowance at lower rates of payment than residents of metropolitan France.

Third, some benefits paid both lower amounts, and also had different types of eligibility requirements, for DOM residents; these included the regular family allowance, certain maternity benefits, and a family-oriented housing allowance. Finally, some benefits—including pre-and post-natal allowances and loans to young families—were denied to DOM residents altogether. "Without a doubt," stated Bertile (*Journal Officiel* 1984: 6642), "we will be told that the demographics are not the same in metropolitan France and in the Overseas Departments. That has been the pretext used by right-wing governments for not distributing pre- and post-natal benefits in the overseas departments . . . " Bertile reminded other representatives, however, that the new family policy was not only guided by pronatalism, but also by the ideal of "national solidarity." Thus, he argued, all family benefits should be extended to the Overseas Departments as part of this second goal. Following these debates, the French government renewed its verbal commitment to equalize family benefits between the DOM and the metropole; but disparities continued.

Beginning in 1986, a period of governmental "cohabitation" commenced, whereby France had a socialist president (Mitterrand) and a more conservative prime minister (Jacques Chirac of the Rally for the Republic party). Chirac's policies focused more on attracting capital investment to the DOM; he abandoned the policy of aligning social legislation (Hintjens 1991). But in April 1988, President Mitterrand restated his pledge to equalize social benefits, writing in his *Letter to All the French:* "How could I fail to think of the populations of our distant departments who are still waiting for social equality?" (quoted in Rollat 1993). Thereafter, the government began a new wave of efforts aimed both at equalizing social policy and also at fostering economic development in the DOM, where unemployment was high and the economies weak and dependent on financial transfers from France.

In 1991, the government presented legislation dealing with "diverse social measures" that included changes in health insurance coverage for both the metropole and DOM as well as a plan for aligning family allowances in the DOM with those in the metropole (Saux 1991b). According to this plan, family allowances would be equalized by 1995. However, by the early 1990s, attitudes of DOM politicians had shifted somewhat from the 1980s. To the surprise of many socialist legislators, some DOM lawmakers opposed the new plan. In their view, economic development should be a higher priority than social benefits. In the National Assembly, Representative Lucette Michaux-Chevry argued "Dignity for the Overseas Departments comes from work, not from public aid or charity." She also criticized the "assimilationist" approach of the bill: "There is a conflict between the generous wishes of the government and our wish to retain the specificities of France, Réunion or the Caribbean Islands" (Saux 1991a). Similar sentiments were voiced in the Senate debate (Saux 1991b). Some legislators took particular issue with a part of the new plan that would terminate the family allowance for first children in the DOM. The distinctly pronatalist style of the French family policy provided more assistance for families with two, and especially three or more, children. Representatives from Guadeloupe and Réunion (see *Journal Officiel,* June 5, 1991) argued that fertility in the DOM was declining, which was good; the changes in family policy might cause DOM residents to have more children, which they felt was not desirable. In addition, perhaps resistance to the new program on the part of some DOM politicians sprang from a long-standing conflict between the need to be ideologically "separatist" on the one hand, and the political need to gain welfare benefits for DOM residents—which they needed to get votes back in their districts (Hintjens 1991: 58). Whatever the case, the representatives from the DOM banded together to change two parts of the legislation they felt went counter to the interests of DOM residents (the elimination of a family allowance for first children and the reduction of state funding for school cafeterias) and the legislation passed. Currently, residents of the DOM may receive allowances for a first child that residents of the metropole receive only for the second or third child.

An important backdrop to the above events should be noted. In mainland France, no distinction has been made between citizens and non-citizens regarding family benefits. The question thus arises as to why the French government would provide legal (non-citizen) immigrants in France with full family benefits while denying some benefits to French citizens of the DOM. Some politicians do favor limiting certain family benefits to citizens, but efforts to do so have thus far been unsuccessful. My speculative explanation for this looks to both France's history as an immigrant receiving country and recent demographic trends pertaining to the immigrant population. Historically, compared to other European countries, France's naturalization laws have been generous in that it has been relatively easy for children of immigrants to become citizens (see Body-Gendrot 1995). Currently, about one in five French citizens has at least one immigrant grandparent (Bernard 1997b). But according to Body-Gendrot (1995: 246), "As soon as they become part of the nation, individuals cannot claim for themselves or for their ethnic group any specific treatment that would loosen the links of the implicit contract they have, as individuals, with the French national sovereignty. This ideology is based upon an indissoluble bond between citizenship and nationality, a French specificity." Historically, the major institutions of French society—including the army, the educational system, the church, and the welfare system—have been integral to this model of assimilation and integration. Providing all types of welfare benefits to immigrants, including family benefits, has facilitated this process. A family policy that distinguished between citizens and non-citizens would seemingly run counter to the ideology of assimilation and integration.

This said, however, in the era of economic growth of the post war years until 1974 (when worker immigration was halted), most immigration to France consisted not of families, but of men who were either single or who left their families behind in the country of origin. Immigration of families was first allowed in 1976; but governments subsequently began restricting family immigration (Bernard 1997a). In 1996, only 14,000 people immigrated to France under the rubric of family reunification. This is important in that the slowing of family immigration has weakened calls—by some centrists as well as by the far right—to restrict some family benefits to French nationals. Seventy-five percent of all family allowances going to legal immigrants go to support a child who is a French national or will soon be one (Bernard 1997b). Providing family benefits to non-citizens does continue to be a somewhat controversial issue, if less so than in the past. A 1998 poll showed that 67 percent of respondents favored providing family allowances to immigrants, up from 48 percent in 1991 (*Le Monde* 1998).

Israeli Veterans' Allowances

Since the founding of Israel, in 1948, the question of how to keep the state *Jewish* in the face of a rapidly growing Arab citizenry has been of central importance for Zionist policy makers. While Israel's Law of Return has brought millions of immigrants, Jewish fertility, with the exception of the ultra-orthodox Jews, has always been lower than Arab fertility and has been steadily declining for decades. In his 1971 autobiography, Israel's first Prime Minister, David Ben-Gurion (1971: 837), wrote, "One of the most vital elements in the equation of survival is the fact that the Jewish birth rate is much lower than that of our neighbours and is decreasing annually." In addition, differential fertility within the state of Israel was worrisome to Jewish leaders. Jewish fertility in Israel has always been much lower than that of Muslim Israeli citizens (see table 2). Nonetheless, Ben-Gurion argued that the government should *not* institute a pronatalist policy: "since the problem of the birth rate does not affect all the inhabitants but only the Jewish community, it cannot be solved by the government. Israel provides equal rights for all its citizens, without distinction of race and nationality" (p. 838). Instead of a state policy, Ben-Gurion preferred private initiatives within the Jewish community to increase fertility.

Although many Israeli lawmakers expressed reservations similar to those of Ben-Gurion, in 1968 "The Fund for Encouraging Fertility" was created in the

Table 18.2
Total Fertility Rate of Jews and Moslems in Israel, 1955-1995

	1955	1960	1965	1970	1975	1980	1985	1990	1995
Jews	3.64	3.49	3.47	3.41	3.21	2.76	2.85	2.69	2.53
Moslems	7.96	9.31	9.87	8.95	7.75	5.98	4.86	4.70	4.69

Adapted from Goldscheider 1996 and from Israel, Central Bureau of Statistics, 1999.

Ministry of Housing to provide housing loans to large families with relatives who served in the Israeli Defense Forces (IDF) (Tzur and Davids 1984; Yuval-Davis 1989). This scheme excluded almost all Arabs, who were not required to serve in the IDF, as Jews were, and who rarely volunteered to do so (Doron and Kramer 1991). The same targeting mechanism was incorporated to extend family allowances almost exclusively to Jews. This exclusion of Arabs was no oversight; policy makers obviously intended these programs for Jews only (Rosenhek 1999).

Child allowances were instituted in Israel in 1959 and provided cash allowances to families with four or more children. Later the program was extended to cover any number of children. Both Jewish and Arab families received these allowances. The stated goals of the original legislation were: "1) to lighten social conditions of weak parts of population; 2) to check the negative trends in demographic developments; [and] 3) to remove some anomalies in the field of employment and the distribution of wages within enterprises in relation to the family situation of workers" (Doron and Kramer 1991: 122).

An additional benefit, the Veterans' Family Allowance Scheme, enacted in 1970, provided for child allowances to large families in which at least one member had served in the Israeli Defense Forces or another national security service. Families could receive this allowance on top of other child allowances they might already have been receiving. Rules for eligibility were liberal—anyone with a parent, grandparent, brother, or sister who served in the IDF could benefit (Schiff 1978). The allowance was distributed by the National Insurance Institute and funded by the state treasury. The Veterans' Family Allowance Program was expanded in 1971 to include all recent immigrants regardless of military service; this program was financed mainly by the Jewish Agency, a semi-private organization. In 1974 the Veterans' Family Allowances were extended to third children.

While Arab citizens of Israel benefited from the regular family allowances, they were almost always excluded from the Veterans' Allowances (with the exceptions of Christian and Bedouin Arabs, who sometimes served in the Israeli army); Arab residents of the Occupied Territories of the West Bank and Gaza were not eligible for family benefits. While the Veterans' Allowance Scheme was popular among most Jewish Israelis, Arab leaders and some Jewish leftists vehemently opposed the Veteran's Allowances, which they saw as racist. At the other end of the political spectrum, some right-wing, Jewish nationalists opposed state-funding of allowances; they wanted the Jewish Agency to oversee all family allowances and provide them only to Jews (Yuval-Davis 1989). Despite opposition, however (as is discussed below), the Veterans' Allowance Scheme remained in effect and in 1994 it was extended to all citizens, Arab and Jewish, regardless of prior military service.

Arab leaders in Israel had always viewed the Veterans' Allowance as racist and discriminatory. During the 1980s, regular child allowances were reduced somewhat; at the same time, however, Veterans' Allowances increased slightly (Doron and Kramer 1991). Arab leaders complained that Jews could receive up to twice as much as Arabs for the third child and more than twice as much for subsequent children (Izenberg 1992). The discriminatory nature of the Veterans' Allowance seemed heightened by the fact that, when the huge wave of Soviet Jewish immigrants arrived in the early 1990s, these allowances were provided to immigrants as well. National Insurance Institute policy was to " ... recognize immigrants as residents with rights equal to those of veterans as soon as possible after their arrival" (Ministry of Labour and Social Affairs, Demographic Center 1994: 54).

Jewish opposition to extending the Veterans' Allowance to Arabs was great and those who supported the status quo rationalized the unequal system. For example, in response to allegations that the National Insurance Institute discriminated against Arabs, director of the National Insurance Institute, Mordechai Zipori, argued that the system was reasonable because Arabs didn't pay their fair share for insurance anyway. Zipori stated, "What they (Israeli Arabs) get is out of all proportion to what they pay. ... " (quoted in Black 1989). Doron and Kramer (1991: 139) predicted that "The debate on this issue will continue, but within the context of the historical Arab-Israel conflict there seems to be insufficient popular support in Israel to expect a change in this policy."

Doron and Kramer's prediction proved wrong, however. In order to seal an alliance with Arab political parties, which he needed to support his coalition Labor government, Prime Minister Yitzhak Rabin promised to close the gap in child allowance payments between Jews and Arabs. In July 1992, to "test Rabin's intentions," Arab Democratic Party representative Abdul Wahab Darawshe drafted a bill in the Knesset calling for equal child allowance payments regardless of whether or not family members had served in the army (Izenberg 1992). In late 1992, at the same time that child allowance rules were changed to remove the means test for first and second children, the Cabinet voted to abolish the Veterans' Allowance and equalize the amount paid to families regardless of former military service. Explaining the decision, Israel's finance minister stated, "Citizens who have served in the army should receive some financial benefit, but it should not be through child allowances" (quoted in Odenheimer 1992).

The Rabin government encountered intense resistance to the proposed equalization. Because the child allowance change was attached to the government's 1993 Economic Arrangements Bill, which had to be approved by the Knesset, those opposing the decision tried hard to block the budget bill altogether when it came up for a vote. Likud leaders protested that the child allowance changes had not been discussed in committee and they tried to have that part of the bill removed on procedural grounds. Tempers in the Knesset were so hot over the child allowance equalization that a fistfight almost broke out. While Likud representative Dan Tichon argued that the procedure through which the child allowance changes had been added to the budget bill had been inappropriate, representative Rehavam Ze'evi called out: "The (proposal) is an incentive for making more Arab children. They will live off us forever. They will give birth to seventy children; they do anyway . ... they will give birth to fifty, sixty, seventy children and we will pay them discharged soldiers' grants" (quoted in Izenberg 1993). Another representative responded, calling Ze'evi a racist; the situation then degenerated until the Deputy Speaker called a recess.[6]

The budget bill passed, however, aided in part by the fact that some ultra-Orthodox representatives threw in their support. The ultra-Orthodox Jews, whose political power has been rising because they are growing in number (mainly due to their relatively high fertility), wanted the Veterans' Allowance extended to all citizens. Because the ultra-Orthodox do not serve in the army, and were therefore excluded from the Veterans' Allowance along with the Arabs, they stood to benefit from the new arrangement.

In Israel, then, practical politics played an important role in the extension of the Veterans' Family Allowances to Arab citizens. It should also be noted that the arrival in Israel, between 1989 and 1992, of over 400,000 Soviet Jews was important as well (Goldscheider 1996). This immigration wave altered the demographic composition of Israel, substantially slowing the decline in the Jewish population as a percentage of the total population. (table 18.3 shows the percentage of Jews and Moslems in the total population.) Concern over low Jewish fertility faded as absorbing these immigrants became a central task of social welfare services.

Discussion/Conclusions

The recent extension of family benefits in France and Israel to formerly excluded groups could be explained in anyone of several ways. One is that fewer lawmakers in these nations subscribe to a pronatalist agenda and more favor a social equity model. It would be understandable if fewer policy makers supported family benefits for pronatalist reasons. Researchers have been hard pressed to show that pronatalist initiatives are successful in raising fertility. Demeny (1987: 350) claims that the evaluation literature has been "less than unanimous in its conclusions" but that the "modal finding is that the effects [of fertility policies] are negligible."[7] It may also be relevant that fertility has dropped significantly among these minority populations in France and Israel. Perhaps it is easier to rationalize extending the family benefits given that their efficacy in raising birth rates is questionable and the minority populations' birth rates have been falling anyway. And while some leaders may have preferred to retract family benefits across the board, once the public comes to expect certain benefits, it becomes difficult for politicians to take them away.

A second possibility is that many supporters of family policies retain a nationalist, pronatalist orientation but that more lawmakers are seeing the national community as including the minority citizens as "one of us." In both France and Israel there have always been those who take an inclusive view of the national

Table 18.3
Religious Composition of the Population of Israel, 1980, 1990, 1998

	1980	1990	1998
Population – total (in thousands)	3,921.7	4,821.7	6,041.4
Percent of total			
Jews	83.7	81.9	79.2
Moslems	12.7	14.1	14.9
Christians	2.3	2.4	2.1
Druze	1.3	1.7	1.6
Religion unclassified	–	–	2.1

Israel, Central Bureau of Statistics, 1999.

community, seeing the nation less as an ethnic community and more as a political community. During the 1980s and 1990s, several leaders, such as Mitterrand, expressed this view. But, as discussed above, there is vocal opposition to this position by some members of the dominant populations in each country.

Finally, a third possible interpretation of the extension of family benefits to formerly excluded groups is that, in general, lawmakers and citizens still want to see more births to the majority or dominant population and have extended the allowances for practical political reasons only. If this is the case, one might expect to see other types of attempts to raise birth rates, perhaps not via family policy but through either private initiatives or new types of public programs.

Whichever the case, however, the extension of family benefits to previously excluded groups may indicate a trend toward more inclusiveness in family policy. What can we learn from the cases of France and Israel? Does the extension of benefits mean French and Israeli family policies are losing their pronatalist orientations and moving toward more of a social welfare model? In both cases, the answer is complex and the political and demographic ground is continually shifting. Certainly some lawmakers in both countries remain concerned about low fertility. Yet, in one important way, the answer to the above question is "yes." Though leaders may be extending benefits to minority populations for practical domestic-political or geo-political reasons one consequence is that, if they are going to do this, politicians must downplay the importance of pronatalism in favor of social welfare. It would be impossible for Israeli Jewish politicians, for example, to justify encouraging more births to Arabs. In France, lawmakers may not find it easy to justify encouraging births to residents of the French DOM, a high percentage of who are poor and already dependent on welfare. The ideology behind the policy has to be reinvented; the discourse shifts from stressing demography to emphasizing social welfare. This does not mean that pronatalist ideology has faded altogether. On the contrary, among certain factions it may remain quite strong. What it *does* mean is that the link between pronatalism and family policy diminishes. Family allowances that were once considered part of a "population policy" become more strictly associated with social welfare policy.

A relational understanding of "family policy" and "pronatalist policy" helps illuminate connections and contradictions between demographic policies and modem welfare state programs that benefit families with children. An inherent tension exists between the goals of pronatalism and the provision of social benefits to raise fertility in that proponents of pronatalism often prefer to raise births only to specific racial/ethnic groups; yet in modem democracies, it is difficult to rationalize and maintain social policies that explicitly discriminate on the basis of race or ethnicity. Although welfare states have been shown to reproduce race, class, and gender inequalities (Quadagno 1994; Rosenhek 1999), the mechanisms through which this has occurred are rarely overtly discriminatory. While immigrants are sometimes denied benefits on the grounds that they are not full members of the nation-state, citizens are generally *technically* eligible for social benefits regardless of their gender, or their racial, ethnic, or regional status. Thus, using social policy to affect demographic trends may eventually compel or foster a movement away from any demographic goals and towards a social welfare imperative.

Notes

1. As is always true with a generalization such as this, there are exceptions. Certainly, not all advocates of pronatalist policies are motivated by racism, ethnocentrism, or extreme nationalism. However, many (and perhaps most) pronatalist initiatives throughout the twentieth century can be said to implicitly or explicitly target certain groups.
2. Departments resemble American states. I do not address the French overseas *territories,* which have a somewhat different status from the overseas *departments.* Martinique, Guadeloupe, Guyane, and Réunion were formerly French colonies that became French departments shortly after World War II.
3. A national community may be imagined in various ways (see Anderson 1995). For example, "France" can be imagined as "white and Christian" or as "multi-cultural and multi-racial" In this case, I am referring to less inclusive nationalists.
4. It is important to note that prior to the 1939 Family Code, employers had set up family allowances through a system of *caisses de compensation* or compensation funds. Businesses, though sometimes justifying these funds with Catholic or pronatalist rhetoric, had their own, economic reasons for providing family allowances (see Pedersen 1993).
5. In France, family policy generally divides along party lines. Socialists tend to emphasize social solidarity; more right-leaning parties often emphasize population increase through pronatalist programs. This is a general tendency; some on the left, while favoring social solidarity, are also pronatalist and no doubt some on the right oppose pronatalism.
6. Hadash MK Tawfik Zayyad and MKs Gonen Segev (Tsomet) and Rehavam Ze'evi (Moledet) argued over the child allowances.

Ze'evi said: "The (proposal) is an incentive for making more Arab children. They will live off us forever. They will give birth to 70 children; they do anyway . . . they will give birth to fifty, sixty, seventy children and we will pay them discharged soldiers' grants."
Zayyad responded: "You're a racist. You should be in jail"
Ze'evi: "You're a red fascist."
Segev: "The entire Arab people are fascists and killers."
Zayyad: "You and Ze'evi ought to be in jail"
Segev: "You are a nation of killing."

The exchange continued in that vein, ending this way:
Ze'evi: "You are a toilet."
Zayyad: "You are shit in a toilet. You son-of-a-bitch"
(cited in Izenberg 1993: 14).

7. There apparently remains among some national leaders, however, a belief in the effectiveness of pronatalist policies. Pronatalist Jacques Chirac (1999), proclaimed in a recent speech at the yearly ceremony awarding the "Medal of the French Family" to mothers of many children that "If demographers are not in agreement when it comes to measuring the exact effect of family policy on fertility, they generally admit the importance of its role."

References

Aldrich, R. 1996. *Greater France: A History of French Overseas Expansion.* New York: St. Martin's Press.

Anderson, B. 1995. *Imagined Communities: Reflections on the Origin and Spread of Nationalism,* revised ed. New York: Verso.

Ben-Gurion, D. 1971. *Israel: A Personal History.* New York: Funk and Wagnalls.

Bernard, P. 1997a. "Consacré par la droite en 1976, le regroupement familial n'a cessé d'être restraint depuis lors." *Le Monde* (16 December).

Bernard, P. 1997b. "L'immigration, fardeau ou bénédiction?" *Le Monde* (1 April).

Black, J. 1989. "Arabs fail to share the NII burden." *Jerusalem Post* (8 June).

Bock, G. 1984. "Racism and sexism in Nazi Germany: Motherhood, compulsory sterilization, and the state." In R. Bridenthal, A. Grossmann and M. Kaplan (eds.), *When Biology Became Destiny: Women in Weimar and Nazi Germany* 271-296. New York: Monthly Review Press.

Bock, G., and P. Thane (eds.). 1991. *Women and the Rise of the European Welfare States, 1880s - 1950s.* New York: Routledge.

Body-Gendrot, S. 1995. "Models of immigrant integration in France and the United States." In M. P. Smith and J. R. Faegin (eds.), *The Bubbling Cauldron*, 244-262. University of Minnesota Press, MN.

Cathala, L. 1991. "Un entretien avec M. Laurent Cathala." *Le Monde* (1 October).

Castles, S., and M. J. Miller. 1998. *The Age of Migration: International Population Movements in the Modern World.* New York: Guilford Press.

Central Bureau of Statistics. 1999. *Statistical Abstract of Israel.* www.cbs.gov.il/shnaton50/shnatone50.htm#3 (viewed March 2000).

Chimere-Dan, O. 1993. "Population policy in South Africa." *Studies in Family Planning* 24: 31-39.

Chirac, J. 1999. "Lors de la remise de la médaille de la famille française." Speech at Elysée Palace (31 May). www.elysee.fr/disc/disc.htm (viewed February 2000).

Debré, M. 1974. *Une politique pour la Réunion.* Paris: Plon.

Demeny, P. 1987. "Pronatalist policies in low-fertility countries: Patterns, performance, and prospects." in K. Davis, M. S. Bernstam and R. Ricardo-Campbell (eds.), *Below-Replacement Fertility in Industrial Societies: Causes, Consequences, Policies*, 335-358. New York: Cambridge University Press.

Doron, A., and R. M. Kramer. 1991. *The Welfare State in Israel: The Evolution of Social Security Policy and Practice.* Boulder, CO: Westview Press.

Gauthier, A. H. 1996. *The State and the Family.* Oxford: Clarendon Press.

Gautier, A. 1986. "Politique familiale et familles monoparentales en métropole et dans les DOM depuis 1946." *Nouvelles Questions Féministes* 13: 89-110.

Ginsburg, N. 1992. *Divisions of Welfare: A Critical Introduction to Comparative Social Policy.* Newbury Park: Sage.

Glass, D. 1940. *Population Policies and Social Movements.* Oxford: Clarendon Press.

Goldscheider, C. 1996. *Israel's Changing Society: Population, Ethnicity, and Development.* Boulder, CO: West view Press.

Heng, G., and J. Devan. 1992. "State fatherhood: The politics of nationalism, sexuality, and race in Singapore." In A. Parker, M. Russo, D. Sommer and P. Yaeger (eds.), *Nationalisms and Sexualities*, 343-364. New York: Routledge.

Hintjens, H. M. 1991. "Regional reform in the French periphery: The overseas departments of Réunion, Martinique and Guadeloupe." *Regional Politics and Policy* 1: 51-73.

Hintjens, H. M. 1992. "France's love children? The French overseas departments." In H. M. Hintjens and M. D. D. Newitt (eds.), *The Political Economy of Small Tropical Islands: The Importance of Being Small*, 64-75. Exeter: University of Exeter Press.

Izenberg, D. 1992. "Proposed child allowance bill meant to test Rabin's intentions." *Jerusalem Post* (15 July).

Izenberg, D. 1993. "Tempers boil over Knesset budget debate." *Jerusalem Post* (23 December).

Jonsson, L. 1974. "Sweden." In B. Berelson (ed.), *Population Policy in Developed Countries*, 113-148. New York: McGraw-Hill.

Journal Officiel 1984. "Assemblée Nationale, 7e Législature, 1e Séance." (5 December) 6663-6686.

Journal Officiel 1984. "Assemblée Nationale, 7e Législature, 2e and 3e Séance." (4 December) 6617-6661.

Journal Officiel 1991. "Assemblée Nationale, 9e Législature, 76e Séance." (5 June) 3814.

King, L., 1998. "France needs children': Pronatalism, nationalism and women's equity." *The Sociological Quarterly* 39: 33-52.

Kligman, G. 1992. "The politics of reproduction in Ceausescu's Romania: A case study in political culture." *East European Politics and Societies* 6: 364-418.

Le Monde 1998. "68% des Français contre la préférence nationale." *Le Monde* (15 June).

Le Pen, J. M. 1984. *Les Français d'Abord.* Paris: Michel Lafon Carrere.

Lee, S. M., G. Alvarez and J. Palen. 1991. "Fertility decline and pronatalist policy in Singapore." *International Family Planning Perspectives* 17: 65-73.

Lenoir, R. 1991. "Family policy in France since 1938." In J. Ambler (ed.), *The French Welfare State: Surviving Social and Ideological Change*, 144-186. New York: New York University Press.

Marshall, T. M. 1950. *Citizenship and Social Class, and Other Essays.* Cambridge: Cambridge University Press.

Ministry of Labor and Social Affairs, Demographic Center. 1994. "The population of Israel." Report prepared for the International Conference on Population and Development.
Murray, D. 1997. "The cultural citizen: Negations or race and language in the making of Martiniquais." *Anthropological Quarterly* 70: 79-90.
Myrdal, G. 1940. *Population, a Problem for Democracy.* Cambridge, MA: Harvard University Press.
Odenheimer, A. 1992. "Families with 3 kids can receive NII money." *Jerusalem Post* (7 December).
Ohlander, A. S. 1992. "The invisible child? The struggle over social democratic family policy." In K. Misgeld, K. Molin and K. Åmark (eds.), *Creating Social Democracy: A Century of the Social Democratic Labor Party in Sweden*, 213-236. University Park: Pennsylvania State University Press.
Pedersen, S. 1993. *Family, Dependence, and the Origins of the Welfare State: Britain and France,* 1914-1945. New York: Cambridge University Press.
Quadagno, J. 1994. *The Color of Welfare.* New York: Oxford University Press.
Rallu, J. L. 1997a. "La population des départements d'outre-mer: Évolution récente, migrations et activité." *Population* 52: 699-728.
Rallu, J. L. 1997b. "Population, migration et emploi dans les départements d'outre-mer." *Populations et Sociétés* 329.
Rollat, A. 1993. "Le défi de l'outre-mer." *Le Monde* (23 January): 11.
Rosenhek, Z. 1999. "The exclusionary logic of the welfare state: Palestinian citizens in the Israeli welfare state." *International Sociology* 14: 195-215.
Saux, J. L. 1991a. "M. Bianco défend un projet de maîtrise des dépenses de santé." *Le Monde* (6 June): 9.
Saux, J. L. 1991b. "Les élus d'outre-mer s'interrogent sur la volonté généreuse' du gouvernement." *Le Monde* (7 June): 10-11.
Schiff, G. 1978. "The politics of population in Israel." In *Forum on the Jewish People, Zionism and Israel* 28-29: 173-192.
Spengler, J. J. 1979. *France Faces Depopulation: Postlude Edition, 1936-1976.* Durham, NC: Duke University Press.
Teitelbaum, M. S., and J. M. Winter. 1985. *The Fear of Population Decline.* Orlando, FL: Academic Press.
Tzur, R., and L. Davids. 1984. "Recent population concerns and government action in Israel." *Middle East Focus* 7: 14-27.
United Nations, Department for Economic and Social Information and Policy Analysis. 1996. *Global Population Policy Data Base,* 1995. New York: United Nations.
Yuval-Davis, N. 1989. "National reproduction and 'the demographic race' in Israel." In N. Yuval Davis and F. Anthias (eds.), *Woman-Nation-State*, 92-109. London: MacMillan.

19

Jerusalem's Population, 1995-2020: Demography, Multiculturalism, and Urban Policies

Sergio DellaPergola

Introduction

This chapter presents selected findings from a new set of population projections for the city of Jerusalem over the period 1995-2020 (DellaPergola and Rebhun 1999). The project was initiated at the request of the Jerusalem Municipality's Division for Strategic Planning and Research in the framework of a new multi-disciplinary Strategic Masterplan aimed at developing a broad conceptual and executive framework for Jerusalem urban policies in future decades (Hershkovitz et al. 2000). The committing body as a general background to the broader project suggested three basic working assumptions: a) Jerusalem at peace; b) Jerusalem within present Municipal boundaries; and c) Jerusalem united under Israeli sovereignty. Besides suggesting this general scenario, the Municipality did not interfere with the technical or substantive contents of the present research. An independent team of researchers and consultants directed by the author performed data processing and analysis.

Attention about Jerusalem's population trends evidently transcends the specific case study. Jerusalem represents a main locus of interest in a global perspective focusing on urban administration, planning, and power allocation under conditions of social and cultural diversity and latent or explicit conflict (Guttmann and Klein 1980; Stotkin 1996; Sharkansky 1996; al-Qaq 1997; Kotek 1997; Roman 1997; Kliot and Mansfield 1997; Klein 1999). The city's observed demographic developments, their projected consequences, and possible policy implications reach far beyond the local arena and powerfully evoke broader questions of regional and urban conflict resolution in the Middle East as well as in other parts of the world.

In historical perspective Jerusalem is known to be one of the world's most important and intensive religious and cultural capitals. The city's architecture unveils over 3,000 years of history, with its impressive constructions and excavations of antiquity, the walled Old City, its late-nineteenth and early-twentieth century expansion in the open space, and the large scale developments of the late-twentieth century (Kroyanker 1975-1985). The complex cultural configuration of Jerusalem's population constitutes one of its most fascinating resources and contributes to making the city a unique pole of attraction to the whole inhabitants of Israel and the Middle East, as well as to Jews, Christians, and Muslims worldwide.

Jerusalem's inhabitants comprise a unique combination of diverse human types. Extreme variation appears in population characteristics such as ethnicity—Jews, Arabs and others; religion—Jewish, Muslim, and Christian of several denominations; cultural orientation—from militantly religious to militantly anti-religious; countries of birth and origin—featuring a great variety of sub-ethnic identities; socioeconomic status (SES)—covering the entire range from affluent to poor; and civic status—from full-scale citizen to permanent or temporary resident to refugee. These various traits often overlap among the same individuals, creating a human mosaic of sharply differentiated subpopulations. While each territorial section of the city usually hosts very different types of people, the prevailing tendency is for similar people to aggregate in quite homogeneous residential neighborhoods. Although culturally different groups and communities may be separated by very little physical distance from one another, Jerusalem's prevailing character is that of a social mosaic with rather rigid delineation between different subpopulations.

Overall, Jerusalem is not high in the ranking of Israeli cities by socioeconomic indicators. In 1995 it was included in the fourth lowest decile in a multivariate classification of Israeli local authorities by major social indicators (Choshen and Shahar 1998, table VI/2). The city's economy is dominated by employment in government, research, community, personal, and other services, including a large concentration in public administration (Hershkovitz et al. 1998). The significant presence of traditionalist groups with large families is a factor associated with lower standards of living for these households, and with substantial social gaps within the urban population as a whole.

More significantly, Jerusalem's social and cultural diversity occurs in, and is the product of, a regional context imbued with long-standing, and still unresolved, political and religious tensions (Lapidoth and Hirsch 1994). The continuing disagreement as to Jerusalem's definitive status renders the governance and planning of the city a very complex and sensitive task. Widely differing needs, interests, and expectations—both from inside and outside the city, nationally, regionally, and globally—should be taken into account and carefully weighed in order to maintain a basic equilibrium between competing constituencies and to allow for the harmonious and orderly development of the city as a whole.

In such a multicultural and politically charged context, demographic behaviors tend to be significantly correlated with ethnic identities, religious orientations, and socioeconomic stratification. Indeed, the demographic development of Jerusalem is comprised of quite extreme variations in the overall growth rates of its component subpopulations. Such gaps reflect variation in each of the main demographic determinants of population growth: mortality, fertility, and local, national, and international geographical mobility.

This chapter provides a summary description of variations observed in some of these demographic variables among Jerusalem's population, with special attention to fertility and geographical mobility. Our analysis relates to eight major subpopulations, reflecting various combinations of religio-cultural and socioeconomic factors. Selected results of population projections are presented, reflecting a range of different hypotheses regarding the future demographic development in Jerusalem. Attention is paid to expected changes in population size and age composition—particularly regarding the balance of Jews versus Arabs and others. Within the Jewish population, attention is devoted to the balance of the *Haredi* (from the Hebrew root *harad* = fearful, that is, the more religiously observant and residentially segregated) sections versus the rest. Some implications of the current and expected demographic trends for policy decisions are briefly outlined in the chapter's conclusions.

Jerusalem's Territory and Population Growth

Jerusalem's municipal borders have changed repeatedly in modem history (Gilbert 1977; Gonen 1992; Kimhi 1992; Lapidoth and Hirsch 1994). This mainly reflected the military, political, and administrative events that have shaped the history of Mandatory Palestine between 1918 and 1948, of the State of Israel and its planning authorities since its independence in 1948, and of the Hashemite Kingdom of Jordan between 1948 and 1967. During the last years of the British Mandate (1944-1948), the District of Jerusalem included a very substantial portion of land around the main built-up city. Within the city itself, mostly as a consequence of the disturbances of 1929 and 1936, there emerged a demographic-functional division between two large and rather contiguous territorial areas, one Jewish and one Arab (Schmelz 1973). The 1947 United Nations General Assembly Resolution on the partition of Palestine proposed quite extensive boundaries for the City of Jerusalem. The designated territory was to include the neighboring city of Bethlehem and would become a *corpus separatum* under a special international regime to be administered by the UN (Lapidoth and Hirsch 1994: 6-11). The 1948 war and the 1949 armistice agreements led to the severing of Jerusalem's western sector, under Israeli rule, from the rest of the former Jerusalem district including most of the outer, rural and urbanized parts, under (Trans-) Jordanian rule. The city itself was divided between the western Israeli side, and the eastern Jordanian side with a narrow north-south belt of no-man's-land separating the two.

Between 1948 and 1964, the borders of Israeli (West) Jerusalem were three times somewhat expanded to provide for the city's growing population. Following the Arab-Israeli war of June 1967, the main built-up areas of Jerusalem were reunited under Israeli rule. Soon after, the Israeli government expanded the Jerusalem municipal borders to incorporate a belt of territory to the North, East, and South of the main built-up area, previously held by the Jordanians. This expansion left out substantial portions of both the Jerusalem District as established by the British Mandate in 1944 and the Jerusalem City area as established by the UN in 1947. The latter areas remained under Israel Defense Force (IDF) administration. The enlarged city borders were further expanded westward (i.e. within pre-1967 Israeli territory) in 1985 and more significantly in 1993, determining a total municipal surface of 126 square km.

Following initial implementation of the 1994 Oslo agreements, the IDF turned over parts of the territory it controlled out of and around Jerusalem (as well as other parts of the neighboring West Bank and of the Gaza area) to the direct rule of the Palestinian Authority. Thus, at the time of this writing, the metropolitan area[1] comprised of Jerusalem and its surroundings, and its population was in fact divided between three different authorities: the State of Israel, the Israel Military Administration (and since 1981 its Civil Administration), and the Palestinian Authority. Three major implications followed. First, the status of residents was quite different in terms of citizenship and political rights. Most Arab residents of East Jerusalem had preferred not to accept the option to become Israeli citizens. They could therefore vote in elections for the local municipal authority but not for the Israeli parliament (the Knesset). Second, significant numbers of West Bank Palestinians were employed in the Israeli economy and daily commuted to Jerusalem city and elsewhere. However, freedom of movement between the Palestinian parts of the Jerusalem metropolitan area and the city itself was occasionally limited, especially in response to or as a device to prevent acts of terrorism. Third, the degree of economic development and the standard of living in various parts of Jerusalem's metropolitan area, namely the Jewish and Arab neighborhoods of Jerusalem city, were quite different. Although under unified municipal rule since 1967, the different parts of Jerusalem that had been under Israeli and Jordanian rule before 1967 still displayed clearly different levels of urban development in 1995. A rough contextual indication of the difference is provided by data on average monthly wages for employees in 1996: U.S. $1,536 in Israel, versus U.S. $373 in the West Bank and Gaza (Central Bureau of Statistics 1998a, T. 12.24, 9.13; Palestinian Central Bureau of Statistics 1998, T. 39).

Because of these political and territorial changes, reapportionment, and divisions, and of the sharp migration flows that sometimes accompanied them, the comparison over time of Jerusalem's population size and movements is not easy. However, thanks especially to the systematic research of U.O. Schmelz (1987a, 1987b, 1994) based on British, Israeli, and Jordanian sources, it is possible to quite faithfully reconstruct Jerusalem's population development within a constant territorial framework substantially similar to the contemporary municipal borders (see table 19.1). Within such fixed terms of reference, Jerusalem's population grew from 186,500 in 1946 to 267,800 in 1967, and to 633,700 at the end of 1998 (Central Bureau of Statistics 1999; Choshen and Shahar 1998). The percentage of Jews out of total inhabitants grew from 53.4 percent in 1946 to a peak of 73.5 percent at the end of 1967, and subsequently gradually declined to 68.4 percent in 1998.

These data refer to the *de jure* resident population. It should be noted that based on yearly updates of the 1983 Israeli population census, Jerusalem's total population at the end of 1995 was estimated at 591,400, of which 417,000 Jewish (70.5 percent), 158,600 Muslim (26.8 percent), and 15,800 Christian and other (2.7 percent). According to the Israeli census of November 4, 1995 (published after the completion of our study), Jerusalem's population was 617,000, of which 417,100 (67.6 percent) Jewish, 182,700 (29.6 percent) Muslim, 14,100 (2.3 percent) Christian, and 3,100 (0.5 percent) other and undetermined (Israel CBS, 1998b, T. 1). These figures reportedly over-covered several thousand persons who were present *(de facto)* on census-day but were not city residents. Consequently, the Israeli Central Bureau of Statistics officially revised the figures for the city's total resident population on December 31, 1995, to 602,700, of which 420,900 (69.8 percent) Jewish and 181,800 (30.2 percent) Arabs and others (Central Bureau of Statistics 1999).

Table 19.1
Jerusalem Population, 1946-1998 (According to 1993 Borders)

Year	Total	Jews	Arabs and others	% Jewish
31.12.1946	186,500	99,600	86,900	53.4
22.5.1961[a]	243,900	165,100	78,800	67.7
27.9.1967	267,800	196,800	71,000	73.5
20.5.1972[a]	313,900	230,300	83,600	73.4
4.6.1983[a]	428,700	306,300	122,400	71.4
31.12.1995, original	591,400	417,000	174,400	70.5
4.11.1995[a]	617,000	417,100	199,900	67.6
31.12.1995, revised	602,700	420,900	181,800	69.8
31.12.1997	622,100	429,100	193,000	69.0
31.12.1998	633,700	433,600	200,100	68.4

[a] Israel population census.
Sources: Schmelz, 1994; Israel CBS, 1998b; Choshen and Shahar, 1998.

Observation of Jerusalem population distribution in 1995 by main ethno-religious groups according to the territorial division that prevailed between 1948 and 1967 still reveals the major partition between the predominantly Jewish Western side and the predominantly Arab and other Eastern side (see figure 19.1). On the other hand, the Jewish population underwent an intensive process of expansion through the creation of new neighborhoods and the development of large-scale housing projects in the areas incorporated since 1967. Of the total population estimate of 591,400 in 1995, 263,900 (44.6 percent) lived in the former Western side, 316,900 (53.6 percent) lived in the former Eastern side, and the exact address for 10,600 residents (1.8 percent) was not sufficiently documented (see table 19.2). Of the total Jewish population in 1995, 62.2 percent lived in the Western side and 35.9 percent in the Eastern side. Of the total Arab and other population, 97.9 percent lived in the Eastern side and 0.6 percent in the Western side. Accordingly, while nearly all inhabitants in the former Israeli Western side lived in Jewish areas (99.6 percent), residents in the former Jordanian Eastern side comprised 52.2 percent in veteran Arab and other areas and 47.8 percent in more recently established Jewish areas. These patterns of urban settlement clearly expressed the Israeli policy framework of a unified Jerusalem under Israeli sovereignty, but generated vehement political objection on the Palestinian side (Choshen et al. 1998).

Projections: Data and Assumptions

Base Population

Our study reflects the available estimates of Jerusalem's population size and characteristics on December 31, 1995. Two factors of bias should be mentioned in this respect. In the first place since, as noted, results of the Israeli census of November 4, 1995 were not yet available, we had to rely on population estimates that were subsequently somewhat revised. A second biasing factor in our database derives from the fact that our analysis was conducted at the micro-geographic rather than at the individual level. We initially analyzed and classified Jerusalem's population according to the characteristics of small territorial units (see below). A first partition was made according to whether the population in each area was predominantly composed of Jews or Arabs and others. The Arabs are in their vast majority Palestinians, mostly Muslims with a minority belonging to different Christian denominations. The "others" mostly comprise Christians belonging to various ethnic or national groups, besides a few Druze. The total population of predominantly Jewish areas was 422,000 (71.4 percent) and that of predominantly Arab and other areas was 169,000 (38.6 percent).

Hence the population figures reported in our study tend to slightly over-represent the Jewish component: whereas we evaluate the population of predo-

Figure 19.1
Jerusalem, by Types of Area, 1995

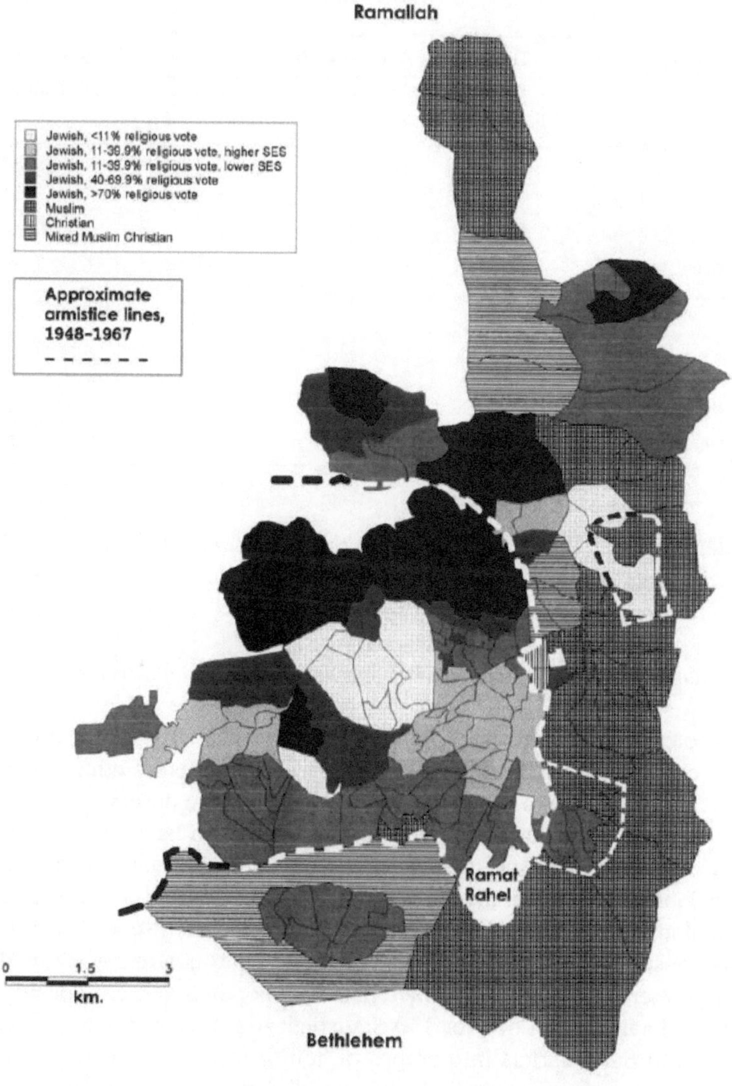

minantly Jewish areas at 71.4 percent of the 1995 city total, the actual percentage of Jewish residents within Jerusalem's municipal borders was 69.8 percent (according to the CBS post-census revision). While these differences do not seriously affect the main results and implications of our study, it is important

Table 19.2
Jerusalem Population Distribution, 1995, According to June 1967 Borders (Percents)

Type of area in 1995	Total 1995	According to 1967 borders: West side (under Israel)	According to 1967 borders: East side (under Jordan)	Residence in 1995 unknown
N	591,449	263,933	316,931	10,585
Column %				
Total	100.0	100.0	100.0	100.0
Jewish	71.4	99.6	47.8	76.6
Arab and Other	29.6	0.4	52.2	23.4
Row %				
Total	100.0	44.6	53.6	1.8
Jewish	100.0	62.2	35.9	1.9
Arab and Other	100.0	0.6	97.9	1.5

to reiterate that all our findings relate to *the inhabitants of neighborhoods with certain characteristics* (e.g., Jewish), and not to *the individual holders of those same characteristics* (e.g., Jews).

Jerusalem's Ethno-Religio-Cultural Subpopulations: Definition and Size

As noted, the goal of our study was to capture the demographic diversity of urban residential neighborhoods characterized by different ethnic, religious, cultural and socioeconomic patterns, and to project the observed trends to the short- and mid-term. Jerusalem, like all major cities in Israel, has a hierarchic system of geographical-statistical divisions for which essential demographic data are available. The broader division comprises eight quarters. The initial level of geographical-statistical detail chosen for our analysis was that of Jerusalem's thirty-five sub-quarters. Where the population of sub-quarters was found to be socially heterogeneous, the characteristics of population were considered at the more detailed level of over 130 Statistical Areas. Hence, where appropriate, we split Sub-quarters into groups of homogeneous contiguous Statistical Areas. In the end, we identified fifty-two different geographical areas, plus two groupings of individuals whose exact place of residence was insufficiently known. Each of these fifty-four urban partitions had internally homogeneous and clearly identified characteristics according to three classification criteria: a) the predominantly Jewish or Arab and other identification of the area residents; b) the degree of religiosity of Jewish areas; and c) the average SES of Jewish areas with intermediate levels of religiosity.

The distinction between Jewish and Arab/other residential neighborhoods was very clear in 1995—with a predominance of 95-100 percent of either type in each instance. There were no difficulties in classifying neighborhoods accordingly. Of the fifty-four areas in our study, forty-one were classified as Jewish, with a total population of 422,000; and thirteen were classified as Arab and other, with a population of 169,000.

The degree of religiosity of Jewish areas was determined according to the frequency of votes for religious parties in the Knesset elections of 1996 (see also Schmelz, 1989). A full range of variation prevails in this respect between areas where nearly 90 percent of the vote was cast for religious parties *(Agudat Israel,* the Askenazic or mostly Central-Eastern-European-origin *Haredi* party; *Shas,* the Sephardic or mostly Asian-African-origin religious party; and *Mafdal,* the National Religious Party), and areas with barely 10 percent of the vote showing the same preferences. The average vote for religious parties in the Jewish areas of Jerusalem was just above 40 percent in 1996. Of the forty-one Jewish areas, a percentage of votes for religious parties of 70 percent or higher was recorded in nine, with a combined population of 124,000; this percentage ranged between 40 percent and 69.9 percent in eight areas, with a population of 45,000; percentages between 11 percent and 39.9 percent were recorded in twenty areas, with a population of 226,000; and four areas had percentages below 11 percent, with a population of 27,000.

The large group of Jewish areas with intermediate percentages of voting for religious parties was further split into areas of higher and lower SES, based on several indicators such as average size of dwellings, frequency of help received from municipal social services within a given area, and voting preferences among nonreligious political parties (another reasonable proxy for social status in the Israeli context). This subdivision of the twenty relevant areas resulted in thirteen of lower SES, with a combined population of 171,000; and seven of higher SES, with a population of 55,000.

Of the thirteen Arab and other areas, seven were predominantly Muslim, with a population of 128,000; two predominantly Christian, with a population of 7,000; and four mixed (though with a Muslim majority in each instance), with a population of 34,000. More than half of the Christians lived in mixed areas other than in the predominantly Christian areas located in Jerusalem's Old City.

These preliminary analyses of the composition of the Jerusalem population resulted in a classification in eight major types, five Jewish and three Arab and other. While our main criteria of classification follow clearly specified ethnic and religious lines, a unified socioeconomic scale can be roughly construed for the whole eight-fold partition. Overall, Jewish areas have a higher SES level than Arab and other areas. Moreover, in Jewish areas, SES levels tend to be negatively correlated with religious voting, and in Arab and other areas SES levels tend to be positively correlated with the percentage of Christians

Table 19.3
Jerusalem Areas, by Major Ethno-Religious Divisions, Percent Voting for Jewish Religious Parties in 1990, Socioeconomic Status, Fertility Levels, and Population in 1995

Type of area	Number of projection areas	Estimated Total Fertility Rate	Population 1995	
			N	%
Total	**54**		**591,000**	**100.0**
Jewish, total	**41**	**3.78**	**422,000**	**71.4**
> 70% religious vote	9	6.37	124,000	21.0
40–69.9% religious vote	8	4.44	45,000	7.6
11–39.9% religious, lower SES	13	2.51	171,000	28.9
11–39.9% religious, higher SES	7	2.51	55,000	9.3
< 11% religious vote	4	1.44	27,000	4.6
Arab and other, total	**13**	**4.90**	**169,000**	**28.6**
Muslim	7	5.29	128,000	21.7
Christian	2	2.79	7,000	1.2
Mixed	4	3.90	34,000	5.8

among the total population. Table 19.3 describes the eight-fold partition of Jerusalem adopted in our study, showing the number of projection areas for various combinations of ethnicity, Jewish religious vote, and SES, as well as fertility level and population size for each type of area. The remainder of this paper mostly refers to these eight partitions. As shown in figure 19.1, these partitions are not necessarily contiguous in geographical terms, but they are highly significant in socio-cultural terms, and expectedly also with regard to demographic processes.

Method and General Assumptions

Population estimates for small urban areas must face problems related to the accuracy of baseline data on size and age composition, especially for those areas which comprise high proportions of students and other temporary residents (Lunn et al. 1998). Such is indeed the case in various parts of Jerusalem. Moreover, it is quite difficult to develop full and different sets of all the assumptions needed for a population projection at the extremely detailed local level.

A different problem concerns a possible discrepancy between projected population figures and the actual physical capability of the city or any of its component areas. Such a discrepancy may be very significant, rendering the results of a population projection actually "impossible." With regard to this last problem, the stated goal of our projections was to illustrate the potential direction of currently visible demographic trends, regardless of physical constraints. The data projected do not in any way constitute a statutory planning scenario (e.g., Sidi et al. 1997) but rather a yardstick against which urban planning may develop. One of the objectives of urban planning may indeed be an attempt to significantly modify the expected results of current demographic processes.

The projections presented here for Jerusalem were separately executed for fifty-four separate micro-areas and aggregated for the eight main subpopulations described above. Population estimates by area, sex, and five-year age groups were projected with the method of component-cohort-specific rates of change.[2]

The components of demographic change and the main assumptions considered are specified in table 19.4. Various combinations of assumptions concerning mortality, fertility, and geographical mobility were implemented. The starting assumption in the current set of projections was continuation of subpopulation-age-sex-specific patterns as they prevailed by the mid-1990s. The background and rationale for these and further assumptions are elaborated in the following sections. The resulting five main projection models display different combinations of relevant demographic variables. In each model, all specified assumptions were simultaneously implemented across the eight subpopulations of the projection. It is obviously possible to create a large number of further scenarios by differently re-combining the various assumptions for each subpopulation.

Mortality Levels

Health and survivorship standards in Israel featured over the years a steady process of general improvement through reduction of absolute gaps between

Table 19.4
Assumptions for Jerusalem Population Projections, 1995-2020

<table>
<tr><th>Variable</th><th>Model 1</th><th>Model 2</th><th>Model 3</th><th>Model 4</th><th>Model 5</th></tr>
<tr><td>1. Life expectancy</td><td colspan="5">Continuing linear increase as in recent years</td></tr>
<tr><td>2. Fertility</td><td colspan="2">As in 1995</td><td>Moderate linear decline</td><td>As in 1995</td><td>Moderate linear decline</td></tr>
<tr><td>3. Internal migration</td><td>None</td><td colspan="4">As in 1995</td></tr>
<tr><td>4. International migration</td><td colspan="3">None</td><td colspan="2">As in 1995</td></tr>
</table>

subpopulations (DellaPergola 1993). Survivorship rates were higher among Jews than among Arabs and others but that edge tended to decline over time. Among the Jewish population socioeconomic status was positively related to higher life-expectancy, but religiosity—while negatively related with socioeconomic status—determined independent and significant rising effects (Friedlander et al., see chapter 11). Jerusalem's population rates featured overall higher than average levels of life-expectancy as compared with other Israeli localities. Geographic origin determined mixed effects of declining intensity. Mortality of Jews of European origin—overall of a higher than average socioeconomic status—was intermediate between the lower one of Jews of Asian origin and the higher one of Jews of African origin—both of a lower than average socioeconomic status (Eisenbach 1994). In view of these findings it was reasonable to assume similar age-specific mortality levels across different Jewish residential areas. In our projections, based on the latest available life-table (Central Bureau of Statistics 1999) we posited the same initial level of life-expectancy (75.9 for men and 79.1 for women) for all of Jerusalem's Jewish divisions. A slightly lower level (73.8 for men and 77.1 for women) was assumed for all Arab and other divisions. Mortality levels were expected to continue their declining course. Extending the Israeli experience of the last several decades, we assumed an increase of one year of life-expectancy at birth for each five-year period, or a total increase of five years of life-expectancy by 2020 across all subpopulations.

The Role of Fertility in Jerusalem's Population

Fertility Measures

Population projections require, among other data, detailed information about ongoing and expected fertility patterns. At the time of this writing, no recent or accurate measure of fertility was available for the various Jerusalem subpopulations that constitute the object of this study. Data needed to compute a TFR for each small geographic division ideally would include census data on population composition by sex and age, and current vital statistics on births by age of mothers in the same geographical divisions. Currently available birth records do specify certain socially relevant characteristics of mothers, such as residential address, religion and/or ethnicity, and age, but they do not provide information on other personal characteristics, such as the degree of religiosity. As to available population estimates, they exist at the aggregate level of geographical divisions, and do provide information on age and sex, but not on religiosity. Census data, but not inter-censal population estimates like the ones we used, provide information on socioeconomic characteristics. TFRs for specific subpopulations can therefore only be inferred through indirect methods of operationalization.

Detailed evaluation of current fertility levels requires linkage of recent vital statistics on births to the population characteristics of the areas of residence of mothers (Schmelz 1989). As noted above, though, when we undertook our study, the available 1995 population database for small areas derived from repeated up dating of the 1983 census. The amount of error due to mismatches between the two different sources on births and on population would subject the findings to serious bias. Using accurate TFRs computed shortly after the 1983 census as a baseline for adjusted TFRs around 1995 would solve this problem. While feasible within a relatively short time lag from 1983 (Municipality of Jerusalem 1992), this procedure would be unsatisfactory in the light of the amount of change undergone by Israeli society over that twelve-year span. Another solution would be to use the Israel Labor Force Survey, which provides information on the number of own children at home, by personal characteristics of parents (Berman and Klinov 1997; Berman 1998). Information on the educational experience of husbands and wives, namely past or ongoing enrolment in *Yeshiva* (religious) education, may provide an indirect criterion for identifying the more religious. However, a national sample does not allow the computation of a set of TFRs for small urban geographical areas.

In order to estimate a set of TFRs by detailed geographical divisions in 1995 we relied on an indirect method using adjusted child-woman ratios (CWR, number of children aged 0-4 divided by number of women aged 15-49)—a rough measure of fertility based on population age composition. First, CWRs were computed from available data on the population's age composition for each of Jerusalem's geographical divisions. Next, standard CWRs were computed from model life-tables for populations with life expectancies equal to those estimated for the actual populations (Coale et al. 1983). According to model life-table assumptions of a stationary population, at a growth rate of 0 a Net Reproduction Rate (NRR) equal to 1 corresponds to a TFR of 2.1. The comparisons of actual CWRs to model life-table CWRs provide a measure of the difference between actual fertility and the fertility expected under the hypothetical conditions of a model stationary population, namely a multiplier or a de-multiplier of the standard 2.1 TFR (Bachi 1967).[3] The TFRs thus obtained are evidently no more than an approximation, though they have the advantage of consistency.

Fertility Levels and Differentials: Data and Determinants

Fertility levels and differentials represent one of the leading determinants of population growth in Jerusalem. As a general characterization, fertility levels in Jerusalem were comparatively high and sharply different across subpopulations in the broader context of comparatively high and stable fertility in Israel and in the Palestinian Territories. We estimated in 1995 a TFR of 3.78 for the total population of Jerusalem's Jewish areas, versus a national average of 2.53 for Jews in Israel, and 4.90 for Jerusalem's Arab and other parts, versus a national Israeli average of 4.09 for Arabs and others (of which: Muslims, 4.69; Christians,

2.44) (Central Bureau of Statistics 1999). In all empirically observed fertility schedules the highest levels are obtained at age 25-29. Our TFR estimates for the various Jerusalem subpopulations reached high average values of 6.37 in the more religiously oriented areas of Jewish population,[4] and 5.29 in predominantly Muslim areas, and lower values of 1.44 in the least religiously oriented areas of Jewish population, and 2.79 in predominantly Christian areas (see table 19.3). These estimates imply widely different growth rates among the respective subpopulations in Jerusalem. The city's fertility levels were quite above the average for both Jews and Arabs in Israel and below the average for Muslims in the Palestinian Territories. In 1995 the TFR was evaluated at 5.44 for the West Bank and 7.41 for the Gaza area, and at 6.16 for Muslims and 2.59 for Christians for both areas together (Palestinian Central Bureau of Statistics 1997).

Although still seeking for definitive explanation, fertility levels in Israel—namely among *Haredi* Jews and Muslims—and in the Palestinian Territories and their relation to cultural and socioeconomic determinants have attracted scholarly attention (Bachi 1976; Eisenbach 1986; Goldscheider and Friedlander 1986; Schmelz 1989; Peritz and Baras 1992; Abu Libdeh et al. 1993; Friedlander and Feldmann, see chapter 2; Anson and Meir, see chapter 3). While the chain of causal relations in fertility levels is sufficiently known (Van de Kaa 1996; Pritchett 1994), recent fertility trends in Jerusalem and the rationale for assuming future changes call for more systematic evaluation.

In the context of our study, fertility variables can be organized in a five-tier sequence. First, *proximate determinants* (Bongaarts 1978)—the immediately preceding bio-demographic causal factors of fertility—instrumentally affect the chance of initiating a new pregnancy and of completing one with a live birth. Second, interventions to enhance or depress the effects of proximate determinants actually reflect *household-level* or *micro-socioeconomic* strategies. These synthesize the value-oriented desirability of children in general and of a child of specific parity in particular, the cost-related feasibility of childbearing and child rearing, and household availability of relevant means, resources and tools (Spengler 1966).

The dilemmas and negotiations of individual households inherent in the potential conflicts between identity and sentiment, on the one hand, and economic rationality, on the other hand, are better evaluated in their *community context*—the third explanatory level. Perceptions broadly shared with one's close environment tend to influence individual family growth behaviors. The role of community influences is especially important in a socio-cultural environment diverse such as Jerusalem's. In this respect five groups of factors call for special attention:

1. *Traditional culture and organization,* or a group's religious and social norms concerning fertility as well as community frameworks and institutions

established for implementing those norms, is a natural source of inter-group differences. Traditional Judaism, Islam, and Christianity, each in their own distinctive ways, carry an explicit pro-natal stance. In traditional Judaism, more explicitly than in other religious frameworks, the principle goes together with definite prescriptions affecting each of fertility's proximate variables (DellaPergola 1988). Traditional Judaism also gives high priority in children's prolonged religious education, but community investments to the same effect may reduce its cost to individual families. Community mechanisms of communication, social control and sanction explain why the more religious individuals generally conform more strictly to each religious group's declared fertility precepts.

2. *Minority/majority status* reflects in the first place past situations of actual legal discrimination or, more relevant to the contemporary experience, community-based subjective perceptions of dependence/dominance relative to the majority of society or other minorities within it. Such perceptions may psychologically affect group propensities to expand or restrain (Goldscheider 1971; Rallu et al. 1997). Minorities may feel pressured to concentrate on the better quality of fewer children to overcome the odds of possible discrimination. Minorities may also consciously try to maximize their natural increase as a mechanism to expand their share of the total population. In Jerusalem, the latter may be the case for communities that feel their lifestyle endangered, such as the *Haredim,* or whose advocacy for political goals requires the support of numbers, such as the Palestinians (Steinberg 1989).

3. *Social class stratification,* namely occupational status and specialization, implies significant differences in perceived interests and access to resources. Shared perceptions of the role of children as potential providers or dependents tend to generate widely different strategies of family growth (Lesthaeghe and Wilson 1986). Other things being equal, social mobility of individuals within a subpopulation or of a whole subpopulation relative to the rest of society may translate into significant fertility change.

4. *Knowledge* obtained through formal education or other channels affects fertility especially via community level awareness of fertility control opportunities and understanding of their mode of operation. In this respect, it would be mistaken to equate religious traditionalism with lack of information. Traditionalism in contemporary societies tends to shift from repudiation of modernity to selectively choosing from modernity those elements compatible with or even supportive of traditional goals (Hammel 1990).

5. *Biological constraints,* such as inherited diseases and other health-related factors, often tied to strict community homogamy, affected fertility differentials in the past but loose importance in contemporary more open and heterogamic societies (Bonné-Tamir and Adam 1992).

National or collective policy interventions provide a fourth explanatory level. Israel's social policies do reflect some general concern with family formation and growth (regardless of the citizens' religion or ethnicity). Means for birth control, while not encouraged are easily available. Abortion is strictly regulated but feasible through public health facilities. The actual impact of Israel's pro-natalist stance tends to be moderate and mostly felt by specific subpopulations.

1. *Direct governmental provisions* such as transfer payments (allowances to children below eighteen) pertain to all relevant households. The Israeli Social Security system offers moderately benign provisions to working women in the case of maternity. Comparatively easy availability of child-care and educational facilities is a facilitating (or rather not a preventing) factor in family growth in Israel. The high cost of housing is the main constraint perceived by families wishing to increase their number of children (Ziegler 1995).

2. *Indirect governmental provisions* are especially significant at the community level. Collective exemption from otherwise universal, three-year compulsory military service applies in Israel to Muslim and Christian Arabs (though not to the Druze community), as well as to the majority of the *Haredi* Jewish population. Military exemption facilitates lower ages at marriage and a longer exposure to the chance of childbearing. Moreover, transfer payments at the community level, in particular public financing of community-specific educational networks or housing projects may significantly reduce the given community's cost of children.

3. *Non-governmental provisions* of a similar nature may derive from the intervention of groups and agencies from Diasporas abroad, whether Jewish or Palestinian, or from other private sources of cultural and political support locally. The main effect on fertility of relevant services and subsidies provided operates, again, through reducing the cost of children.

A fifth explanatory level reflects the continual flow of civilization, in particular political, socioeconomic, cultural and technological change, subsumed under the general definition of *modernization,* and its enhanced *global effects* on local populations through diffused media and communication networks. Broad transformations of macro-economic patterns, standards of living, contents and boundaries of community identities and individual *mentalités* may significantly affect demographic patterns (Inglehart 1997; Lesthaeghe and Moors 1995). The comparative evidence points to predominantly lowering effects on fertility levels. However, technological advances are of special interest inasmuch a previous generation of scientific research greatly enhanced fertility control, while more recent advances have focused on overcoming fecundity impairments.

Given such complex and multi-level package of explanatory determinants of fertility, its overall effects in a multicultural context like Jerusalem's are expectedly mixed. Because of: a) the high resilience of the socio-cultural components related to higher fertility, b) the possibly contradictory and compensatory trends of fertility change among different groups and communities, and c) compensatory trends within each subpopulation, it is reasonable to expect future fertility changes to occur at a slow pace. On the other hand, each subpopulation tends to recombine differently the various factors leading to high and low fertility levels, resulting in an extremely wide range of differentiation.

In our projections, one initial assumption concerned the possible continuation of current fertility levels for each of the eight subpopulations. The main alternative scenario suggests a gradual moderate reduction in fertility levels of about 5 percent per five-year period, or 18 percent over the whole period 1995-2020. These changes were posited across subpopulations, in accordance with the expected continuation of current fertility differentials. It should be noted that a certain amount of fertility variation appears within each of Jerusalem's eight main types of areas. In order to avoid undue variation possibly connected with the insufficient quality of the fertility estimates for small populations, projections were computed using the average TFR for each of the eight subpopulations, rather than for the fifty-four detailed projection areas.

Jerusalem Migration Balance

Assumptions tested in the projections included a possible absence of migration, or rather the prevalence of zero migration balances, versus a continuation of the current impact of inter-city, intra-city, and international migration. In each instance such impact was measured through age-sex-specific rates for each of fifty-four projection areas.

Inter-City

Migration into, out of and within Jerusalem is a powerful factor of demographic change, affecting population size and composition. Since the early 1980s, and more intensely since the early 1990s, Jerusalem has experienced a negative balance of migration with other localities in Israel. During the mid-1990s, around 9-10,000 persons moved to Jerusalem annually from other places in Israel, and about 15-16,000 left the city for other places. The ensuing negative balance fluctuated around -5,000-6,000 persons, nearly all residents of the Jewish parts of the city. Over 80 percent of this internal migration deficit occurred to the benefit of other localities within the Jerusalem District (the Israeli administrative division comprising Jerusalem city) and the neighboring Judea and Samaria District (the administrative jurisdiction for the Israeli inhabitants of the West Bank). Such mobility patterns, from the central city to suburban areas where housing tends to be less expensive, are typical of most large metropolitan areas and therefore cannot be construed as especially related to the particular socio-cultural, economic or political configuration of Jerusalem. Nonetheless, the impact of inter-city mobility on Jerusalem's population size and composition is significant.

Of the negative inter-city migration balance of over 5,500 in 1995, about 24 percent came from the economically more established Jewish parts of the city that comprised 17 percent of the Jewish population. On the other hand, 30 percent of the negative balance came from the more religious Jewish areas reflecting the weight of these areas that comprised 29 percent of Jerusalem's population. Notably, the share of these same areas in the negative population balance was 73 percent among young adults aged 20-24, 38 percent among those aged 15-19, and 41 percent among children aged 0-4. This geographical mobility implied significant consequences for the future demographic development in Jerusalem, as a considerable part of the reproductive potential of the more religious Jewish subpopulation was transferred elsewhere, though not at great geographic distance.

Overall, inter-city migration tended to be a factor of aging for the Jewish population, as the age composition of the migration deficit was significantly younger than that of the resident population. As to the Arab and other parts of Jerusalem, the available data pointed to little or no propensity to leave, whereas other evidence indicated a continuing propensity to migrate into the city, especially into the Muslim areas (Central Bureau of Statistics 1999). On the other hand, historical evidence points to a significant trend for Christian Arabs to leave the city for other locations in the area, and to other countries (Bachi 1976).

Intra-City

Changes of address within Jerusalem constituted a further element of population transformation. Data for 1995 relating to about 31,000 intra-city moves show a predominant tendency to move from one location to another within the same type of neighborhood, as defined in our eight-fold typology of subpopulations. This pattern comprised 58 percent of all moves, but 61 percent of moves originating from the very religious Jewish areas of Jerusalem, 72 percent of moves originating from areas with intermediate religious voting and lower socioeconomic status, and 77 percent of moves from predominantly Muslim areas. Overall, the full matrix of intra-city moves determined net population gains in Jewish areas with intermediate frequencies of religious voting and a lower socioeconomic status. In 1995, these areas experienced a net gain of over 2,000 migrants, about one quarter of who came from highly religious areas. All other types of neighborhood, Jewish as well as Arab and others had negative intra-city migration balances. Intra-city movement between Jewish and Arab and other areas resulted in a net transfer of 200 to the Jewish areas.

These residential changes do not necessarily point to an expansion of the more religious population into neighborhoods with different characteristics. If this were true, the character of residential areas might shift from one cultural type to another, eventually determining a new citywide balance. However, it is also possible that people moving out of the more religious neighborhoods may eventually adapt their lifestyle to that of their new places of residence. While the former process is impressionistically more visible, the latter has been more significantly documented in historical perspective (Levy et al. 1993).

International Migration

Immigration to Israel *(aliyah)* and the absorption of part of it in Jerusalem consistently was a significant factor affecting population growth and territorial distribution. The impact of immigration varied over time, as did the geographical composition of countries of origin (DellaPergola 1998). Throughout the 1980s Jerusalem was absorbing approximately 2,500 immigrants each year. This increased in 1990 and 1991 to about 14,000 a year (Hershkovitz et al. 1998). During the mid-1990s Jerusalem received a yearly average of nearly 5,000 new immigrants or 7 percent of the countrywide total- a lower figure than Jerusalem's share out of the total Israeli population. In recent years, mostly secular Jewish households from the Former Soviet Union (FSU) and comparatively more traditional Jews from North America and other western countries comprised the dominant share of new immigrants to Jerusalem. Many of these new immigrants settled in areas characterized by intermediate religious voting and lower SES. Our projection assumptions duly considered the fact that the overall volume of immigration to Israel is bound to diminish with the progressive exhaustion of the main Jewish population reservoir in the FSU.

Population Prospective

Size and Share of Subpopulations

Table 19.5 summarizes the total population projected for Jerusalem in the year 2020 according to the alternative hypotheses inherent in our five models. We recall that in 1995 Jerusalem's population was estimated at 591,400, of which 422,400 in the Jewish areas (71.4 percent) and 169,000 in the Arab and other parts (28.6 percent). According to the projections, the city total might grow to a figure between 845,000 (Model 3) and 1,088,000 (Model 1) by 2020. Of these, 487,000 to 707,000 (57 percent to 65 percent) would live in the Jewish parts of the city and 358,000 to 384,000 (35 percent to 43 percent) would live in the Arab and other parts.

The various subpopulations distinguished in the projections are assumed to develop at different paces, in accordance with currently observed trends and the further assumptions in each model. The strongest decline in the share of Jewish population out of Jerusalem's total would occur with a zero balance of international migration, in the presence of a negative Jewish internal migration balance and no change in fertility (Model 2). Minimum decline would occur in the case of lack of migrations, with natural increase continuing at steady fertility levels (Model 1). The share of the more religious parts out of Jerusalem's total Jewish population would be highest under complete lack of migrations with steady fertility levels (Model 1), and lowest in the case of a continuation of present trends in internal and international migrations with a lowering in fertility (Model 5).

The bottom part of table 19.5 illustrates the incidence expected of each of the different components of population change according to the various assumptions adopted in the five projections. Since these projections extrapolate over time the known effects of current trends, the balance of inter-city migration would expectedly continue to be negative and significantly subtract inhabitants from Jerusalem. Such prospective migration deficit might cumulate to a total loss of 192,000 inhabitants over the period 1995-2020, all of them from Jerusalem's Jewish areas. On the other hand, international migration might bring an additional 106,000 inhabitants, practically all in the Jewish areas. The impact of a decline in fertility (which we assumed to be moderate) might cause a reduction

Table 19.5
Summary of Jerusalem Population Projections, 1995-2020

Projection model	Type of area			% in Jewish areas out of total population	% in areas with high religious voting out of total in Jewish areas
	Total	Jewish	Arab and other		
Base population 1995	**591,400**	**422,400**	**169,000**	**71.4**	**29.4**
Population in 2020:					
1. Natural increase only, steady fertility	1,088,000	707,000	381,000	65.0	42.3
2. With internal migration, steady fertility	896,000	512,000	384,000	57.1	35.7
3. With internal migration, declining fertility	845,000	487,000	358,000	57.6	35.3
4. With international migration, steady fertility	1,002,000	618,000	384,000	61.7	32.8
5. With international migration, declining fertility	947,000	589,000	358,000	62.2	32.3
Summary of effects (difference):					
Internal migration (Models 2 – 1)	–192,000	–195,000	+3,000		
International migration (Models 4 – 2)	+106,000	+106,000	0		
Fertility decline (Models 5 – 4)	–55,000	–29,000	–26,000		

of 55,000 people, split nearly equally between the Jewish and the Arab and other parts of the city.

Model 5, which incorporates more assumptions, also appears as a more likely scenario than others do. In the following we focus on this particular scenario and present selected additional findings from it. The changing weights of Jerusalem's different subpopulations may significantly alter the overall profile of the city. As already noted, the population is expected to grow at a faster rate in Jerusalem's Arab and other areas than in the Jewish areas. High fertility among Jerusalem's Muslim population and the negative inter-city migration balance among Jews are the main determinants of these expected changes. Of the total population increase of 356,000 people up to 2020, over 53 percent are bound to occur in the Arab and other city parts (see table 19.6).

Within the Jewish population, the major increase in absolute terms is expected to affect especially the neighborhoods with intermediate religious voting and lower SES. Their share is also expected to increase significantly from 40-41 percent to 47 percent of the total population of Jewish areas. Increase in the population of the more religious parts of the city is expected too, but to a lesser extent. The share of these areas should increase from 29 percent in 1995 to 32 percent in 2020. As noted, a large part of the high natural increase of this subpopulation is drawn out of Jerusalem in the process of inter-city migration. A decline is expected in the share of Jewish population in the strongly though not extremely religious parts of the city (where voting for religious parties reaches 40-70 percent). A highly significant finding is the prospective decline, both in absolute and relative terms, of the more economically established subpopulations, associated with intermediate or low voting for religious parties. If present demographic trends continue, the latter two categories combined are expected to lose 14,000 people, while their joint share of the Jewish population would diminish from 19 percent in 1995 to 11 percent in 2020.

In Jerusalem's Arab and other parts, the Muslim predominance is bound to increase even more than at present relative to the Christian and religiously mixed areas.

Age Composition

Jerusalem's population composition by age is comparatively young. In 1995, about 35 percent of the total population were aged 0-14, versus 8 percent aged sixty-five and over. A moderate process of aging is expected to occur by 2020, when (according to projection Model 5) the proportion at ages 0-14 would decline to 31 percent and that of the elderly would increase to 9 percent.

The age profiles of the several Jerusalem sub populations analyzed here are displayed in figure 19.2. The left-hand part refers to the situation in 1995, and the right-hand part to the 2020 projection. Partly because the present set of projections reflects an assumption of moderately declining fertility, a common

Table 19.6
Jerusalem Population, by Type of Area, 1995-2020 (Model 5: Declining Fertility, Continuing Internal and International Migration)

Type of area	1995		2020		Difference	
	Number	%	Number	%	Number	%
Total	**591,000**	**100.0**	**947,000**	**100.0**	**+356,000**	**100.0**
Jewish	422,000	71.4	589,000	62.2	+167,000	46.9
Arab and other	169,000	28.6	358,000	37.8	+189,000	53.1
Jewish, total	**422,000**	**100.0**	**589,000**	**100.0**	**+167,000**	**100.0**
> 70% religious vote	124,000	29.4	190,000	32.3	+66,000	39.5
40–69.9% religious vote	45,000	10.7	53,000	9.0	+8,000	4.8
11–39.9% religious, lower SES	171,000	40.5	278,000	47.2	+107,000	64.1
11–39.9% religious, higher SES	55,000	13.0	45,000	7.6	−10,000	−6.0
< 11% religious vote	27,000	6.4	23,000	3.9	−4,000	−2.4
Arab and other, total	**169,000**	**100.0**	**358,000**	**100.0**	**+189,000**	**100.0**
Muslim	128,000	75.8	286,000	79.9	+158,000	83.6
Christian	7,000	4.1	9,000	2.5	+2,000	1.0
Mixed	34,000	20.1	63,000	17.6	+29,000	15.4

trend toward population aging is clearly visible in the graphs. The striking age-structural differences provide a cross-section of the whole gamut of positions along a continuum of demographic transition. Differences in demographic behaviors and their translation in terms of population composition are a frequent feature in developing or more developed societies, often reflecting rural-urban residential differentials. What is less usual in these data is that each of the population groups examined has experienced exposure to an urban environment, ranging from relatively recent to extremely prolonged. Interesting parallelisms appear from comparing the different subpopulations. Highly religious Jewish and Muslim parts of Jerusalem have populations with quite similar young age compositions, as the consequence of continuing high fertility. The stronger effects of migration, though, are visible in the Jewish religious areas. Structural similarity also appears between the Jewish areas with intermediate religious voting and a lower SES, and the Christian areas. The marked to extreme aging of the Jewish subpopulations with lower religious voting and higher SES closely resembles the age profile of contemporary Jewish communities out of Israel, which have experienced delayed marriage and low fertility over the last several decades (DellaPergola 1999).

Table 19.7 illustrates the expected changes in the age composition of Jerusalem's total population, and outlines the changing share in Jewish areas out of the total in each age group. Similarly, the table shows the share of Jews in highly religious areas of the total population in Jewish areas in each age group. The proportion in Jewish areas out of the total population tends to decrease steadily with the passage from older to younger age groups. In 1995 it represented 88 percent at age seventy-five and over, and gradually decreased to 64 percent of the 0-4 age group. These structural differences reflect higher mortality among certain subpopulations in the past, different fertility rates among Jews, Arabs and others, as well as inter-city migration patterns, especially regarding young adults and their children. The age composition of new immigrants from abroad is older on average than that of the receiving population, though it appears to be significantly younger than that of Jewish communities in the countries of origin (DellaPergola 1999). In 2020, even stronger variation should appear in the percentages living in Jewish areas out of the total population in each age group. This share would approach 54 percent among children aged 0-4, and 56 percent among all other age groups below twenty-five. At the other end of the age spectrum, Jews would comprise 83 percent of the elderly above seventy-five.

With regard to the percentage of population in the more intensely religious areas out of the total Jewish population, in 1995 they constituted 44 percent of the 0-4 age group, and their share gradually decreased with age, reaching 22 percent of the Jewish population aged seventy-five and over. This situation is expected to remain similar in 2020, with some further increase in the weight of the more religious sections of the total of children and younger adults. The proportion of the more religious section of the total Jewish population would be 45-47 percent below age ten, 40-42 percent at ages 10-19, around 30 percent at ages 20-24, and would decline further to a minimum of 18 percent among the over seventy-five age group.

Table 19.7
Jerusalem Population by Age Groups and Types of Area, 1995-2020 (Model 5: Declining Fertility, Continuing Internal and International Migration)

Age	Total population distribution		% in Jewish areas out of total in age-group		% in areas with high religious voting out of total in Jewish area		Total population growth
	1995	2020	1995	2020	1995	2020	1995–2020
Total n.	**591,000**	**947,000**					**356,000**
Total %	**100.0**	**100.0**	**71.4**	**62.2**	**29.4**	**32.3**	**100.0**
0–4	13.3	11.3	63.8	53.8	44.0	46.9	8.1
5–9	11.6	10.5	68.3	55.7	42.4	45.3	8.7
10–14	10.2	9.6	67.2	55.8	37.7	42.5	8.7
15–19	8.9	9.1	65.3	56.4	32.9	40.3	9.3
20–24	8.2	8.3	66.7	56.1	23.3	32.1	8.6
25–44	25.9	25.7	73.2	64.0	24.3	29.1	25.4
45–64	13.9	16.3	79.4	69.2	18.9	22.3	20.4
65–74	4.7	5.5	84.9	78.6	19.2	19.8	6.8
75+	3.3	3.6	87.6	83.4	21.7	17.9	4.0

Table 19.8
Percentages of Change in Jerusalem Projected Population, 1995-2020, by Type of Area and Age (Model 5: Declining Fertility, Continuing Internal and International Migration)

Type of area	0–4	5–9	10–14	15–19	20–24	25–44	45–64	65–74	75+	Total
Total	**36.3**	**45.0**	**51.4**	**62.8**	**63.4**	**59.0**	**88.1**	**87.9**	**72.0**	**60.1**
Jewish, total	**15.1**	**18.3**	**25.6**	**40.5**	**37.3**	**38.9**	**64.1**	**74.0**	**63.8**	**39.4**
> 70% religious vote	22.8	26.2	41.7	71.8	89.2	66.2	93.5	79.6	35.1	53.2
40–69.9% religious vote	–2.1	5.2	20.2	47.0	37.7	9.5	41.3	–7.3	24.2	17.5
11–39.9% rel., lo. SES	27.5	28.8	28.2	38.8	47.3	60.4	95.2	157.3	134.9	61.9
11–39.9% rel., hi. SES	–27.5	–23.2	–17.0	–14.4	–30.7	–18.1	–23.0	–15.3	15.5	–17.7
< 11% religious vote	–44.5	–41.9	–43.0	–41.3	–46.4	–38.5	40.7	38.8	69.5	–14.7
Arab and other, total	**73.8**	**102.5**	**104.5**	**104.9**	**115.7**	**113.9**	**180.4**	**166.1**	**130.0**	**112.0**
Muslim	81.5	112.7	119.1	113.8	127.3	126.3	216.5	206.0	183.4	124.5
Christian	8.8	18.5	27.4	17.2	6.4	27.4	33.7	31.8	38.9	24.1
Mixed	46.7	70.5	59.5	82.0	91.7	89.2	131.3	129.3	78.8	83.3

The amount of population growth expected in Jerusalem by 2020 and its age distribution are shown in the column furthest to the right in table 19.7. This would consist of 356,000 people, including 91,000 children aged below 15, 64,000 aged 15-24, 90,000 aged 25-44, 72,000 aged 45-64, and 39,000 aged sixty-five and over.

Percent-wise, the additional population expected in Jerusalem will be distributed quite differently than the population of 1995. Relative to the 1995 baseline, by the year 2020 the city's total population should grow by 60 percent (according to Model 5, see table 19.8). However, sharp differences in the pace of growth characterize different combinations of subpopulations and age groups. While the overall increase is expected to be greatest at ages 45-64 and 65-74 (88 percent) and smallest at age 0-4 (36 percent), inter-group variation patterns are especially noteworthy. In the highly religious Jewish areas, significant population increases are expected over the whole labor force age-span. Among the Jewish areas with lower religious voting and better SES, actual population decreases are expected at most ages, excluding the elderly, with prospective declines of over 40 percent among children and youth in Jewish areas with very low religious voting. The most extreme rates of increase are projected in Jerusalem's Muslim areas, whose population is expected to more than double above age five, with peaks of over 200 percent growth at ages forty-five to sixty-four and sixty-five to seventy-four.

These data on the prospective transformations of Jerusalem's population by age-composition carry enormous policy implications. Careful attention is called for the types, amounts and location of investments needed in the fields of education, employment, housing, health services, community facilities, and care for the elderly.

Figure 19.2
Jerusalem Population, by Types of Area and Age, 1995-2020 (Percentages)

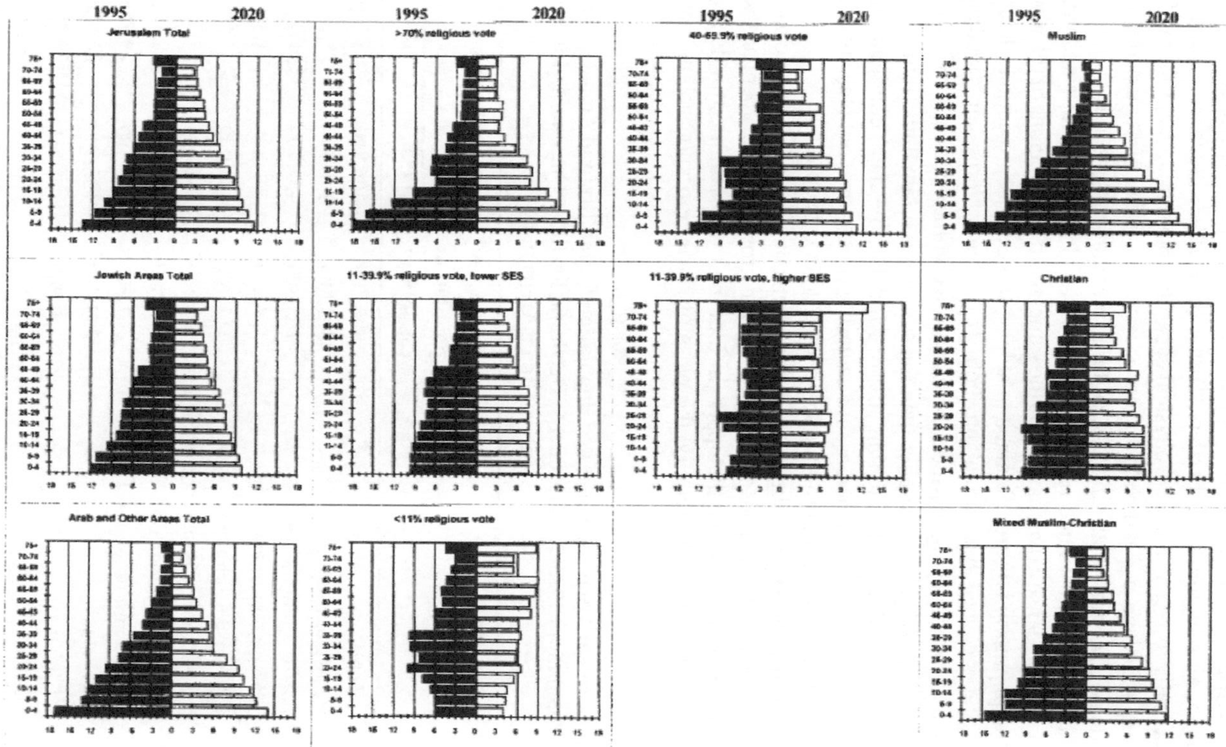

Spatial Constraints

Jerusalem's maximum carrying capacity has been evaluated at about 900,000 inhabitants (within 1993 borders: Turner et al. 1997). Such an evaluation does not really reflect an absolute physical capability but rather an optimum of private and public land-use and built-up versus open spaces for residential, institutional, industrial, commercial, religious, cultural, recreational, and transportation needs. That optimum estimate reflects among other things cultural standards about population density that may not be the same in different regions of the world. The total population figures obtained in at least some of the projections discussed in this paper exceed that optimal threshold. In particular, Jerusalem's total projected population according to Model 5—the more complex and in our view the more likely-is nearly 50,000 higher than the suggested optimal maximum (see table 19.9). According to (quite unrealistic) Model 1, the mere continuation of the current pace of natural increase for each subpopulation would lead to exceeding the stated ecological optimum by nearly 200,000 people.

The problem is in reality more acute when considering that some parts of Jerusalem still offer ample space for population growth, while other parts will very soon, or already do face the upper limit of their opportunities for demographic expansion. Not unexpectedly, the parts of Jerusalem approaching population

Table 19.9
Jersusalem Areas, by Suggested Population Capability, and Actual or Projected Population, 1995-2020 (Model 5: Declining Fertility, Continuing Internal and International Migration)

Type of area	Suggested population capability[a]	Difference population – capability	
		1995	2020[b]
Total	**898,300**	**–306,900**	**48,200**
Jewish, total	**531,000**	**–108,500**	**57,700**
> 70% religious vote	158,300	–34,400	31,600
40–69.9% religious vote	54,400	–9,200	–1,300
11–39.9% religious, lower SES	213,000	–41,600	64,500
11–39.9% religious, higher SES	63,500	–8,400	–18,200
< 11% religious vote	41,800	–14,900	–18,800
Arab and other, total	**367,300**	**–198,400**	**–9,500**
Muslim	263,300	–135,700	22,900
Christian	6,900	–0	1,700
Mixed	97,100	–62,700	–34,000

[a] Turner et al. (1997).
[b] Areas where population would exceed capability are shaded.

saturation are those with the highest rates of growth: Jewish areas with more intensely religious population, Jewish areas with intermediate levels of religious voting and lower SES, and predominantly Muslim areas. Areas where expected demographic trends leave space for further population expansion beyond 2020 include the Jewish areas with intermediate or low religious voting and a higher SES, and the areas with a mixed Muslim-Christian population.

Overview and Conclusions

Discussion

From the demographic data and scenarios outlined in this paper, it is quite clear that the total population of Jerusalem is bound to increase quite substantially in future decades. At the same time, the many imponderables—political, economic, social—concerning the future of Jerusalem render the demographic scenarios presented here as only part of a broader range of possible developments (Morley and Schachar 1986). Notably, the question of the definitive international status of Jerusalem has been deferred to the final stage of negotiations between the Government of Israel and the Palestinian Authority.

Population trends are tightly correlated with employment and housing opportunities existing locally, with the offer and quality of public services available, and with the general character of the metropolitan area centered in Jerusalem and around it. Although characteristics of the Jerusalem metropolitan area were not discussed in this paper, it should be noted that Jerusalem-based institutions provide employment and educational, health, and other services to a much broader population spread over the whole metropolitan area. However the two fundamental criteria by which the future of Jerusalem will be determined concern the cultural balance between different subpopulations that coexist in the city, and the quality of life in relation to the physical environment. Ideally in the unique ethnic, social, and cultural situation outlined here—and more generally in any major city characterized by significant internal diversity—population size and composition would reflect the harmonious weighing and balancing of different socio-demographic forces. Special attention should be given to the equilibrium between population and physical constraints on the one hand, and preservation of the existing equilibrium between the various existing subpopulations on the other hand.

In reality, the different growth rates of the various subpopulations, each related to a particular set of determinants, tend to produce significant departures from the current socio-cultural and ecological equilibrium, which may in turn lead to further departures from a preferred course of socio-demographic development. Regarding the ecological constraints, the population growth projected by 2020 tends to exceed the suggested city's optimum physical capability. The new and still uninhabited areas of Jerusalem incorporated after 1993 may provide some solution to the issues outlined here. Yet, among future scenarios to be taken into account, the possibility exists that a certain type of subpopulation whose territorial resources have dried up would try to expand its presence into areas that naturally represent future areas of expansion for a different sub population. Under the present configuration of a segmented population, this may be a determinant of possible future tensions, unless a deeper and mutual process of acculturation, integration, and, perhaps, even assimilation, takes place across Jerusalem's various subpopulations. But such a process appears for now either unrealistic or, at least, the object for steady national and municipal policies.

Regarding Jerusalem's socio-cultural characteristics, enhanced growth of one particular subpopulation and the consequent relative shrinking of another subpopulation might induce members of the latter to feel endangered, through a complex interplay of perceptions and realities. This has stimulated in the past, as it might in the future, selective emigration from the city, thus further affecting the share of each particular subpopulation among the total. One important consequence of these population movements, actually observed in the past and further expected according to our projections, is a lowering of the average socioeconomic status of the population living in Jerusalem. In this context, the expected decline in the weight of Jewish areas of the overall population, especially among children and younger adults, calls for careful consideration. In the much longer term, the population projections presented here suggest a possible shift of the majority of Jerusalem's population from the Jewish parts to the Arab and other parts. On the other hand, perhaps contrary to diffuse public perceptions, the projections do point to only moderate increase in the weight of the highly religious sections of the Jewish population in relation to the total Jewish population in 2020, as against the situation in 1995.

As one of the main causes for differential population growth continues to be differential fertility, the question which naturally arises is whether and how existing gaps can be significantly reduced, leading in the much longer run to more balanced rates of growth among the various subpopulations. The answers seem to be intriguingly undetermined. A necessary, though perhaps insufficient factor would be the toning down of political and cultural tensions between the main subpopulations involved in the Jerusalem mosaic, particularly between Israelis and Palestinians, and between the Jewish *Haredi* minority and the majority of the Jewish population. Less militancy in the public and community sphere and greater concentration on the promotion of interests in the private and individual sphere might stimulate the transition and convergence toward average (though in any case not very low) family size. It can hence be hypothesized that normalization would bring about a lowering of tensions and, as a consequence of less community militancy, lower fertility among the Muslim and the Jewish *Haredi* subpopulations in particular. On the other hand it can be reasonably argued that as a consequence of political normalization and of the ensuing transferal of resources from national security to private needs, the population's standard of living and household income would improve. As long as the strongly ideological cultural framework typical to high fertility subpopulations prevails, augmented economic family resources might generate, at least in the first stage, better opportunities to cover the cost of child rearing, hence higher fertility.

In demographic perspective, a further significant consequence of political normalization, and of the enhanced freedom of movement, circulation and access it would ensure, might be a greater propensity among the population of the Arab and other parts of Jerusalem to seek a better quality of life out of Jerusalem city. Some movement of Palestinians might develop from high density housing in Jerusalem's Old City and eastern parts toward the suburban belt, as has been the established pattern among the Jewish population since the 1980s. The emergence of such a trend would be both conducive to better living conditions for the concerned population, and to a more balanced growth among the various Jerusalem subpopulations. Clearly, a prerequisite for such demographic transitions is the solution or at least normalization of the major issues of contention in the Middle East conflict, namely the establishment of mutually agreed and formally sanctioned patterns in the relationship between Israel and the Palestinian Authority in Jerusalem and around it. The uneasy relationships between different constituencies within the Jewish population also call for arbitration to regulate mutual relations in a collegial mode. These are obviously central issues for national and not only for municipal strategic policies.

Some Policy Implications

One basic assumption emerging from the preceding discussion and a leading principle for urban policy planning in the complex environment of Jerusalem and of similarly heterogeneous cities appears to be the overarching interest in coherence, peace, and stability. A fundamental element of such stability relates to the demographic development of the different and potentially conflicting ethno-religious subpopulations simultaneously present on the territory. Diffused perceptions of demographic trends bound to upset each subpopulation's share out of the total may generate an endless chain of reactions and counter-reactions potentially disruptive of the overall urban equilibrium. A balanced ethno-demographic development can thus be posited as one of the main strategic goals for urban policies in Jerusalem and comparable cases. An outline of the major policy options emerging from the preceding discussion is presented in table 19.10 that specifies some of the broader contextual factors and the main operative variables of demographic change affecting the city's population size and composition with an emphasis of ethnic and religious subpopulations.

Some control over population size and distribution may be achieved, at least in theory, through manipulating the various operative variables responsible for demographic change, as well as through further administrative policy-making instruments. Inter-city and international migration balances, as well as fertility levels are highly sensitive to life quality opportunities in the urban context. Policies affecting employment, housing, physical environment, municipal services, and personal and collective security may have significant effects on in-migration and out-migration propensities. Fertility levels and differentials may also be expected to respond to these various intervening factors. While causal mechanisms linking life quality opportunities and demographic response affecting the size and composition of urban population are easily specified and understood, clearly no full control can be expected over the amount and direction of actual response. Even the most successful policies can only expect to partial results, whatever the goals be in the demographic development of a heterogeneous urban population.

The major challenge lies in the relationship between demographic behaviors and the deeper roots of existing conflicts in the urban context. Defusing of political and cultural tensions may be the more fundamental prerequisite

Table 19.10
Main Types of Possible Policy Interventions Aimed at Affecting Jerusalem's Population Size and Composition

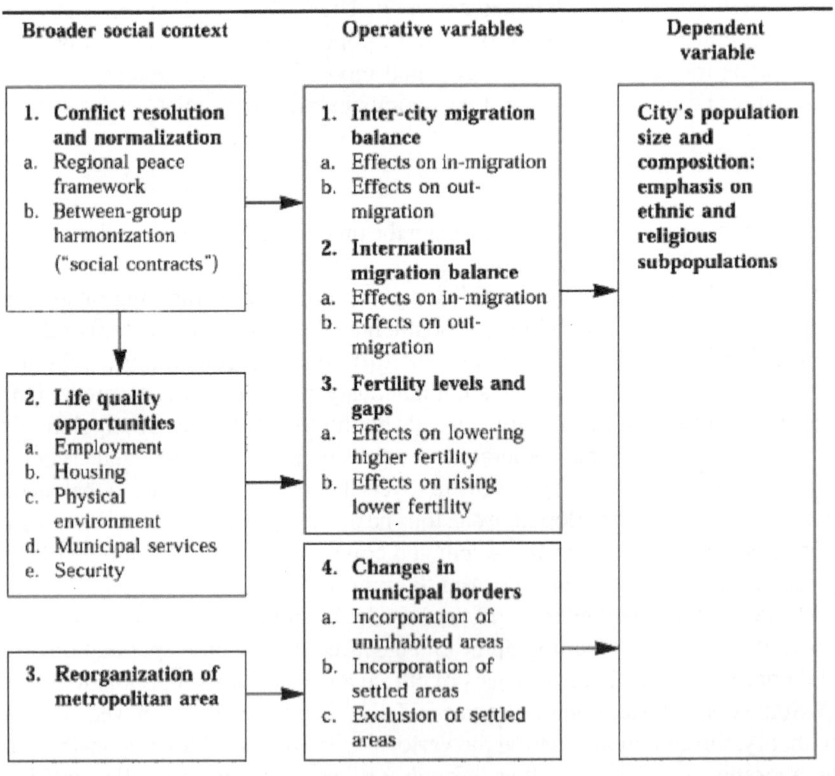

for the cooling down of demographic trends, namely with regard to fertility levels and geographical mobility. In the case of Jerusalem this operates at the multiple level of the Israeli-Palestinian conflict, and of religio-cultural conflicts within each of the Jewish and of the Arab parties. Normalization involves, in the first place, mutual agreement on a regional peace framework including a clear definition of national boundaries between Israel and the Palestinian Authority. Such agreement would enable provisions for a semi-autonomous administration of different neighborhoods in Jerusalem, combining one unified municipal authority with functional divisions in accordance with the major ethno-religious subpopulations. A further need lies in the harmonization between the different religio-cultural sectors within each of the two major Jewish and Arab parties, namely the Jewish *Haredi* minority versus the majority of Jewish population, or the Christian minority versus the Muslim majority. A sort of new "social contract" has been advocated aimed at establishing more mutually respectful rules of political discourse. This would facilitate agreements or non-interference on topics of potential conflict possibly leading, again, to functional semi-autonomy in specific neighborhoods. Some of the provisions mentioned here form part of the extensive Strategic Masterplan that constitutes the broader framework to our population projections (Hershkovitz et al. 2000).

A different approach to the issue of controlling urban population size and composition from the point of view of ethno-demographic equilibrium concerns possible manipulations of city borders, in the framework of a reorganization of Jerusalem's metropolitan area. For example, the specific goal of preserving a given balance between Jewish and Arab and other city residents facing the changes outlined in our projections can conceivably be achieved by expanding the municipal territory and incorporating new areas to the west of Jerusalem. Such territorial expansion may include either existing localities of the suburban belt with their Jewish population or empty territory comprising potential points of destination for future out-migration from Jerusalem. A symmetric solution would be to exclude from the current Jerusalem territory some of the areas now densely inhabited by Arabs and others, transferring them to a separate municipal administration with varying amounts of connection to the Palestinian Authority. While this would imply partial return to the Jerusalem configuration that preceded the 1967 unification, all responsible parties concerned agree that by no means will Jerusalem return to the pre-1967 situation of a city center crossed by a wall with hostile combat forces on the two sides of it.

Population projections, successful or not at depicting the reality in Jerusalem in the year 2020, are useful in that they expose the overwhelming challenges to urban planning and public policies. How to make the complex of value-laden and more pragmatic considerations part of a coherent and functioning program will be crucially connected with the future Jerusalem demographic equation. Jerusalem planners should seize the opportunity to create a model example of a truly multicultural society and to distance themselves from what might otherwise turn into a serious planning and policy concern. The findings discussed in this study of Jerusalem's population shed light on the critical importance of the mutual relationship between demography and socio-political developments.

Acknowledgements

A previous version of this paper was originally presented at the European Population Conference, The Hague, 1999. The larger research of which this paper is an outcome was coordinated by Dr. Sarah Hershkovitz, Head, Division for Strategic Planning and Research, Jerusalem Municipality. The author is especially indebted to Dr. Uzi Rebhun who coordinated the project's demographic-social team and prepared most of the population projections. Thanks are due to the many people who participated at various stages of consulting and administration in this project: Uri Aviram, Israel Bar-Gil, Moni Ben Ari, Uri Ben Asher, Hagit Bezalel, David Cassuto, Maya Choshen, Ra'anan Dinur, Avraham Diskin, Menahem Friedman, Chaya Gamshee, Shalom Goldstein, Amiram Gonen, Arieh Hecht, Avi Heifetz, Sarah Hershkovitz, Ya'akov Kop, Yosef Landau, Judith Laster, Nehemiah Levzion, Nafaz Nazel, Ehud Olmert, Sarit Rafiah, Paul Ritterband, Avino'am Rosenak, Nissim Salomon, Joe Savitzky, Laura Schneider, Avraham Schwartz, Dvorah Shalev, Alice Shalvi, Nadim Sheeban, Moshe Sicron, Nira Sidi, Zion Turgeman, Mike Turner, Batia Vashitz, Michael Weil, Mahfouz Zahir, and the anonymous reviewers. Judith Even edited the English text. Leah DellaPergola provided graphic help. Responsibility for the contents of this paper solely rests with the author.

Notes

1. "Metropolitan area" is intended here in a generic descriptive sense. There exists no official definition of a "Jerusalem Metropolitan Area," though the matter has been discussed by experts and administrators.
2. All projections were executed with the help of the *People 3.0* software package.
3. The pertinent relation is $NRR = (P_{0-4}/^{f} P_{15-49})/(L_{0,4}/^{f} L_{15,49})$, where P values refer to an actual population, L values refer to the age composition of a stationary population in an appropriate life-table, the superscript f indicates females, and the subscripts indicate relevant age groups.
4. Based on much narrower definitional criteria of the target population Berman (1998) estimated the TPR of the ultra-orthodox Jewish population in Israel at 7.61 in 1995/1996.

References

Abu Libdeh, H., G. Ovensen and H. Brunborg. 1993. "Population characteristics and trends." In M. Heiberg and G. Ovensen (eds.), *Palestinian Society in Gaza, West Bank and Arab Jerusalem: A Survey of Living Conditions*, 35-97. Oslo: PAPO.

al-Qaq, Z. 1997. "Post-1967 Palestinian strategies for Jerusalem?" In *Brussels-Jerusalem: Conflict Management and Conflict Resolution in Divided Cities*, 339-368. Jerusalem: IPCRI Israel/Palestine Centre for Research and Information; and Brussels: VUB, Centre for Interdisciplinary Study of Brussels.

Bachi, R. 1967. *An Introduction to Demography,* compiled by J. Yam. Jerusalem: Akademon.

Bachi, R. 1976. *The Population of Israel.* CICRED Series. Jerusalem: Demographic Center and the Institute of Contemporary Jewry, Hebrew University of Jerusalem.

Berman, E. 1998. *Sect, Subsidy and Sacrifice: An Economist View of Ultra-Orthodox Jews.* Jerusalem: Jerusalem Institute for Israel Studies.

Berman, E., and R. Klinov. 1997. "Human capital investment and nonparticipation: Evidence from a sample with infinite horizons (or: Jewish father stops going to work)." Research paper No. 97.05. Jerusalem: Maurice Falk Institute for Economic Research in Israel.

Bonné-Tamir, B., and A. Adam (eds.). 1992. *Genetic Diversity among Jews: Disease Markers at the DNA Level.* New York: Oxford University Press.

Bongaarts, J. 1978. "A framework for analyzing the proximate determinants of fertility." *Population and Development Review* 4: 105-133.

Central Bureau of Statistics. 1998a. *Population and Vital Statistics 1997.* Jerusalem: Central Bureau of Statistics.

Central Bureau of Statistics. 1998b. *Demographic Characteristics of the Population in Localities and Statistical Areas.* 1995 Census of Population and Housing Publications, No.7, Vol. A. Jerusalem: Central Bureau of Statistics.

Central Bureau of Statistics. 1999. *Statistical Abstract of Israel.* Jerusalem: Central Bureau of Statistics.

Choshen, M., R. Khamaisi , M. Hirsch and R. Nasarallha. 1998. *Planning, Building and Development in the Jerusalem Area.* Jerusalem: Jerusalem Institute for Israel Studies and Arab Studies Society.

Choshen, M., and N. Shahar (eds.). 1998. *Statistical Yearbook of Jerusalem.* Jerusalem: Municipality of Jerusalem and the Jerusalem Institute for Israel Studies.

Coale, A., P. Demeny and B. Vaughan. 1983. *Regional Model Life Tables and Stable Populations,* 2nd edition. New York: Academic Press.

DellaPergola, S. 1988. "Some effects of religion on population trends: The case of the Jews." In P. Delooz (ed.), *Religions and Population Policies, Pro Mundi Vita Studies* 5: 40-48.

DellaPergola, S. 1993. "Demographic changes in Israel in the early 1990s." In Y. Kop (ed.), *Israel's Social Services 1992-93*, 57-115. Jerusalem: Center for Social Policy Studies in Israel.

DellaPergola, S. 1998. "The global context of migration to Israel." In E. Leshem and J. T. Shuval (eds.), *Immigration to Israel: Sociological Perspectives*, 51-92. New Brunswick: Transaction.

DellaPergola, S. 1999. "World Jewry beyond 2000: the demographic prospects." Oxford Centre for Hebrew and Jewish Studies, Occasional Papers 2, Oxford.

DellaPergola, S., and U. Rebhun. 1999. "Summary of Jerusalem population projections 1995-2020." Strategic Masterplan for Jerusalem 2020. Jerusalem: Jerusalem Municipality (in Hebrew).

Eisenbach, Z. 1986. "Family planning among the Muslim population of Israel." In U.O. Schmelz and G. Nathan (eds.), *Studies in the Population of Israel, in Honor of Roberto Bachi*, 1-14. Jerusalem: Magnes Press.

Eisenbach, Z. 1994. "Socioeconomic differences in the mortality of elderly people in Israel, 1983-88: Analysis of individual data." In D. Friedlander and Y. Tamir (eds.), *Socioeconomic Characteristics and Old Age Mortality in Israel*, 59-90. Jerusalem: JDC-Brookdale Institute of Gerontology and Human Development and the Department of Demography, Hebrew University of Jerusalem (in Hebrew).

Gilbert, M. 1977. *Jerusalem Illustrated History Atlas.* Jerusalem: Steimatzky.

Goldscheider, C. 1971. *Population, Modernization and Social Structure.* Boston, MA: Little Brown.

Goldscheider, C., and D. Friedlander. 1986. "Reproductive norms in Israel." In U.O. Schmelz, G. Nathan (eds.), *Studies in the Population of Israel, in Honor of Roberto Bachi*, 15-35. Jerusalem: Magnes Press.

Gonen, A. 1992. "Continuity and change in the geography of Jewish middle class in the Jerusalem metropolitan area." In *Urban Geography in Israel 1967-1997*, 127-160. Jerusalem: Jerusalem Institute for Israel Studies.

Guttmann, E., and C. Klein. 1980. "The institutional structure of heterogeneous cities: Brussels, Montreal and Belfast." In J. Kreamer (ed.), *Jerusalem: Problems and Prospects*, 178-207. New York: Praeger.

Hammel, E.A. 1990. "A theory of culture for demography." *Population and Development Review* 16: 455-481.

Hershkovitz, S., S. Fairmont-Rafiah and M. Oval. 1998. *Jerusalem: Urban Characteristics, Major Trends in the City's Development and Municipal Services.* Jerusalem: Municipality of Jerusalem, Division for Strategic Planning and Research.

Hershkovitz, S. et al., 2000. *Strategic Masterplan for Jerusalem 2020.* Jerusalem: Municipality of Jerusalem, Division for Strategic Planning and Research.

Inglehart, R. 1997. *Modernization and Postmodernization: Cultural, Economic and Political Change in 43 Societies.* Princeton, NJ: Princeton University Press.

Kimhi, I. 1992. "Demographic, economic and metropolitan development." in *Urban Geography in Israel 1967-1997.* In *Urban Geography in Israel 1967-1997*, 5-32. Jerusalem: Jerusalem Institute for Israel Studies.

Klein, M. 1999. *Doves over Jerusalem's Sky: The Peace Process and the City 1977-1999.* Jerusalem: Jerusalem Institute for Israel Studies (in Hebrew).

Kliot, N., and Y. Mansfield. 1997. "The political landscape of partition: the case of Cyprus." *Political Geography* 16: 495-521.

Kotek, J. 1997. "Frontier cities: a major stake at world level." In *Brussels-Jerusalem: Conflict Management and Conflict Resolution in Divided Cities*, 165-172. Jerusalem: IPCRI Israel/Palestine Centre for Research and Information; and Brussels: VUB, Centre for Interdisciplinary Study of Brussels.

Kroyanker, D. 1975-1985. *Jerusalem Planning and Development,* 5 vols. Jerusalem: Jerusalem Institute for Israel Studies.

Lapidoth, R., and M. Hirsch (eds). 1994. *The Jerusalem Question and its Resolution: Selected Documents*. Dordrecht/Boston/London: Martinus Nijhoff.

Lesthaeghe, R., and G. Moors. 1995. "Is there a new conservatism that will bring back the old family? Ideational trends and the stages of family formation in Germany, France, Belgium and the Netherlands, 1981-1990." In *Evolution or Revolution in European Population: European Population Conference, Milano 1995*, Vol. 1, 225-266. Milano: FrancoAngeli.

Lesthaeghe, R., and C. Wilson. 1986. "Modes of production, secularization and the pace of fertility." In A.J. Coale and S. Cotts Watkins (eds.), *The Decline of Fertility in Europe.* Princeton, NJ: Princeton University Press.

Levy, S., H. Levinsohn and E. Katz. 1993. *Beliefs, Observances and Social Interaction among Israeli Jews.* Jerusalem: The Louis Guttman Israel Institute of Applied Social Research.

Lunn, D.J., S.N. Simpson, I. Diamond and L. Middleton. 1998. "The accuracy of age-specific population estimates for small areas in Britain." *Population Studies* 52: 327-344.

Morley, D., and A. Shachar (eds.). 1986. *Planning in Turbulence.* Jerusalem: Magnes Press.

Municipality of Jerusalem. 1992. *Jerusalem Urban Projections 1995, 2000, 2010,* by C. Feldmann and D. Friedlander, Jerusalem Area Transportation Masterplan. Jerusalem: Municipality of Jerusalem and Ministry of Transport.

Palestinian Central Bureau of Statistics. 1997. *The Demographic Survey in the West Bank and Gaza Strip.* Final Report, Ramallah: Palestinian Central Bureau of Statistics.

Palestinian Central Bureau of Statistics, 1998. *Labor Force Survey, Annual Report: 1996.* Ramallah: Palestinian Central Bureau of Statistics.

Peritz, E., and M. Baras (eds) 1992. *Studies in the Fertility of Israel.* Jerusalem: Hebrew University.

Pritchett, L.H. 1994. "Desired fertility and the impact of population policies." *Population and Development Review* 20: 1-55.

Rallu, J.L., Y. Courbage, and V. Piché (eds). 1997. *Old and New Minorities.* Montrouge: John Libbey Eurotext; and Paris: INED.

Roman, M. 1997. "Comparing Jerusalem and Brussels: A conceptual framework." In *Brussels-Jerusalem: Conflict Management and Conflict Resolution in Divided Cities*, 173-180. Jerusalem: IPCRI Israel/Palestine Centre for Research and Information; and Brussels: VUB, Centre for Interdisciplinary Study of Brussels.

Schmelz, U.O. 1973. "The evolution of Jerusalem's population." In D.H.K. Amiran, Arieh Shachar and I. Kimhi (eds.), *Urban Geography of Jerusalem: Companion Volume to the Atlas of Jerusalem*, 53-75. Berlin and New York: Walter de Gruyter.

Schmelz, U.O. 1987a. *Modern Jerusalem's Demographic Evolution.* Jerusalem: Hebrew University, Institute of Contemporary Jewry, and the Jerusalem Institute for Israel Studies.

Schmelz, U.O. 1987b. "The population of reunited Jerusalem, 1967-1985." *American Jewish Year Book 1987* 87: 39-113.

Schmelz, U.O. 1989. "Religiosity and fertility among the Jews of Jerusalem." In U.O. Schmelz and S. DellaPergola (eds.), *Papers in Jewish Demography 1985*, 157-185. Jerusalem: Institute of Contemporary Jewry, Hebrew University.

Schmelz, U.O. 1994. "The Jewish population in Jerusalem, 1949-1967." In A. Brali (ed.), *Divided Jerusalem, 1948-1967*, 133-165. Jerusalem: Yad Izhak Ben Zvi (in Hebrew).

Sidi, N., C. Kuhn, U. Ben Asher, M. Edinger, Z. Segal and B. Korot. 1997. *Policy for Jerusalem Development, 1997-2005.* Jerusalem: Municipality of Jerusalem, Division for City Planning, Department for Planning Policy.

Stotkin, R. 1996. *Gunfighter Nation: The Myth of the Frontier in the 20th Century America.* New York: Atheneum.

Sharkansky, I. 1996. *Governing Jerusalem.* Detroit: Wayne State University Press.

Spengler, J.J. 1966. "Values and fertility analysis." *Demography* 3: 109-130.

Steinberg, M., 1989. 'The demographic dimension of the struggle with Israel as seen by the PLO." *Jerusalem Journal of International Relations* 11: 27-51.

Turner, M. et al. 1997. *Data on Population and Housing Capability.* Jerusalem: Jerusalem Municipality, Jerusalem Strategic Masterplan, Physical Planning Team (in Hebrew).

Van de Kaa, D.J. 1996. "Anchored narratives: The story and findings of half a century of research into the determinants of fertility." *Population Studies* 50: 389-432.

Ziegler, I. 1995. "Family Growth in Israel and the 'Critical Child'." Ph.D. dissertation, Hebrew University of Jerusalem.